Neurorehabilitation in Neuro-Oncology

Michelangelo Bartolo
Riccardo Soffietti · Martin Klein
Editors

Neurorehabilitation in Neuro-Oncology

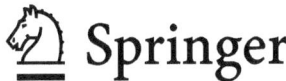 Springer

Editors
Michelangelo Bartolo
Department of Rehabilitation
Neurorehabilitation Unit, Habilita S.p.A.
Zingonia/Ciserano, Bergamo
Italy

Riccardo Soffietti
University and City of Health and Science
Department Neuro-Oncology
Turin, Torino
Italy

Martin Klein
Department of Medical Psychology
VU University Medical Center Department
of Medical Psychology
Amsterdam
The Netherlands

ISBN 978-3-319-95683-1   ISBN 978-3-319-95684-8   (eBook)
https://doi.org/10.1007/978-3-319-95684-8

Library of Congress Control Number: 2019930720

This Springer imprint is published by the registered company Springer Nature Switzerland AG
The registered company address is: Gewerbestrasse 11, 6330 Cham, Switzerland

Foreword

A diagnosis of cancer radically alters the patient's approach to daily life. Due to advances in therapeutic strategies, the number of neuro-oncological survivors is increasing, so that consequently the impact of neuro-oncological rehabilitation of these patients gains in importance. The multidisciplinary approach not only involves physical function, fatigue, and pain but also sexual function, cognitive function, depression, employment, nutrition, and participation.

Good evidence exists for the use of physical therapy in reducing paresis and fatigue after cancer treatment, improving upper and lower extremity function and trunk control. The interventions involving pain, sexual function, cognitive function, and eventual return to employment are equally important. The effect of neurorehabilitation in these parameters is not clearly demonstrated, and more research should be undertaken.

Leopold Saltuari
Department of Neurology
Hochzirl Hospital
Zirl, Austria

Preface

The physical, cognitive, and psychosocial disorders of patients with brain tumors are numerous: in addition to neurological disorders, patients are confronted with limitations in sensory, motor, and cognitive functions as well as depression, anxiety, and fatigue as common consequences of brain tumors and their treatments. Since these disturbances may negatively affect patient's quality of life by producing long-term disability, patients may benefit from rehabilitative interventions.

The rehabilitation in the field of neuro-oncology has to be modified over time in line with the different needs in different stages of disease the patient is confronted with. In the early disease stages, rehabilitation aims at restoring functions after cancer therapies or preventing functional deterioration, while in the advanced disease stages, neurorehabilitation run in parallel to palliative care aims to favor patients' independence, prevent complications, and ultimately improve quality of life.

Chapters devoted to neuro-oncological neurorehabilitation from different disciplines are rarely included in a single volume in the field of clinical oncology, although a holistic approach to persons affected by brain tumors should in a modern vision also include the therapeutic opportunities offered by neurorehabilitation.

This book aims to provide a comprehensive, practical, and state-of-the-art guide to neurorehabilitation strategies of persons affected by tumors of the nervous system by addressing the latest developments from different subfields comprising current neuro-oncological rehabilitation.

The book is structured in two main parts: the first part is devoted to the basics of brain tumors and the main clinical features of tumors of the nervous system as well as to the essentials of therapeutic options; the second part is focused on rehabilitative issues and provides the tools for a holistic care of persons affected by a neuro-oncological disease.

With this book, we hope to provide a useful contribution to the work of all health professionals who are involved in the multidisciplinary care of persons affected by central nervous system tumors.

We would like to thank Springer Nature Switzerland AG, especially Mr. Andrea Ridolfi and Ms. Beauty Christobel Gunasekaran for their excellent contribution.

We thank in advance any reader who will report errors, omissions, or just has suggestions.

Zingonia di Ciserano, Italy   Michelangelo Bartolo
Turin, Italy   Riccardo Soffietti
Amsterdam, The Netherlands   Martin Klein

Contents

Introduction

Michelangelo Bartolo

Cancer has become one of the leading causes of death. If recent trends in the incidence of major cancers and population growth are seen globally in the future [1, 2], it is predicted there will be 23.6 million new cancer cases worldwide annually by 2030 [3].

Over the last 30 years, there has been an increasing incidence of brain tumours in many countries. At the same time, progress in the multimodal treatment has modestly improved survival rate. This has resulted in an increased number of brain tumours patients living longer with residual neurological deficits [4–6]. Moreover, since one third of primary brain tumours are considered malignant and aggressive, and advanced treatment strategies that show better outcomes gain ground, also late effects of treatment are increasingly been recognised as crucial. In fact postsurgical morbidity, acute, subacute, and late radiation effects on normal brain tissue, chemotherapy induced toxicity, as well as the effects of high-dose corticosteroids and anticonvulsants can all have adverse effects [7, 8].

More than 50% of brain tumour patients show three or more concurrent symptoms and/or deficits [9], evidently depending on tumour size, tumour location and lateralisation, and the invasive nature of the tumour; the most common symptoms include seizures, functional impairment, cognitive deficits, weakness, visual-perceptual deficits, sensory loss, and bowel and bladder dysfunction. Other neurologic deficits in decreasing incidence are cranial nerve palsies, dysarthria, dysphagia, and ataxia [7, 10–12]. Tumour-related fatigue remains one of the most frequent and bothersome adverse events reported by brain cancer patients during and after treatment, as it reduces the ability to complete medical treatments, and undermines the quality of life (QoL) [8].

A diagnosis of cancer is expected to cause a psychological burden by itself, but psychological factors, such as stress, anxiety, and depression can also negatively

M. Bartolo (✉)
Department of Rehabilitation, Neurorehabilitation Unit, HABILITA, Bergamo, Italy
e-mail: michelangelobartolo@habilita.it

© Springer Nature Switzerland AG 2019
M. Bartolo et al. (eds.), *Neurorehabilitation in Neuro-Oncology*,
https://doi.org/10.1007/978-3-319-95684-8_1

impact the disability and the person [13]. These aspects must be carefully considered in the global evaluation of the person and treatment planning because these aspects may represent confounding factors, e.g. emotional disturbances may cause impairment on neuropsychological testing that otherwise would be attributed to therapy or tumour.

Overall, these symptoms may cause significant disability similar to those seen in patients commonly admitted to rehabilitation programmes and have a relevant impact on patients' daily life, hindering their ability to function independently and to maintain usual family and social roles, influencing ultimately their QoL as well as the QoL of their family members [14]. Consequently, patient-centred care, focusing on improving QoL in patients with brain tumours, has become relevant. In recent years, many clinical trials evaluating new treatment options for brain tumour patients incorporated QoL as a relevant secondary or even primary outcome measure in addition to overall survival and progression-free survival [15]. In fact, assessment of QoL has become mandatory in all European Organisation for Research and Treatment of Cancer (EORTC) Brain Tumour Group clinical trials.

Actually, considering the limited survival of neuro-oncological patients, it is increasingly recognised that the choice of treatment also should entail careful consideration of its effects on the health-related quality of life (HRQoL) during the remaining survival time, being HRQoL an independent prognostic factor in both primary and metastatic brain tumours [16].

The conceptual framework proposed by the World Health Organisation: International Classification of Functioning, Disability and Health (ICF) [17] suggests that health problems may impact on many areas of a person's life and describes three different levels of impact of a health condition. The first level concerns the domain of impairment (i.e. basic level describing a problem in body function or structure as a result of disease or injury, e.g. a memory problem). The second level relates to limitations in activities or tasks that a person can perform (consequences of the impairment in daily life, e.g. the patient cannot find his car keys). The third level gauges the extent to which a person can participate in societal interactions (e.g. the patient cannot go to a birthday party of a distant friend). The ICF importantly also includes the impact of the environment on the person and describes functioning from both an individual and societal perspective [18], providing a suitable approach to explore the functional difficulties experienced by people living with cancer. According to the ICF, HRQoL as a multidimensional concept covering physical, psychological, and social domains, as well as symptoms induced by the disease and its treatment, represents a more integrated way to measure patients' functioning and well-being.

In this scenario, as cancer is viewed as a chronic disease, rehabilitation process becomes of paramount relevance in brain tumour patients when compared to other malignancies because of their extremely high rate of associated disability. Several studies focused on the issue of the functional outcome of brain tumour patients, showing that rehabilitative treatment offers significant benefit to these patients, comparable to functional gain reported for patients affected by other neurological diseases, like stroke and traumatic brain injury [7, 11, 14]; preliminary data also demonstrate the effectiveness of cognitive rehabilitation in this population [19, 20]. A recent meta-analysis showed that physical exercise and psychological support are also useful for reducing tumour-related fatigue during and after treatment, with significantly better efficacy than drug therapy [21].

According to the "simultaneous care" model [22], rehabilitation should have a role in cancer patients both in early stage of disease, for restoring function after cancer therapy, and in the advanced stage of disease as important part of palliative care with the aim to maintain patients' independence as long as possible. Early initiation of rehabilitative and palliative care integrated with standard anticancer therapy seems to be effective for symptom management, resulting in the improvement of the QoL.

However, despite the high incidence of neurological and functional deficits in brain tumour patients and preliminary data supporting rehabilitation, in this population rehabilitation treatments are not as well established as it is for patients with other neurological conditions, probably because neuro-oncological patients are not considered good candidates to rehabilitative intervention due to their poor prognosis associated with continuing tumour growth despite intensive treatment. Literature evidence, in fact, demonstrates that rehabilitation services are difficult to access for brain tumour patients, poorly utilised and referrals were sporadic and consequential, indicative of poor awareness of rehabilitation for people with cancer among potential referrers [23].

Nevertheless, we can identify several key points that need to be addressed to develop successful care provision models that contribute to continuity of care and autonomy of the person with disability due to oncological disease, including:

(a) training for the health professionals, who should adopt an integrative approach to the person rather than providing a performance or service;
(b) implementation and dissemination of the methodology for a coordinated delivery of multidisciplinary rehabilitation, in consideration of the complexity of patient's needs (clinical, functional, cognitive, psychological, spiritual), using a holistic biopsychosocial model of care, as defined by the ICF. The management of brain tumours represents by definition a model for multidisciplinarity because of the multitude of problems which are encountered that require a multidisciplinary approach with health care providers skilled in a variety of disciplines;
(c) customisation of the rehabilitation project and programmes, defining mid- and long-term (when possible) goals, shared with the patient and caregiver, meaningful and realistic;
(d) develop ad-hoc tools to measure efficacy, efficiency, quality, and appropriateness of the interventions. The tools should take into account the person, including biological, medical, functional, and psycho-cognitive variables, as well as social interaction, participation, and QoL;
(e) continuity of care, offering dedicated care pathways that include rehabilitative care in all the stages of the disease (*simultaneous care*);

(f) focus on patient's and caregiver's QoL, adding more appropriate evaluation tools other than traditional outcome measures such as overall survival and progression-free survival.

The actual gap seems to be mostly educational and there is a great need to enhance training and knowledge for health professionals involved in the care management of neuro-oncological patients [24]. Health professionals need to meet the challenges posed by this disease and its disabilities, considering rehabilitation treatments an opportunity to obtain the best possible outcomes for these persons.

References

1. Bray F, Jemal A, Grey N, Ferlay J, Forman D. Global cancer transitions according to the Human Development Index (2008–2030): a population-based study. Lancet Oncol. 2012;13(8):790–801.
2. Ferlay J, Soerjomataram I, Dikshit R, Eser S, Mathers C, Rebelo M, et al. Cancer incidence and mortality worldwide: sources, methods and major patterns in GLOBOCAN 2012. Int J Cancer. 2015;136(5):E359–86.
3. De Santis CE, Lin CC, Mariotto AB, Siegel RL, Stein KD, Kramer JL, et al. Cancer treatment and survivorship statistics, 2014. CA Cancer J Clin. 2014;64(4):252–71.
4. Kirshblum S, O'Dell MW, Ho C, Barr K. Rehabilitation of persons with central nervous system tumors. Cancer. 2001;92:1029–38.
5. Rose JH, Kypriotakis G, Bowman KF, Einstadter D, O'Toole EE, Mechekano R, et al. Patterns of adaptation in patients living long term with advanced care. Cancer. 2009;115(18):4298–310.
6. Thorne SE, Oliffe JL, Oglov V, Gelmon K. Communication challenges for chronic metastatic cancer in an era of novel therapeutics. Qual Health Res. 2013;23(7):863–75.
7. Vargo M. Brain tumor rehabilitation. Am J Phys Med Rehabil. 2011;90(Suppl):S50–62.
8. Asher A, Fu JB, Bailey C, Hughes JK. Fatigue among patients with brain tumors. CNS Oncol. 2016;5(2):91–100.
9. Mukand JA, Blackinton DD, Crincoli MG, Lee JJ, Santos BB. Incidence of neurologic deficits and rehabilitation of patients with brain tumors. Am J Phys Med Rehabil. 2001;80(5):346–50.
10. Osoba D, Aaronson NK, Muller M, Sneeuw K, Hsu MA, Yung WK, et al. Effect of neurological dysfunction on health-related quality of life in patients with high-grade glioma. J Neurooncol. 1997;34(3):263–78.
11. Giordana MT, Clara E. Functional rehabilitation and brain tumour patients. A review of outcome. Neurol Sci. 2006;27:240–4.
12. Posti JP, Bori M, Kauko T, Sankinen M, Nordberg J, Rahi M, et al. Presenting symptoms of glioma in adults. Acta Neurol Scand. 2015;131(2):88–93.
13. Lezak MD, Howieson DB, Bigler ED, Tranel D. Neuropsychological assessment. 5th ed. Oxford: Oxford University Press; 2012.
14. Bartolo M, Zucchella C, Pace A, Lanzetta G, Vecchione C, Bartolo M, et al. Early rehabilitation after surgery improves functional outcome in inpatients with brain tumours. J Neurooncol. 2012;107(3):537–44.
15. Mauer ME, Bottomley A, Taphoorn MJ. Evaluating health-related quality of life and symptom burden in brain tumour patients: instruments for use in experimental trials and clinical practice. Curr Opin Neurol. 2008;21(6):745–53.
16. Meyers CA, Hess KR, Yung WK, Levin VA. Cognitive function as a predictor of survival in patients with recurrent malignant glioma. J Clin Oncol. 2000;18(3):646–50.
17. World Health Organization. International classification of functioning, disability, and health (ICF). Geneva: WHO; 2001.

18. Bickenbach J, Rubinelli S, Stucki G. Being a person with disabilities or experiencing disability: two perspectives on the social response to disability. J Rehabil Med. 2017;49(7):543–9.
19. Zucchella C, Capone A, Codella V, De Nunzio AM, Vecchione C, Sandrini G, et al. Cognitive rehabilitation for early post-surgery inpatients affected by primary brain tumor: a randomized, controlled trial. J Neurooncol. 2013;114(1):93–100.
20. Gehring K, Sitskoorn MM, Gundy CM, Sikkes SA, Klein M, Postma TJ, et al. Cognitive rehabilitation in patients with gliomas: a randomized controlled trial. J Clin Oncol. 2009;27(22):3712–22.
21. Mustian KM, Alfano CM, Heckler C, Kleckner IR, Leach CR, Mohr D, et al. Comparison of pharmaceutical, psychological, and exercise treatments for cancer-related fatigue: a meta-analysis. JAMA Oncol. 2017;3(7):961–8.
22. Meyers FJ, Linder J. Simultaneous care: disease treatment and palliative care throughout illness. J Clin Oncol. 2003;21:1412–5.
23. McCartney A, Butler C, Acreman S. Exploring access to rehabilitation services from allied health professionals for patients with primary high-grade brain tumours. Palliat Med. 2011;25(8):788–96.
24. Bartolo M, Zucchella C, Pace A, De Nunzio AM, Serrao M, Sandrini G, et al. Improving neuro-oncological patients care: basic and practical concepts for nurse specialist in neuro-rehabilitation. J Exp Clin Cancer Res. 2012;31:82.

Basics of Brain Tumor Biology for Clinicians

Hans-Georg Wirsching and Michael Weller

2.1 Brain Tumor Risk

Hereditary cancer syndromes are overall rare and account for a small minority of primary brain tumors and of cancers forming brain metastases [1, 2]. Most of these syndromes are caused by defects in DNA repair and tumor suppressor genes. Examples include Li-Fraumeni syndrome caused by mutations in the tumor suppressor genes *TP53* or *CHEK*, which can cause the formation of gliomas and breast cancer; Turcot syndrome caused by mutation of the tumor suppressor gene *APC,* or of the DNA mismatch repair genes *MLH1* and *PMS2*, causing the formation of colon cancer, medulloblastoma and, less commonly, gliomas; neurofibromatosis types I and II caused by mutations in the tumor suppressor genes *NF1* and *NF2*, which are associated with the formation of gliomas and breast cancer (*NF1*), and with the formation of multiple meningiomas (*NF2*); the hereditary breast and ovarian cancer (HBOC) syndrome most commonly caused by mutations in the DNA damage response genes *BRCA1* or *BRCA2*; Lynch syndrome, also referred to as hereditary non-polyposis colorectal cancer (HNPCC), which is caused by mutations in any of the mismatch DNA repair genes *MLH1, MSH2, MSH6, PMS1,* or *PMS2,* which is associated with colorectal cancer and, less frequently, with kidney and primary brain cancers.

Other endogenous risk factors for brain tumors include risk alleles associated with the formation of gliomas in genes involved in telomere biology (*TERT, RTEL1*), in the gene encoding the epidermal growth factor receptor, *EGFR*, and in *TP53* [3]. However, the overall low penetrance of each of these risk alleles supports a polygenic pathomechanism of gliomagenesis. Risk alleles for the formation of brain metastases in breast cancer patients have been identified among genes of the phosphoinositide 3-kinase (PI3K)/protein kinase B (AKT) pathway [4]. Allergy is

H.-G. Wirsching · M. Weller (✉)
Department of Neurology, University Hospital and University of Zurich, Zurich, Switzerland
e-mail: michael.weller@usz.ch

© Springer Nature Switzerland AG 2019
M. Bartolo et al. (eds.), *Neurorehabilitation in Neuro-Oncology*,
https://doi.org/10.1007/978-3-319-95684-8_2

associated with a decreased risk for gliomas [5] and probably also for meningiomas [6]. Meningiomas are more common in women than in men (3.5:1) [7]. A tendency to spontaneous growth arrest in post-menopausal women and the presence of progesterone receptors suggest the contribution of hormonal factors to the pathogenesis of at least a subgroup of meningiomas, albeit hormonal treatments of meningioma patients have been futile [8, 9].

Exogenous risk factors for primary brain tumors include ionizing irradiation as the only established exogenous risk factor for the development of gliomas and meningiomas, but the overall contribution of these cases to the incidence of both entities is marginal [10–15]. Exogenous risk factors for the formation of brain metastases have not been identified.

2.2 Hallmarks of Brain Tumors

2.2.1 Brain Tropism

A characteristic feature of primary brain tumors is the fact that beyond anecdotal reports, primary brain tumors do not metastasize to distant organs, i.e., they exhibit a distinct brain tropism [16]. In reverse, the formation of brain metastases from circulating cancer cells also occurs late during the disease course of most cancers, usually following the occurrence of metastases in other organs [17]. This is of note given that the brain is a highly vascularized organ receiving about 20% of the cardiac output, suggesting that the mere stochastic probability of cell-vessel contacts does not determine metastasis formation.

The blood–brain barrier (BBB) causes demarcation of the brain from circulating cancer cells. However, the lack of distant metastases of primary brain tumors is not explained by the cellular barrier function of the BBB, because disruption of the BBB is a key feature of most primary brain tumors, and a priori absent in meningiomas, which likewise rarely metastasize to distant organs. Interactions with parenchymal organ cells are thought to underlie brain tropism of primary brain tumors, but overall the underlying cause is elusive.

2.2.2 Angiogenesis

Extensive vascularization is common to many brain tumors and metastases [18]. Qualitatively, these new blood vessels are often tortuous and leaky with a disrupted BBB, allowing extravasation of larger molecules and yielding an increase in interstitial fluid pressure. The resulting vasogenic edema contributes significantly to the morbidity of patients with brain tumors by causing headache and neurological deficits. Angiogenesis is primarily driven by the vascular endothelial growth factor (VEGF) [18]. Proliferation of abnormal blood vessels is a defining criterion of glioblastoma, the most common malignant primary brain tumor constituting about half of all gliomas [19]. The anti-VEGF antibody bevacizumab effectively reverts vasogenic edema and induces blood vessel normalization in these tumors, thereby alleviating symptom burden [18]. However, overall survival of patients with glioblastomas is not affected by anti-angiogenic therapy, as will be discussed in more detail in Chap. 6.

2.2.3 Immunosuppression

Bone-marrow derived immune cells are rare or absent in the normal brain, rendering the brain an "immune-privileged" organ that is widely protected from innate or adaptive immune reactions. The relatively low incidence of primary brain tumors compared to other cancers is striking in that context, because elimination of abnormal, cancerous cells by the immune system has traditionally been considered a key mechanism preventing cancer development in other organs. Once cancer has developed or seeded in the brain, several mechanisms mediate the evasion of anti-cancer immune responses [20]: (1) secretion of immunosuppressive molecules such as TGFβ-2, PGE, IL-10, and FGL2 by tumor cells, (2) decreased antigen processing and presentation, e.g., through down-regulation of major histocompatibility complex (MHC)-I molecules on tumor cells, (3) recruitment of tumor-associated macrophages and reprogramming towards an immunosuppressive phenotype through secretion of M-CSF, TGFβ-1, and IL-10 by tumor cells, (4) direct inhibition of adaptive immune responses through expression of immune checkpoint molecules such as PD-L1 or PD-L2 on tumor cells and macrophages, and (5) by means of metabolic reprogramming discussed further below. Therapeutic strategies to revert immunosuppression will be discussed in Chap. 6.

2.2.4 Metabolism

The brain utilizes approximately 60% of our daily glucose intake, despite constituting only about 2% of our bodyweight. In the normal brain, most glucose is metabolized by oxidative phosphorylation in the mitochondria, thereby generating up to 36 molecules of adenosine-triphosphate (ATP) per glucose molecule to meet the energetic demands of neurons and other brain cells [21]. Under hypoxic conditions in the cancer milieu cancer cells undergo a metabolic switch towards the less energetic, anaerobic glycolytic glucose metabolism generating only two molecules of ATP per molecule glucose, a process that was termed "Warburg effect" and that is common to most cancers including malignant primary brain tumors [22]. The Warburg effect is however not merely an opportunistic reaction to hypoxia, but yields the production of anabolic building blocks to generate lipids, nucleotides, and proteins to meet the high demand of cancer cells for continued growth. The generation of lactate and other by-products of glycolysis also contributes to the harshness of the tumor microenvironment and inhibition of functions of non-cancer cells, including immune cells [22]. Gliomas moreover secrete large quantities of glutamate as a by-product of glutathione synthesis, a means to counteract oxidative stress. High concentrations of glutamate may also contribute to seizures and tissue destruction through cytotoxicity in neurons [23]. More brain-specific metabolic adaptions of cancer cells that are common to gliomas and brain metastases include preferential metabolism of acetate as a bioenergetics substrate [24].

2.2.5 Cancer Stem-Like Cells

The cellular organization of gliomas and most cancers that form brain metastases is hierarchical [25, 26]. Stem-like cells at the apex of this hierarchy give rise to more differentiated off-spring that form the bulk of the tumor. Glioma stem-like cells are adapted to and induced by hypoxia and nutrient restriction and rest in distinct stem-cell niches that are characterized by such harsh conditions [27, 28]. Moreover, interaction with the tumor vasculature can induce or maintain their phenotype, e.g., by signaling through nitric oxide or notch signaling [29, 30]. De-differentiation of non-stem-like cancer cells and assumption of a stem-like phenotype do also occur [31]. In gliomas, single cell gene expression analyses revealed that the hierarchical concept of "stemness" reflects a continuum of more or less differentiated states rather than clearly distinguishable cell types [32]. Cancer stem-like cells mediate resistance to classical chemo- and radiotherapy, in part by resting in a slow cycling or hibernating state and by preferential activation of the DNA damage response [31]. However, translation of this biological concept of stemness to molecularly targeted therapies, e.g., by inducing differentiation or utilizing drugs that selectively target stem-like cells, has failed in brain tumors [31].

2.2.6 Clonal Evolution and Therapy Resistance

Cancer growth and therapy both yield clonal selection pressure. Solid tumor entities with circumscribed growth are genetically less complex than tumors that infiltrate diffusely and may therefore be more amenable to molecular targeted therapies (discussed in Chap. 6) [33]. Most non-brain tumors and some primary brain tumors initially grow non-infiltrative and will only invade neighboring tissue or form distant metastases upon acquisition of additional genetic aberrations [17, 33]. Historically, this unidirectional model of oncogenesis was exemplified by the unraveling of a distinct sequence of mutations acquired by cells of the colon mucosa that cause the formation of adenomatous lesions and subsequently of infiltrative cancers [34]. However, genomic instability is a key feature of many cancers and causes the simultaneous generation of a vast number of clones. While only one or a few clones may dominate growth of an individual tumor, anti-cancer treatment can drive the selection of a different set of therapy resistant clones that may be present within tumors before the initiation of treatment. This multidirectional model of clonal evolution applies to most late-stage cancers and is a key characteristic of diffusely infiltrating gliomas, the most common malignant primary brain tumors [35, 36].

Recent technological advances in single-cell sequencing have improved our understanding of these biological processes and will aid in unraveling mechanisms of acquired therapy resistance.

2.3 Biological Features of Selected Brain Tumor Entities

2.3.1 Diffusely Infiltrating Astrocytomas and Oligodendrogliomas

The discovery that specific point mutations in genes encoding isocitrate dehydrogenase (IDH)-1 or -2 are present in the majority of diffusely infiltrating gliomas of WHO grades II and III was the foundation for the molecular classification of these tumors [19, 37]. Mutated IDH causes the production of 2-hydroxy-glutarate (2-HG), an oncometabolite thought to inhibit α-ketoglutarate-dependent dioxygenases and demethylases, yielding genome-wide DNA-hypermethylation, a phenomenon termed glioma CpG-island methylator phenotype (G-CIMP) [38–41]. Diffusely infiltrating astrocytomas and oligodendrogliomas comprise three major groups that are classified based on the integration of molecular information and histology [19]: (1) Astrocytomas with wild-type IDH, (2) astrocytomas with mutated IDH, and (3) oligodendrogliomas, which are defined by the co-occurrence of mutated IDH and additional co-deletion of chromosome arms 1p and 19q. The assignment of WHO grade II–IV is done mostly based on histological features of malignancy.

Details of the classification of diffusely infiltrating gliomas are summarized in Chap. 3 and implications for treatment will be discussed in Chap. 6.

Astrocytoma, IDH Wild-Type Astrocytomas with wild-type IDH comprise mostly glioblastomas (WHO grade IV), the most common malignant primary brain tumors. The incidence of these tumors increases with age and the prognosis is dismal [7]. Astrocytomas with wild-type IDH constitute a biological entity that is fundamentally different from IDH mutated astrocytomas or oligodendrogliomas. These tumors frequently harbor amplifications of chromosome 7 and loss of one copy of chromosome 10. This has clinical implications, because chromosome 10 also harbors *MGMT*, the gene encoding the DNA repair protein O6-methylguanyl DNA methyltransferase. Hypermethylation of the promoter region of *MGMT* predicts response to temozolomide in patients with diffusely infiltrating IDH wild-type astrocytomas, likely because of the lack of a second copy of *MGMT* to compensate for hypermethylation of one allele [42]. The clinical utility of *MGMT* testing will be discussed in more detail in Chap. 6.

Common gene level copy number alterations in astrocytomas with wild-type IDH include homozygous deletion of *PTEN*, homozygous deletion of *CDKN2A* and *CDKN2B*, amplification of genes encoding mitogenic receptor tyrosine kinases such as *EGFR*, *PDGFRA*, or *MET*, and cell cycle promoter genes including *CDK4* and *CDK6* that mediate transition from G1 to S phase or genes encoding p53 inhibitors such as *MDM2* or *MDM4* [33]. Activating *TERT* promoter mutations are also common in IDH wild-type astrocytomas. Less common mutations affect *TP53*, *PIK3CA*, *PIK3R1* (encoding PI3K-regulatory subunit 1), and *NF1* [33]. Attempts to further classify the genetically heterogeneous group of astrocytomas with wild-type IDH included genome-wide methylation arrays. This approach identified five glioblastoma subtypes with wild-type IDH designated receptor tyrosine kinase (RTK)-I, RTK-II, and mesenchymal as well as two profiles that were associated with distinct histone H3 mutations, *H3F3A*$^{G34R/V}$ and *H3F3A*^{K27M} [43]. Gliomas with the latter mutation typically arise in midline structures and have a poor prognosis. Given these distinct clinical and molecular features, diffuse midline glioma with *H3F3A*^{K27M} mutation (WHO grade IV) was included as a novel entity in the revised WHO classification (Chap. 3) [19].

Moreover, gene expression profiling identified three IDH wild-type glioblastoma subtypes designated proneural, classical, and mesenchymal based on similarities to known genesets [44]. Single cells that can be assigned to these whole-tumor derived subtype classifications are present simultaneously in individual tumors [32] and switching of subtypes at recurrence is common [35], thus limiting the clinical utility of such a classification approach.

Astrocytoma, IDH Mutated IDH mutated astrocytomas comprise the vast majority of WHO grade II and grade III diffusely infiltrating astrocytomas. IDH mutated glioblastomas (WHO grade IV) account for approximately 10% of all glioblastomas. Patients with IDH mutated astrocytomas are mostly young adults and the prognosis is more favorable compared to astrocytomas with wild-type IDH [33].

IDH mutation is one of the earliest events during oncogenesis of these tumors [45], but additional aberrations are required to initiate tumor formation in mice [46]. In IDH mutant astrocytomas, other common mutations affect *TP53* and the transcriptional regulator of chromatin remodelling *ATRX* [19]. There are also several genetic molecular features associated with the progression of WHO grade II to grade III and eventually to WHO grade IV. These driver events converge on dysregulation of cell division. Examples include chromosomal deletion of 9p21, which harbors *CDKN2A* and *CDKN2B*, activation of MYC and receptor tyrosine kinase (RTK) signaling, or somatic mutations in genes of inhibitors of the G1/S cell cycle checkpoint such as the retinoblastoma (Rb) pathway, or low methylation at CpG sites that regulate cell cycle progression, e.g., *TP73* [33, 47, 48].

Oligodendroglioma, IDH Mutated, 1p/19q Co-deleted Oligodendrogliomas are defined by co-deletion of chromosome arms 1p and 19q in IDH mutated tumors [19]. They almost generally harbor activating mutations in the promoter region of *TERT*, leading to aberrant telomere lengthening [49]. Other common somatic mutations in oligodendrogliomas include inactivating mutations of the transcriptional repressor gene *CIC*, the MYC suppressor gene *FUBP1*, developmental pathway genes such as *NOTCH1*, epigenetic regulator genes such as *SETD1*, and phosphorinisitol-3-kinase (PI3K) pathway genes such as *PIK3CA* [33].

2.3.2   Gliomas with Circumscribed Growth

Gliomas with circumscribed growth occur mostly in children and young adults [7]. The prognosis of these tumors is generally favorable, but multifocal growth can occur among all of these entities and pleomorphic xanthoastrocytoma and ependymomas can assume a malignant phenotype with infiltrative growth [19, 33].

Pilocytic Astrocytoma   Pilocytic astrocytoma is the most common entity in this category. Pilocytic astrocytoma is considered a "single pathway disease" that rarely harbors genetic alterations other than such that result in activation of mitogen-activated protein kinase (MAPK) signaling [50]. The most common underlying genetic event is the fusion of the proto-oncogene *BRAF* and *KIAA1549*, which is associated with cerebellar tumor location and favorable prognosis [51]. Other genetic aberrations include fusion genes that involve the MAPK-pathway genes *RAF1*, *PTPN11*, or *NTRK2*, or harbor activating mutations in *NF1*, *FGFR1*, *KRAS*, or *BRAF* [50].

Subependymal Giant-Cell Astrocytoma (SEGA)   SEGA is a pathognomonic feature of tuberous sclerosis and typically occurs from mutation or allelic loss of the genes encoding hamartin (*TSC1*) or tuberin (*TSC2*), both of which form the tuberous sclerosis complex, a key regulator of the mammalian target of rapamycin (mTOR)-signaling pathway in healthy cells [52].

Pleomorphic   Xanthoastrocytoma   (PXA)   PXA   almost   generally   harbors *BRAF*^{V600E} mutations, often occurring together with loss of both copies of the cell cycle regulator gene *CDKN2A* [53, 54]. The genetic basis of the occasional transition of PXA to an infiltrative growth pattern is unclear [33].

Ependymomas   Ependymomas constitute a molecularly more heterogeneous group that comprises a total of nine molecular subtypes [55]. Approximately two thirds of all supratentorial ependymomas harbor *RELA-C11orf95* gene fusions. The fusion protein drives aberrant NF-κB signaling and is associated with an unfavorable prognosis [55]. These tumors have been included as a novel entity in the 2016 WHO classification (Chap. 3) [19]. Fusions with the *YAP1* gene have also been identified in supratentorial ependymomas and are associated with better prognosis. Among ependymomas arising in the posterior fossa (PF), the PF-A subtype is characterized by genetic stability and probably driven by epigenetic aberrations [55]. The prognosis of PF-A ependymomas is unfavorable. Another ependymoma subtype designated PF-B is characterized by chromosomal instability and has a more favorable prognosis. Spinal ependymomas often carry *NF2* mutations and rarely recur after resection [55].

2.3.3   Medulloblastoma

The term medulloblastoma comprises at least four clinically and molecularly distinct entities designated Wnt-activated, Shh-activated, group 3, and group 4 [56, 57]. The classification of medulloblastomas into these groups has been integrated in the revised WHO classification of central nervous system tumors of 2016 (see Chap. 3).

Wnt-Activated Medulloblastoma Wnt-activated medulloblastoma occurs in children and, less commonly, in adults. This subtype is described as having frequent oncogenic mutations of the *CTNNB1* gene encoding the Wnt down-stream signaling molecule β-catenin [58] or by germline mutations of the Wnt-signaling inhibitor gene *APC* in patients with Turcot syndrome [59]. Moreover, this subgroup has frequent loss of one copy of chromosome 6. The almost generally favorable prognosis of this group fostered an ongoing discussion on therapy de-escalation [3], which will be discussed in more detail in Chap. 6.

Sonic Hedgehog (Shh)-Activated Medulloblastoma Shh-activated medulloblastoma is common in both, infants and adults, but rarely occurs in children. It is often driven by germline mutations in the Shh-receptor gene *PTCH*, the Shh inhibitor *SUFU*, by activating mutations in the Shh-co-receptor gene *SMO*, or with amplification of the transcription factors mediating down-stream Shh signaling, *GLI1* and *GLI2* [56]. This subtype also comprises most tumors of the desmoplastic/nodular histological medulloblastoma variant. The prognosis of Shh-activated medulloblastoma is intermediate in the majority of cases with wild-type *TP53*, but co-occurrence of *TP53* mutations confers a poor prognosis [56, 60].

Group 3 and Group 4 Medulloblastoma Group 3 and group 4 medulloblastomas occur in infants and children, and only group 3 almost never occurs in adults [56]. There is a predisposition of both subtypes for males versus females. Group 3 is additionally characterized by high incidences of large cell anaplastic histology and of metastasis within the central nervous system [57]. *MYC* amplification and overexpression are characteristic of group 3 and associated with poor prognosis, but almost absent in group 4 [57, 61]. High expression levels of *MYC* and *MYCN* are also found in Wnt- and Shh-activated medulloblastoma, respectively, *MYC* expression of the Wnt-activated subtype is not driven by gene copy number gain. In contrast, group 4 commonly has *MYCN* copy number amplification, but not higher gene expression. The oncogene *OTX* is also commonly amplified and overexpressed in group 3 and group 4, and *CDK6* is commonly amplified in group 4 [57, 61]. Moreover a variety of chromosomal aberrations are characteristic of group 3 and group 4, of which gain of chromosome 1q, loss of chromosome 5q, and loss of chromosome 10q are more common in group 3, and the presence of an isochromosome 17q is more common in group 4 [60]. Gene expression profiles of group 3 and group 4 overlap with genesets involved in retinal and brain development, respectively, but the clinical significance of these traits is elusive [56].

2.3.4   Meningiomas

Meningiomas are the most common intracranial tumors in adults and their incidence is tightly associated with age [7]. They usually arise from meningothelial arachnoidal cells that cover the brain and spinal cord, but can rarely occur in other locations such as intraventricularly, in the brain parenchyma or even in extracranial organs such as the lung [62]. Copy number alterations are overall rare in meningiomas [63]. The most common cytogenetic alteration in meningiomas is the deletion of one copy of chromosome 22 [63]. Chromosome 22 harbors the *NF2* gene, which is the most commonly mutated tumor suppressor gene in these tumors affecting close to half of all meningiomas and about 75% of WHO grade II meningiomas [64, 65]. Vice versa, chromosomal aberrations are also more frequent in *NF2* mutated meningiomas, indicating a role of the *NF2* gene product merlin for chromosomal stability [66]. Chromosomal aberrations occurring independent of *NF2* are associated with recurrence, higher WHO grade and consequently more aggressive disease course [63], and with the small subgroup of meningiomas arising years or decades after radiotherapy of the skull [67, 68]. Mutations that recurrently coincide with *NF2* mutations affect genes encoding epigenetic modifiers (*KDM5C, KDM6A, SMARCB1*) [63]. Recurrent mutations in *NF2* non-mutated meningiomas activate members of the PI3K/Akt/mTor pathway (*AKT1, PIK3CA, mTOR*) and of the Shh pathway (*SMO*) [63]. Mutations in *POLR2A*, which encodes the DNA-directed RNA polymerase II subunit RPB1, seem to be confined to WHO grade I meningiomas and are associated with meningothelial histology and location at the tuberculum sellae [69]. Mutations of the transcription factor gene *KLF4* are present in approximately half of all meningiomas with wild-type *NF2* and often co-occur with mutations in the gene encoding tumor necrosis factor receptor-associated factor 7 (*TRAF7*) [70, 71]. WHO grade II and grade III meningiomas have been reported to harbor mutations in *TP53, CDKN2A,* and *CDKN2B* [63, 66]. There is also an association of the rare rhabdoid histological variant of anaplastic meningioma (WHO grade III) with mutations in the *BAP1* gene [72], which encodes a deubiquitinase that functions as a histone modifier. Implications of these biological features of meningiomas for treatment strategies are discussed in Chap. 6.

2.3.5   Brain Metastases

The cancers that most commonly metastasize to the brain are lung and breast cancer, melanoma, and, to a lesser extent, renal cell carcinoma and colorectal cancer. In order to form metastases, cancers need to undergo epithelial-to-mesenchymal transition, invade, extravasate, evade the immune system, initiate angiogenesis, and adapt to organ-specific functions [17]. Molecular signatures of brain metastases have been proposed [73–75], e.g., to identify circulating tumor cells with potency to form brain metastases and enable treatment at an early stage. Examples of brain-metastasis specific genes include *ST6GALNAC5*, which encodes a brain-specific endothelial adhesion molecule that is required to transition through the BBB [75]. Other examples include upregulation of cyclic oxygenase 2, acquisition of the ability to metabolize acetate, or the expression of various *EGFR* ligands [24, 75]. Of note, many molecular traits are shared between brain metastases and malignant primary brain tumors, indicating how brain-specific factors entail certain characteristics of cancer cells that are shared between primary brain tumors and brain metastases. However, to date precise molecular programs leading to the formation of brain metastases have not been defined.

References

1. Garber JE, Offit K. Hereditary cancer predisposition syndromes. J Clin Oncol. 2005;23(2):276–92.
2. Ohgaki H, Kim YH, Steinbach JP. Nervous system tumors associated with familial tumor syndromes. Curr Opin Neurol. 2010;23(6):583–91.
3. Ostrom QT, Bauchet L, Davis FG, Deltour I, Fisher JL, Langer CE, et al. The epidemiology of glioma in adults: a "state of the science" review. Neuro-Oncology. 2014;16(7):896–913.
4. Le Rhun E, Bertrand N, Dumont A, Tresch E, Le Deley MC, Mailliez A, et al. Identification of single nucleotide polymorphisms of the PI3K-AKT-mTOR pathway as a risk factor of central nervous system metastasis in metastatic breast cancer. Eur J Cancer. 2017;87:189–98.
5. Linos E, Raine T, Alonso A, Michaud D. Atopy and risk of brain tumors: a meta-analysis. J Natl Cancer Inst. 2007;99(20):1544–50.
6. Claus EB, Calvocoressi L, Bondy ML, Schildkraut JM, Wiemels JL, Wrensch M. Family and personal medical history and risk of meningioma. J Neurosurg. 2011;115(6):1072–7.
7. Ostrom QT, Gittleman H, Liao P, Vecchione-Koval T, Wolinsky Y, Kruchko C, et al. CBTRUS Statistical Report: primary brain and other central nervous system tumors diagnosed in the United States in 2010–2014. Neuro Oncol. 2017;19(suppl_5):v1–v88.
8. Claus EB, Calvocoressi L, Bondy ML, Wrensch M, Wiemels JL, Schildkraut JM. Exogenous hormone use, reproductive factors, and risk of intracranial meningioma in females. J Neurosurg. 2013;118(3):649–56.
9. Ji Y, Rankin C, Grunberg S, Sherrod AE, Ahmadi J, Townsend JJ, et al. Double-blind phase III randomized trial of the Antiprogestin agent mifepristone in the treatment of unresectable meningioma: SWOG S9005. J Clin Oncol. 2015;33(34):4093–8.
10. Neglia JP, Robison LL, Stovall M, Liu Y, Packer RJ, Hammond S, et al. New primary neoplasms of the central nervous system in survivors of childhood cancer: a report from the Childhood Cancer Survivor Study. J Natl Cancer Inst. 2006;98(21):1528–37.
11. Ron E, Modan B, Boice JD Jr, Alfandary E, Stovall M, Chetrit A, et al. Tumors of the brain and nervous system after radiotherapy in childhood. N Engl J Med. 1988;319(16):1033–9.
12. Sadetzki S, Chetrit A, Freedman L, Stovall M, Modan B, Novikov I. Long-term follow-up for brain tumor development after childhood exposure to ionizing radiation for tinea capitis. Radiat Res. 2005;163(4):424–32.
13. Pearce MS, Salotti JA, Little MP, McHugh K, Lee C, Kim KP, et al. Radiation exposure from CT scans in childhood and subsequent risk of leukaemia and brain tumours: a retrospective cohort study. Lancet. 2012;380(9840):499–505.
14. Davis F, Il'yasova D, Rankin K, McCarthy B, Bigner DD. Medical diagnostic radiation exposures and risk of gliomas. Radiat Res. 2011;175(6):790–6.
15. Mathews JD, Forsythe AV, Brady Z, Butler MW, Goergen SK, Byrnes GB, et al. Cancer risk in 680,000 people exposed to computed tomography scans in childhood or adolescence: data linkage study of 11 million Australians. BMJ. 2013;346:f2360.
16. Schweitzer T, Vince GH, Herbold C, Roosen K, Tonn JC. Extraneural metastases of primary brain tumors. J Neuro-Oncol. 2001;53(2):107–14.
17. Chiang AC, Massague J. Molecular basis of metastasis. N Engl J Med. 2008;359(26):2814–23.
18. Jain RK, di Tomaso E, Duda DG, Loeffler JS, Sorensen AG, Batchelor TT. Angiogenesis in brain tumours. Nat Rev Neurosci. 2007;8(8):610–22.
19. Louis DN, Perry A, Reifenberger G, von Deimling A, Figarella-Branger D, Cavenee WK, et al. The 2016 World Health Organization classification of tumors of the central nervous system: a summary. Acta Neuropathol. 2016;131(6):803–20.
20. Nduom EK, Weller M, Heimberger AB. Immunosuppressive mechanisms in glioblastoma. Neuro Oncol. 2015;17(Suppl 7):vii9–vii14.
21. Brady S, et al. Basic neurochemistry: molecular, cellular, and medical aspects. 7th ed. Amsterdam: Elsevier; 2006.

22. Agnihotri S, Zadeh G. Metabolic reprogramming in glioblastoma: the influence of cancer metabolism on epigenetics and unanswered questions. Neuro-Oncology. 2016;18(2):160–72.
23. Huberfeld G, Vecht CJ. Seizures and gliomas--towards a single therapeutic approach. Nat Rev Neurol. 2016;12(4):204–16.
24. Mashimo T, Pichumani K, Vemireddy V, Hatanpaa KJ, Singh DK, Sirasanagandla S, et al. Acetate is a bioenergetic substrate for human glioblastoma and brain metastases. Cell. 2014;159(7):1603–14.
25. Reya T, Morrison SJ, Clarke MF, Weissman IL. Stem cells, cancer, and cancer stem cells. Nature. 2001;414(6859):105–11.
26. Singh SK, Hawkins C, Clarke ID, Squire JA, Bayani J, Hide T, et al. Identification of human brain tumour initiating cells. Nature. 2004;432(7015):396–401.
27. Flavahan WA, Wu Q, Hitomi M, Rahim N, Kim Y, Sloan AE, et al. Brain tumor initiating cells adapt to restricted nutrition through preferential glucose uptake. Nat Neurosci. 2013;16(10):1373–82.
28. Li Z, Bao S, Wu Q, Wang H, Eyler C, Sathornsumetee S, et al. Hypoxia-inducible factors regulate tumorigenic capacity of glioma stem cells. Cancer Cell. 2009;15(6):501–13.
29. Eyler CE, Wu Q, Yan K, MacSwords JM, Chandler-Militello D, Misuraca KL, et al. Glioma stem cell proliferation and tumor growth are promoted by nitric oxide synthase-2. Cell. 2011;146(1):53–66.
30. Zhu TS, Costello MA, Talsma CE, Flack CG, Crowley JG, Hamm LL, et al. Endothelial cells create a stem cell niche in glioblastoma by providing NOTCH ligands that nurture self-renewal of cancer stem-like cells. Cancer Res. 2011;71(18):6061–72.
31. Lathia JD, Mack SC, Mulkearns-Hubert EE, Valentim CL, Rich JN. Cancer stem cells in glioblastoma. Genes Dev. 2015;29(12):1203–17.
32. Patel AP, Tirosh I, Trombetta JJ, Shalek AK, Gillespie SM, Wakimoto H, et al. Single-cell RNA-seq highlights intratumoral heterogeneity in primary glioblastoma. Science. 2014;344(6190):1396–401.
33. Reifenberger G, Wirsching HG, Knobbe-Thomsen CB, Weller M. Advances in the molecular genetics of gliomas – implications for classification and therapy. Nat Rev Clin Oncol. 2017;14(7):434–52.
34. Vogelstein B, Fearon ER, Hamilton SR, Kern SE, Preisinger AC, Leppert M, et al. Genetic alterations during colorectal-tumor development. N Engl J Med. 1988;319(9):525–32.
35. Wang J, Cazzato E, Ladewig E, Frattini V, Rosenbloom DI, Zairis S, et al. Clonal evolution of glioblastoma under therapy. Nat Genet. 2016;48(7):768–76.
36. Suzuki H, Aoki K, Chiba K, Sato Y, Shiozawa Y, Shiraishi Y, et al. Mutational landscape and clonal architecture in grade II and III gliomas. Nat Genet. 2015;47(5):458–68.
37. Yan H, Parsons DW, Jin G, McLendon R, Rasheed BA, Yuan W, et al. IDH1 and IDH2 mutations in gliomas. N Engl J Med. 2009;360(8):765–73.
38. Turcan S, Rohle D, Goenka A, Walsh LA, Fang F, Yilmaz E, et al. IDH1 mutation is sufficient to establish the glioma hypermethylator phenotype. Nature. 2012;483(7390):479–83.
39. Noushmehr H, Weisenberger DJ, Diefes K, Phillips HS, Pujara K, Berman BP, et al. Identification of a CpG island methylator phenotype that defines a distinct subgroup of glioma. Cancer Cell. 2010;17(5):510–22.
40. Parsons DW, Jones S, Zhang X, Lin JC, Leary RJ, Angenendt P, et al. An integrated genomic analysis of human glioblastoma multiforme. Science. 2008;321(5897):1807–12.
41. Xu W, Yang H, Liu Y, Yang Y, Wang P, Kim SH, et al. Oncometabolite 2-hydroxyglutarate is a competitive inhibitor of alpha-ketoglutarate-dependent dioxygenases. Cancer Cell. 2011;19(1):17–30.
42. Weller M, Stupp R, Reifenberger G, Brandes AA, van den Bent MJ, Wick W, et al. MGMT promoter methylation in malignant gliomas: ready for personalized medicine? Nat Rev Neurol. 2010;6(1):39–51.
43. Sturm D, Witt H, Hovestadt V, Khuong-Quang DA, Jones DT, Konermann C, et al. Hotspot mutations in H3F3A and IDH1 define distinct epigenetic and biological subgroups of glioblastoma. Cancer Cell. 2012;22(4):425–37.

44. Wang Q, Hu B, Hu X, Kim H, Squatrito M, Scarpace L, et al. Tumor evolution of glioma-intrinsic gene expression subtypes associates with immunological changes in the microenvironment. Cancer Cell. 2017;32(1):42–56. e6

45. Mazor T, Pankov A, Johnson BE, Hong C, Hamilton EG, Bell RJA, et al. DNA methylation and somatic mutations converge on the cell cycle and define similar evolutionary histories in brain tumors. Cancer Cell. 2015;28(3):307–17.

46. Sasaki M, Knobbe CB, Munger JC, Lind EF, Brenner D, Brustle A, et al. IDH1(R132H) mutation increases murine haematopoietic progenitors and alters epigenetics. Nature. 2012;488(7413):656–9.

47. Ceccarelli M, Barthel FP, Malta TM, Sabedot TS, Salama SR, Murray BA, et al. Molecular profiling reveals biologically discrete subsets and pathways of progression in diffuse glioma. Cell. 2016;164(3):550–63.

48. Mazor T, Pankov A, Johnson BE, Hong C, Hamilton EG, Bell RJ, et al. DNA methylation and somatic mutations converge on the cell cycle and define similar evolutionary histories in brain tumors. Cancer Cell. 2015;28(3):307–17.

49. Arita H, Narita Y, Fukushima S, Tateishi K, Matsushita Y, Yoshida A, et al. Upregulating mutations in the TERT promoter commonly occur in adult malignant gliomas and are strongly associated with total 1p19q loss. Acta Neuropathol. 2013;126(2):267–76.

50. Jones DT, Hutter B, Jager N, Korshunov A, Kool M, Warnatz HJ, et al. Recurrent somatic alterations of FGFR1 and NTRK2 in pilocytic astrocytoma. Nat Genet. 2013;45(8):927–32.

51. Hawkins C, Walker E, Mohamed N, Zhang C, Jacob K, Shirinian M, et al. BRAF-KIAA1549 fusion predicts better clinical outcome in pediatric low-grade astrocytoma. Clin Cancer Res. 2011;17(14):4790–8.

52. Chan JA, Zhang H, Roberts PS, Jozwiak S, Wieslawa G, Lewin-Kowalik J, et al. Pathogenesis of tuberous sclerosis subependymal giant cell astrocytomas: biallelic inactivation of TSC1 or TSC2 leads to mTOR activation. J Neuropathol Exp Neurol. 2004;63(12):1236–42.

53. Weber RG, Hoischen A, Ehrler M, Zipper P, Kaulich K, Blaschke B, et al. Frequent loss of chromosome 9, homozygous CDKN2A/p14(ARF)/CDKN2B deletion and low TSC1 mRNA expression in pleomorphic xanthoastrocytomas. Oncogene. 2007;26(7):1088–97.

54. Schindler G, Capper D, Meyer J, Janzarik W, Omran H, Herold-Mende C, et al. Analysis of BRAF V600E mutation in 1,320 nervous system tumors reveals high mutation frequencies in pleomorphic xanthoastrocytoma, ganglioglioma and extra-cerebellar pilocytic astrocytoma. Acta Neuropathol. 2011;121(3):397–405.

55. Pajtler KW, Witt H, Sill M, Jones DT, Hovestadt V, Kratochwil F, et al. Molecular classification of ependymal tumors across all CNS compartments, histopathological grades, and age groups. Cancer Cell. 2015;27(5):728–43.

56. Taylor MD, Northcott PA, Korshunov A, Remke M, Cho YJ, Clifford SC, et al. Molecular subgroups of medulloblastoma: the current consensus. Acta Neuropathol. 2012;123(4):465–72.

57. Northcott PA, Korshunov A, Witt H, Hielscher T, Eberhart CG, Mack S, et al. Medulloblastoma comprises four distinct molecular variants. J Clin Oncol. 2011;29(11):1408–14.

58. Zurawel RH, Chiappa SA, Allen C, Raffel C. Sporadic medulloblastomas contain oncogenic beta-catenin mutations. Cancer Res. 1998;58(5):896–9.

59. Hamilton SR, Liu B, Parsons RE, Papadopoulos N, Jen J, Powell SM, et al. The molecular basis of Turcot's syndrome. N Engl J Med. 1995;332(13):839–47.

60. Kool M, Korshunov A, Remke M, Jones DT, Schlanstein M, Northcott PA, et al. Molecular subgroups of medulloblastoma: an international meta-analysis of transcriptome, genetic aberrations, and clinical data of WNT, SHH, group 3, and group 4 medulloblastomas. Acta Neuropathol. 2012;123(4):473–84.

61. Cho YJ, Tsherniak A, Tamayo P, Santagata S, Ligon A, Greulich H, et al. Integrative genomic analysis of medulloblastoma identifies a molecular subgroup that drives poor clinical outcome. J Clin Oncol. 2011;29(11):1424–30.

62. Preusser M, Brastianos PK, Mawrin C. Advances in meningioma genetics: novel therapeutic opportunities. Nat Rev Neurol. 2018;14(2):106–15.

63. Brastianos PK, Horowitz PM, Santagata S, Jones RT, McKenna A, Getz G, et al. Genomic sequencing of meningiomas identifies oncogenic SMO and AKT1 mutations. Nat Genet. 2013;45(3):285–9.
64. Seizinger BR, de la Monte S, Atkins L, Gusella JF, Martuza RL. Molecular genetic approach to human meningioma: loss of genes on chromosome 22. Proc Natl Acad Sci U S A. 1987;84(15):5419–23.
65. Ruttledge MH, Sarrazin J, Rangaratnam S, Phelan CM, Twist E, Merel P, et al. Evidence for the complete inactivation of the NF2 gene in the majority of sporadic meningiomas. Nat Genet. 1994;6(2):180–4.
66. Goutagny S, Yang HW, Zucman-Rossi J, Chan J, Dreyfuss JM, Park PJ, et al. Genomic profiling reveals alternative genetic pathways of meningioma malignant progression dependent on the underlying NF2 status. Clin Cancer Res. 2010;16(16):4155–64.
67. Agnihotri S, Suppiah S, Tonge PD, Jalali S, Danesh A, Bruce JP, et al. Therapeutic radiation for childhood cancer drives structural aberrations of NF2 in meningiomas. Nat Commun. 2017;8(1):186.
68. Sahm F, Toprak UH, Hubschmann D, Kleinheinz K, Buchhalter I, Sill M, et al. Meningiomas induced by low-dose radiation carry structural variants of NF2 and a distinct mutational signature. Acta Neuropathol. 2017;134(1):155–8.
69. Clark VE, Harmanci AS, Bai H, Youngblood MW, Lee TI, Baranoski JF, et al. Recurrent somatic mutations in POLR2A define a distinct subset of meningiomas. Nat Genet. 2016;48(10):1253–9.
70. Clark VE, Erson-Omay EZ, Serin A, Yin J, Cotney J, Ozduman K, et al. Genomic analysis of non-NF2 meningiomas reveals mutations in TRAF7, KLF4, AKT1, and SMO. Science. 2013;339(6123):1077–80.
71. Reuss DE, Piro RM, Jones DT, Simon M, Ketter R, Kool M, et al. Secretory meningiomas are defined by combined KLF4 K409Q and TRAF7 mutations. Acta Neuropathol. 2013;125(3):351–8.
72. Shankar GM, Abedalthagafi M, Vaubel RA, Merrill PH, Nayyar N, Gill CM, et al. Germline and somatic BAP1 mutations in high-grade rhabdoid meningiomas. Neuro-Oncology. 2017;19(4):535–45.
73. Zhang L, Ridgway LD, Wetzel MD, Ngo J, Yin W, Kumar D, et al. The identification and characterization of breast cancer CTCs competent for brain metastasis. Sci Transl Med. 2013;5(180):180ra48.
74. Hanniford D, Zhong J, Koetz L, Gaziel-Sovran A, Lackaye DJ, Shang S, et al. A miRNA-based signature detected in primary melanoma tissue predicts development of brain metastasis. Clin Cancer Res. 2015;21(21):4903–12.
75. Bos PD, Zhang XH, Nadal C, Shu W, Gomis RR, Nguyen DX, et al. Genes that mediate breast cancer metastasis to the brain. Nature. 2009;459(7249):1005–9.

Classification of Tumours of the Central Nervous System

3

Luca Bertero and Paola Cassoni

3.1 Introduction

Tumours of the central nervous system (CNS) may arise from cells and structures properly belonging to the CNS (i.e. primary CNS tumours) or may be secondary tumour sites from other systemic neoplasms. Overall, CNS metastases are more frequent compared to primary CNS tumours, but the latter represent the most frequent solid paediatric tumours (0–14 years) and the first cause of death due to a neoplastic disease in this age range. In adults, incidence of CNS tumours progressively increases, but they remain relatively rare compared to other tumours. Meningioma is the most common primary CNS tumour, while glioblastoma is the most frequent glioma and it usually occurs in older adults [1].

3.2 Classification and Grading

Before the latest edition of WHO classification of central nervous system tumours (published in 2016) [2], CNS neoplasms were classified based on morphological criteria alone, grouping tumours according to their cell lineage (e.g. glial versus neuronal or astrocytic versus oligodendroglial). In the last two decades, however, many significant prognostic factors have been identified, including molecular markers which are strictly related to specific disease entities sharing similar epidemiological, histopathological, clinical and prognostic characteristics. Since the main aim of any tumour classification is to identify well-defined and prognostically relevant entities to optimize patients' care, it was decided to include these molecular alterations directly into the new diagnostic criteria. Thus, according to the latest WHO classification, diagnosis and

L. Bertero (✉) · P. Cassoni
Division of Pathology, Department of Medical Sciences, University of Turin, Turin, Italy
e-mail: luca.bertero@unito.it; paola.cassoni@unito.it

© Springer Nature Switzerland AG 2019
M. Bartolo et al. (eds.), *Neurorehabilitation in Neuro-Oncology*,
https://doi.org/10.1007/978-3-319-95684-8_3

21

classification of primary CNS tumours is now based on integration of both phenotypic (morphological) and genotypic parameters.

Histological grading is a significant prognostic factor for a wide range of tumours. Specific grading parameters vary between neoplasms, but the features evaluated for tumour grading are usually related to its differentiation. In CNS tumours, these include cytological atypia, cellularity, mitotic count and necrosis, but specific criteria are provided for each tumour type by the WHO classification. A grade ranging from I (a tumour which can be potentially cured by surgery) to IV (a highly malignant tumour) is provided for most entities; WHO grades primarily concern the natural history of disease.

A debated point is whether "traditional" histological grading is still relevant in the age of molecular prognostic markers and further studies will help answer this question, possibly identifying new meaningful grading criteria [3, 4].

3.3   Glial Tumours

Gliomas arise from glial-differentiated CNS cells and include astrocytomas, oligodendrogliomas and ependymomas. These tumours express glial markers like the glial fibrillary acidic protein (GFAP) which can be detected by immunohistochemistry.

Gliomas include two main groups of neoplasms based on the growth pattern: (1) Diffuse gliomas: these tumours show a markedly infiltrative growth into the surrounding brain parenchyma. Until the latest WHO classification, these tumours were classified into astrocytomas, oligodendrogliomas and oligoastrocytomas based on their morphological features: now, they are grouped also according to their molecular profile. This group includes grade II, III and IV tumours, without any grade I entity, since they usually recur over time, often showing a progression in terms of histological grade; (2) A second group of primary CNS tumours shows a more circumscribed growth pattern which may help achieve a greater extent of resection. Prognosis is usually better compared to diffuse gliomas. Pilocytic astrocytoma (grade I), pleomorphic xanthoastrocytoma (grade II) and anaplastic pleomorphic xanthoastrocytoma (grade III) are included in this group.

3.3.1   Diffuse Gliomas

Classification of diffuse gliomas is based on the integrated evaluation of morphological and molecular features (Fig. 3.1). The main, recurrent molecular alterations are:

- *IDH1/IDH2* **mutations:** mutations of the *IDH1* or *IDH2* isoforms of isocitrate dehydrogenase (IDH) are present in about 80% of grade II and III gliomas and *IDH1* is the most commonly mutated isoform (>90% of cases). This alteration is

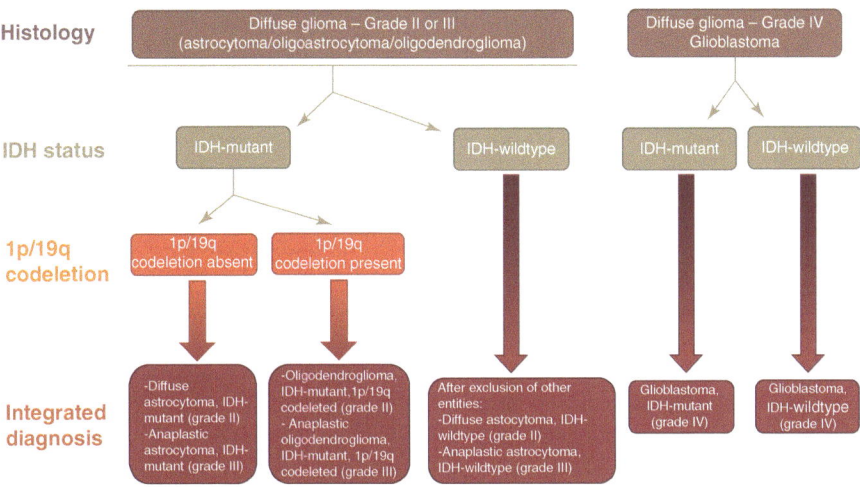

Fig. 3.1   Diagnostic algorithm for integrated histological–molecular diagnosis of diffuse gliomas

an early event during oncogenesis and induces a change of the protein function (the mutated protein leads to the production of 2-hydroxyglutarate, instead of α-ketoglutarate, which inhibits the function of enzymes involved in histone and DNA methylation, possibly leading to tumourigenesis) [5]. Prognosis of *IDH1/IDH2*-mutant gliomas is significantly better compared to *IDH1/IDH2*-wildtype tumours.

– **1p/19q codeletion:** this molecular alteration consists in the complete deletion of both the 1p and 19q chromosomal arms and it is now required for the diagnosis of oligodendroglioma. 1p/19q codeletion is associated with increased sensitivity to chemotherapy with alkylating drugs (like temozolomide). Partial deletions of the same arms do not share the same favourable prognostic/predictive role and they can occur also in other tumours.

– *ATRX* **and** *TERT* **promoter mutations:** these alterations help neoplastic cells to preserve telomeres length, thus evading replication senescence [6]. *ATRX* mutations result in a loss of its expression and are usually present in association with *TP53* mutations in IDH-mutant astrocytomas, while they are mutually exclusive with 1p/19q codeletion. Conversely, *TERT* promoter mutations are characteristic of IDH-mutant, 1p/19q codeleted, oligodendrogliomas. Since *TERT* promoter mutations are also frequent in IDH-wildtype glioblastoma, they are not specific of a disease entity and do not harbour a specific prognostic meaning.

– *EGFR* **alterations,** *CDKN2A* **deletion,** *PTEN* **mutations, 7p gain and 10q loss:** these molecular alterations are common in IDH-wildtype glioblastoma [7].

– *MGMT* **promoter methylation:** this molecular feature is not specific of a single tumour entity, but it is a favourable prognostic/predictive factor, in particular in IDH-wildtype glioblastoma treated with alkylating drugs [8].

– **H3 K27M mutation:** this mutation occurs in histone variants, including H3.3 (*H3F3A*) and H3.1 (*HIST1H3B* and *HIST1H3C*), and is a required feature for the diagnosis of diffuse midline glioma, H3 K27M-mutant, although it can be found in other CNS tumours.

Some of these alterations have to be evaluated for a correct diagnostic assessment of a diffuse glioma, but sometimes this may be not possible or may be not conclusive. In these cases, the diagnosis will be based on morphological features and the tumour will be classified as "not otherwise specified (NOS)" (e.g. "diffuse astrocytoma, grade II, NOS").

3.3.1.1 Diffuse Astrocytoma, IDH-Mutant (Grade II) and Anaplastic Astrocytoma, IDH-Mutant (Grade III)

These tumours usually occur in adults (30–40 years old), are slightly more common in males and usually arise in the frontal lobes. Histologically, diffuse astrocytoma, IDH-mutant (grade II) is characterized by a proliferation of well-differentiated fibrillary astrocytes with mild nuclear atypia (Fig. 3.2), while anaplastic astrocytoma, IDH-mutant (grade III) shows higher cellularity, more prominent nuclear atypia and increased proliferation with mitoses (Fig. 3.3). Microvascular

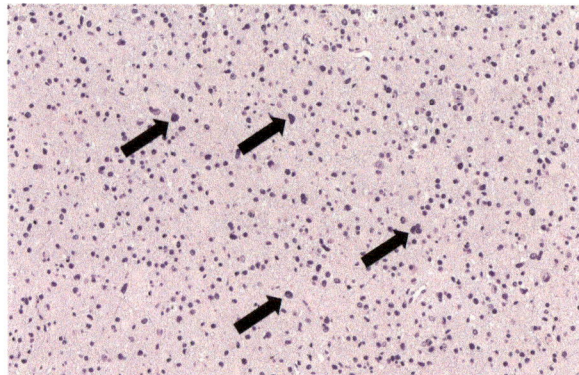

Fig. 3.2 Diffuse astrocytoma, IDH-mutant (grade II). H&E image showing brain parenchyma with increased cellularity. Neoplastic cells display astrocytic morphology and mild nuclear atypia (arrows) without mitoses

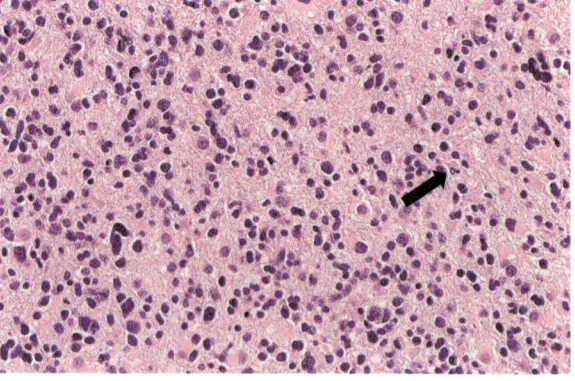

Fig. 3.3 Anaplastic astrocytoma, IDH-mutant (grade III). Compared to Fig. 3.2, cellularity is significantly increased and mitoses are present (arrow)

proliferations and necrosis are absent in both entities. By definition, these tumours harbour *IDH1* or *IDH2* mutations, usually along with *ATRX* and *p53* alterations.

Reported median survival times are 6–8 years and 3–5 years for diffuse astrocytoma and anaplastic astrocytoma, respectively, but these data need to be re-evaluated in homogenous cohorts of IDH-mutant tumours diagnosed according to the new diagnostic criteria.

3.3.1.2 Diffuse Astrocytoma, IDH-Wildtype (Grade II) and Anaplastic Astrocytoma, IDH-Wildtype (Grade III)

Morphologically, these tumours are virtually identical to their IDH-mutant counterparts, but lead to a significantly poorer outcome (<2 years median survival time). Molecular profiling data demonstrated the heterogeneous genetic landscape of these tumours, including a significant number of cases harbouring molecular fingerprints characteristic of glioblastoma, IDH-wildtype, thus providing an explanation for their clinical behaviour [9]. Nevertheless, some cases displayed molecular profiles suggestive of other astrocytic tumours, like pilocytic astrocytoma. A careful, multidisciplinary evaluation is therefore warranted in these cases to devise the best therapeutic management for each patient.

3.3.1.3 Oligodendroglioma, IDH-Mutant and 1p/19q-Codeleted (Grade II) and Anaplastic Oligodendroglioma, IDH-Mutant and 1p/19q Codeleted (Grade III)

Oligodendrogliomas are rarer than astrocytomas, but they share a similar age at diagnosis and the slightly higher prevalence in males. These tumours usually arise in the white matter and the cortex of the cerebral hemispheres, frequently in the frontal lobes. Histologically, oligodendroglioma, IDH-mutant and 1p/19q codeleted, appears as a diffusely infiltrating proliferation of monomorphic cells with round nuclei and perinuclear haloes (fried-egg appearance) on formalin-fixed paraffin-embedded sections (Fig. 3.4). A network of delicate branching capillaries is usually present and microcalcifications are also common. Mitoses are absent or rare. Conversely, brisk mitotic activity, microvascular proliferation and necrosis,

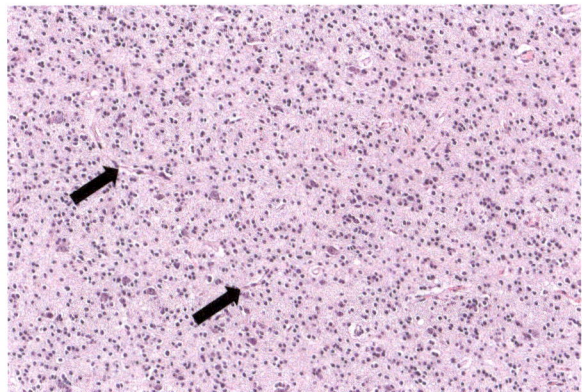

Fig. 3.4 Oligodendroglioma, IDH-mutant, 1p/19q-codeleted (grade II). H&E image showing a diffuse glial neoplasm made up of round cells with a clear perinuclear halo (*fried egg*-like cells) and with small, branching, *chicken wire*-like blood vessels (arrows)

Fig. 3.5 Anaplastic oligodendroglioma, IDH-mutant, 1p/19q-codeleted (grade III). Compared to Fig. 3.4, cellularity and atypia are increased. Microvascular proliferations and mitoses (arrows) are also present

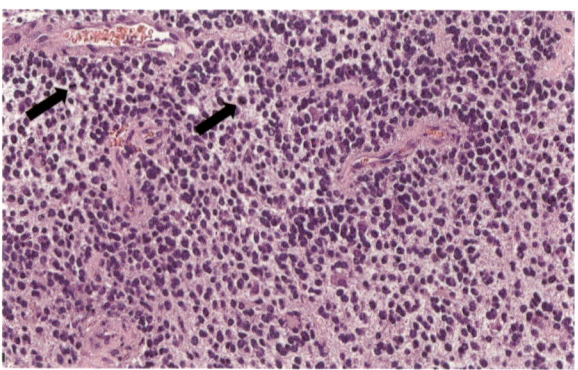

usually along with higher cellularity and more severe nuclear atypia, are diagnostic features of anaplastic oligodendroglioma, IDH-mutant and 1p/19q-codeleted (grade III) (Fig. 3.5). Diagnosis of these tumours requires the presence of either *IDH1* or *IDH2* mutation and 1p/19q codeletion, which are usually associated with *TERT* promoter mutation.

Prognosis is more favourable compared to diffuse astrocytic gliomas (median survival time greater than 10 years following current treatment protocols) [10, 11].

3.3.1.4 Glioblastoma, IDH-Wildtype (Grade IV) and Glioblastoma, IDH-Mutant (Grade IV)

Glioblastoma, IDH-wildtype (grade IV) is the most frequent glioma and usually occurs in older adults (60–70 years) compared to lower-grade diffuse gliomas. Temporal lobes are the most common affected site of IDH-wildtype glioblastoma, whereas IDH-mutant glioblastoma (grade IV) usually arises in frontal lobes, similarly to other IDH-mutant gliomas. Glioblastoma typically shows a rapidly infiltrating growth and contralateral extension through the corpus callosum is common. Microscopically, it appears as a highly cellular lesion, with poorly differentiated, atypical tumour cells and numerous mitoses. Microvascular proliferations and/or necrosis are the necessary diagnostic features (Fig. 3.6). Histopathology of this tumour can vary significantly, even in different areas of the same tumour. IDH-mutant glioblastoma histological features are similar, but necrosis is usually more limited.

Some rare variants of IDH-wildtype glioblastoma are defined: giant cell glioblastoma, gliosarcoma and epithelioid glioblastoma. Giant cell glioblastoma is characterized by the presence of multinucleated giant cells, while gliosarcoma shows a biphasic pattern with glial and mesenchymal differentiation. Epithelioid glioblastoma displays a dominant population of epithelioid or rhabdoid cells and a specific molecular alteration (*BRAF* V600E mutation) is present in about 50% of cases.

Glioblastoma, IDH-wildtype is an aggressive neoplasm with a median survival time of 15–18 months. *MGMT* promoter methylation is a favourable prognostic factor and predicts response to treatment with alkylating drugs [12]. Although limited, prognosis of glioblastoma, IDH-mutant is better (median survival time: 27–31 months) compared to its IDH-wildtype counterpart [13]. This latter tumour

Fig. 3.6 Glioblastoma, IDH-wildtype (grade IV). H&E image shows a glial neoplasm with high cellularity, necrosis and microvascular proliferations

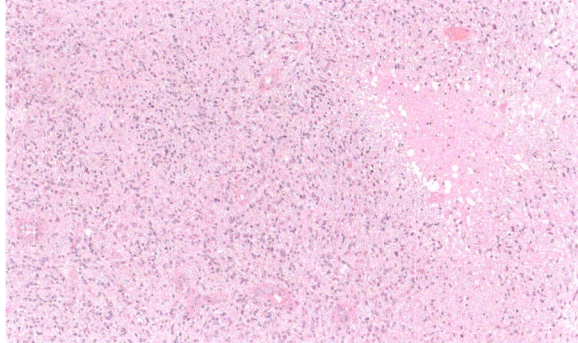

usually harbours the hallmark mutations of IDH-mutant astrocytomas (*IDH1/IDH2*, *ATRX* and *TP53* mutations) plus other molecular alterations which are acquired during disease progression.

3.3.1.5 Diffuse Midline Glioma, H3 K27M-Mutant (Grade IV)

This tumour is more frequent in children (median age at diagnosis: 5–11 years) without sex predilection. Usually, H3 K27M-mutant diffuse midline glioma (grade IV) involves midline structures including brain stem, thalamus and spinal cord. Histologically, it shows an infiltrative growth pattern and, in most cases, an astrocytic morphology. Mitoses are usually present and microvascular proliferation/ necrosis can be present, although they are not required for this diagnosis. Prognosis is poor (<10% of patients alive 2 years after diagnosis).

3.3.2 Other Astrocytic Gliomas

Pilocytic astrocytoma (grade I) usually occurs in children, with a similar incidence in both sexes. It usually arises within infratentorial structures and, histologically, it shows a relatively circumscribed growth, a low to moderate cellularity and a biphasic pattern comprising variable proportions of areas with compacted bipolar cells with Rosenthal fibres (eosinophilic fibrillary aggregates) and areas with multipolar cells, microcysts and occasional eosinophilic granular bodies (Fig. 3.7). Rare mitoses, hyperchromatic and pleomorphic nuclei, along with glomeruloid vascular proliferations can be present and are compatible with the diagnosis of pilocytic astrocytoma. Nevertheless, the presence of marked pleomorphism, brisk mitotic activity and necrosis can be due to an anaplastic change, which has prognostic implications [14]. Pilocytic astrocytomas usually harbour alterations in the MAPK pathway and the *BRAF/KIAA1549* fusion is the most common alteration (present in about 70% of cases). Prognosis is favourable (>95% 10-year overall survival rates after surgical resection alone) [15]. Pilomyxoid astrocytoma is a variant of pilocytic astrocytoma, usually arising in the hypothalamic/chiasmatic region and characterized by an angiocentric arrangement of monomorphous and bipolar tumour cells in a myxoid

Fig. 3.7 Pilocytic astrocytoma (grade I). Glial neoplasm with low to moderate cellularity, astrocytic morphology and the presence of Rosenthal fibres and eosinophilic granular bodies (arrow)

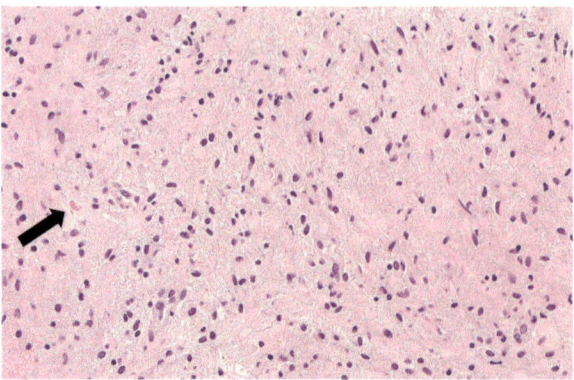

background. Compared to pilocytic astrocytoma, a higher recurrence rate is reported, although a definite WHO grade is not provided considered the limited data available.

Pleomorphic xanthoastrocytoma (grade II) is an astrocytic glioma, usually occurring in children and young adults, with a similar incidence in both sexes. Temporal lobes are the preferential site, commonly with a superficial location. Histopathological findings can vary significantly, including large, pleomorphic and often multinucleated elements, spindle and xanthomatous cells and numerous eosinophilic granular bodies. A characteristic finding is the dense pericellular reticulin network. Neuronal differentiation can be present. A ≥5/10 high power fields mitotic count is necessary for the diagnosis of anaplastic pleomorphic xanthoastrocytoma (grade III). Necrosis may be present in the latter entity, but it is not sufficient for its diagnosis. *BRAF* V600E mutation is often present. Prognosis of pleomorphic xanthoastrocytoma is relatively favourable with 5-year recurrence-free and overall survival rates of about 70% and 90%, respectively. Its anaplastic counterpart is associated with a significantly worse outcome: about 50% 5-year overall survival rate [16].

Subependymal giant cell astrocytoma (grade I) is a benign, slow-growing, astrocytic tumour with a strong association with the tuberous sclerosis syndrome (occurring in 5–15% of these patients). This neoplasm typically develops during the first two decades of life and arises from the lateral walls of the lateral ventricles adjacent to the foramen of Monro. Histologically, it shows a circumscribed growth, with a proliferation of large ganglion cell-like astrocytes (resembling gemistocytic astrocytes) arranged in fascicles, sheets and nests. Calcifications are common and mitotic activity may be present, but this finding does not seem to be associated with an adverse clinical course. Neuronal differentiation may also be present. Prognosis is good if gross total resection is achieved [17].

3.3.3 Ependymomas

Ependymomas are glial tumours which arise from the ependymal cells lining ventricles and the central canal of the spinal cord. This group of tumours encompasses

Fig. 3.8 Ependymoma (grade II). H&E image showing a perivascular pseudorosette (arrow), a histological hallmark of ependymoma

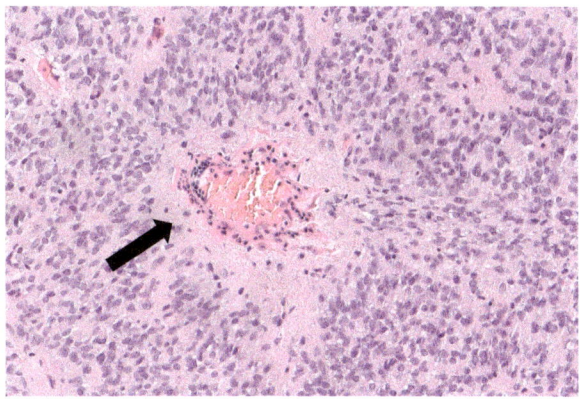

different entities: subependymoma and myxopapillary ependymoma (grade I), ependymoma (grade II) and anaplastic ependymoma (grade III). Different variants of ependymoma are recognized, based on the site of origin (supratentorial, posterior fossa and spine) and the clinico-pathological features. In recent years, molecular profiling identified specific subgroups with relevant prognostic correlations: in particular, supratentorial ependymomas characterized by the RELA gene fusion (grade II or III based on the morphological parameters) harbour a poor prognosis [18]. Although it is not a specific marker, L1CAM expression, detected by immunohisto-chemistry, correlates with the presence of RELA-fusion in supratentorial ependymomas [19].

In children, ependymomas are usually intracranial and they commonly arise from the IV ventricle; conversely, in adults most ependymomas are spinal. Histologically, perivascular pseudorosettes (consisting in neoplastic cells surrounding a fibrillary area centred by a blood vessel) are present in most ependymomas (Fig. 3.8), while true ependymal rosettes are rarer and they consist of tumour cells collected around an acellular lumen.

Prognosis is variable, usually poorer in children; extent of surgical resection, tumour site and molecular genotype have a prognostic significance, whereas the role of histological grade is uncertain [20]. Leptomeningeal dissemination through CSF is a possible complication.

3.4   Neuronal and Mixed Neuronal-Glial Tumours

These tumours are overall rarer than glial neoplasms and consist of entities with a neuronal or a mixed neuronal–glial differentiation. They usually occur in children or young adults and they are typically associated with drug-resistant seizures. Outcome is usually favourable and surgical resection is often curative. Many specific entities are categorized in this group, including dysembryoplastic neuroepithelial tumour (grade I), gangliocytoma (grade I), ganglioglioma (grade I) and anaplastic ganglioglioma (grade III).

3.4.1 Dysembryoplastic Neuroepithelial Tumour (Grade I)

Dysembryoplastic neuroepithelial tumour (grade I) (DNT) is a benign glioneuronal neoplasm usually occurring in children or young adults, with a slight prevalence in males and typically arising in the temporal lobe cortex with a multinodular architecture. A histological hallmark of this tumour is the so-called specific glioneuronal element which consists of columns oriented perpendicularly to the cortical surface, made up of bundles of axons lined by small oligodendrocyte-like cells. Between these columns, a mucinous matrix, including cytologically normal floating neurons, is present. DNTs harbour *BRAF* V600E mutation in about 30% of cases [21]. Outcome is usually excellent and recurrence or progression is exceptional.

3.4.2 Ganglioglioma (Grade I) and Anaplastic Ganglioglioma (Grade III)

Ganglioglioma (grade I) is a well-differentiated, slow-growing, glioneuronal tumour made up of dysplastic ganglion cells and neoplastic glial cells. It usually occurs in children and young adults without a clear prevalence between the sexes. Most common sites are temporal lobes, but it has been reported throughout the CNS. Histologically, it appears as a combination of neuronal and glial elements. Dysplastic ganglion cells appear as large, possibly binucleated, cells with dysmorphic neuronal features and lacking cytoarchitectural organization. Occasional mitoses and small foci of necrosis are allowed. Also for this tumour, *BRAF* V600E mutation is the most common genetic alteration, occurring in a significant number of cases [21–23]. Prognosis is usually good, although recurrence and malignant transformation can occur [24].

In anaplastic ganglioglioma (grade III), a malignant transformation of the glial component is present, including increased cellularity, pleomorphism and increased mitotic count. Vascular proliferation and necrosis can also be present. Available data concerning prognosis of this specific entity are limited and conflicting [24–26].

3.5 Embryonal Tumours

Embryonal tumours usually occur in infants and children and, in most cases, they display an aggressive clinical behaviour, although successful treatment is possible, thanks to multimodal protocols. The classification of this group of neoplasms has been heavily influenced by the molecular profiling data published during last years, which now integrate the traditional histopathological criteria. This group of tumours includes the medulloblastoma (grade IV), the embryonal tumour with multi-layered rosettes, C19MC-altered (grade IV) and the atypical teratoid/rhabdoid tumour (grade IV).

3.5.1 Medulloblastoma (Grade IV)

This is the most frequent CNS embryonal tumour, arising in the cerebellum or in the dorsal brain stem. Up to the latest WHO classification, medulloblastomas (grade IV) were classified in specific morphological variants (i.e. classic medulloblastoma, desmoplastic/nodular medulloblastoma, medulloblastoma with extensive nodularity and large cell/anaplastic medulloblastoma) based on their histological features and prognostic relevance. In recent years, however, recurrent molecular alterations were identified and four groups of genetically defined medulloblastomas have been defined [27]. Their comparison with the morphology-based variants of medulloblastoma showed only a partial overlap.

Histologically, classic medulloblastoma appears as highly cellular tumours with small, round, undifferentiated cells displaying mild-moderate nuclear pleomorphism and a high mitotic count (Fig. 3.9). Intratumoural desmoplasia is absent, although nodular areas of neurocytic differentiation with reduced cell proliferation can be present. The desmoplastic/nodular variant shows a nodular architecture including nodular, reticulin-free areas, and intervening densely cellular areas with an intercellular network of reticulin-positive collagen fibres. Medulloblastoma with extensive nodularity features prominent large reticulin-free nodules of neurocytic cells in a neuropil-like matrix and narrow internodular strands of poorly differentiated neoplastic cells in a desmoplastic matrix. Lastly, large cell/anaplastic medulloblastoma displays markedly pleomorphic, undifferentiated neoplastic cells with prominent nucleoli and a high mitotic count.

Genetically, four main molecular groups of medulloblastomas are recognized. WNT-activated medulloblastomas show activation of the WNT signalling pathway, represent about 10% of all medulloblastomas and usually correspond to the classic medulloblastoma morphological variant. Following the present multimodal treatments, prognosis is excellent and, contrary to SHH-activated medulloblastomas, it is not worsened by *TP53* mutation. SHH-activated medulloblastomas are about 30% of all medulloblastomas and include the desmoplastic/nodular and

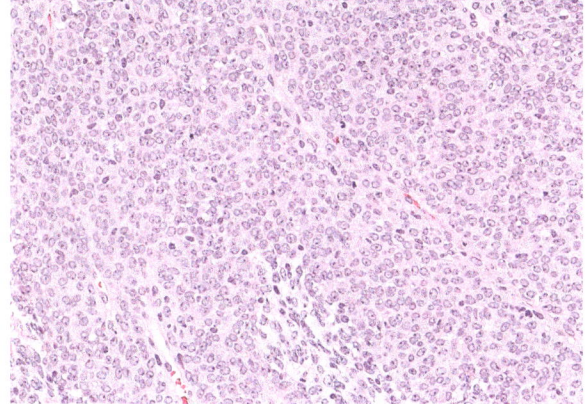

Fig. 3.9 Medulloblastoma (grade IV). Medulloblastoma, histologically defined as classic, consisting of densely packed, undifferentiated cells with high mitotic count

the extensive nodularity subtypes, although the other morphological variants can also resolve as SHH-activated medulloblastomas. Prognosis is significantly impacted by *TP53* status, being poorer in mutated tumours [28]. The group of non-WNT/non-SHH medulloblastomas includes group 3 and group 4 medulloblastomas and represents about 60% of all of these tumours (20% are group 3 and 40% group 4). Morphology is either classic or large cell/anaplastic. Prognosis is relatively poor, especially for group 3 tumours which often show metastases at diagnosis.

A surrogate determination of the molecular group is partially possible by immunohistochemistry [29] and an integrated diagnosis including both the histologically defined and the genetically defined type of medulloblastoma is recommended, since it provides the most comprehensive prognostic–predictive information.

3.5.2 Embryonal Tumour with Multi-Layered Rosettes, C19MC-Altered (Grade IV)

This is an aggressive embryonal tumour with multi-layered rosettes (ETMR) and alterations (including amplification and fusions) of the C19MC locus at 19q13.42 [30, 31]. ETMR, C19MC-altered (grade IV) can arise both in the supratentorial (70% of cases) and in the infratentorial (30%) compartments and usually occur in infants and young children with a similar distribution between sexes. Histological findings can vary significantly and any CNS embryonal tumour, even lacking the distinctive histopathological features, qualifies for this designation if it harbours C19MC amplification or fusion. Prognosis is limited: reported survival times are about 12 months even after multimodal treatments.

3.5.3 Atypical Teratoid/Rhabdoid Tumour (Grade IV)

Atypical teratoid/rhabdoid tumour (AT/RT) (grade IV) is a malignant CNS embryonal tumour occurring most frequently in young children. Histologically, this tumour consists mainly of poorly differentiated cells, often with rhabdoid features (cells with eccentric nuclei, prominent eosinophilic nucleoli, abundant cytoplasms with an eosinophilic globular inclusion and well-defined cell borders). However, these lesions are usually heavily heterogeneous and can show primitive neuroectodermal, mesenchymal and epithelial features. Diagnosis requires demonstration of *SMARCB1* or *SMARCA4* inactivation (leading to negative INI1 and BRG1 immunohistochemistry, respectively): if this molecular alteration is present, diagnosis is allowed even if the distinctive rhabdoid features are absent. Recent data suggest that specific molecular subgroups of this tumour do exist [32, 33]. Overall prognosis is poor, but intensive combined treatments may benefit a subgroup of patients.

3.6   Meningiomas

Meningiomas are the most common CNS primary tumour. They usually occur in adults, more frequently in females and can arise throughout the CNS from the meningothelial cells of the arachnoid layer. Different histological types of meningiomas are recognized by the WHO classification, including entities from grade I (about 70–80% of cases) to III. Grade I meningiomas are usually amenable of cure by surgical resection alone, grade II meningiomas have higher recurrence rates and anaplastic, grade III meningiomas show an aggressive behaviour with possible metastases.

Meningothelial and fibrous are the most common morphological variants among grade I meningiomas: the first shows medium-sized epithelioid neoplastic cells arranged in lobules, partially demarcated by thin collagenous septa (Fig. 3.10), while the latter consists of spindle cells arranged in parallel, storiform and interlacing bundles in a collagen-rich matrix. In both variants, whorls and psammoma bodies (round collections of calcium) are infrequent, although they are frequently observed in transitional meningioma, another common grade I meningioma variant which displays both meningothelial and fibrous patterns as well as transitional features. Independently of other histological features, meningiomas are classified as atypical (grade II) if increased mitotic activity or brain invasion or three out of these five characteristics are observed: increased cellularity, small cells with a high nuclear/cytoplasm ratio, prominent nucleoli, sheeting (i.e. uninterrupted patternless growth) and foci of spontaneous necrosis. Moreover, two specific rare morphological variants are considered grade II tumours: chordoid meningioma and clear cell meningioma. Anaplastic meningiomas (grade III) display overtly malignant cytology (resembling carcinoma, melanoma or high-grade sarcoma) and/or markedly elevated mitotic activity. As per grade II meningiomas, two rare morphological variants are classified as grade III tumours: papillary meningioma and rhabdoid meningioma.

Fig. 3.10 Meningothelial meningioma (grade I). A common variant of meningioma with uniform cells and lobular architecture

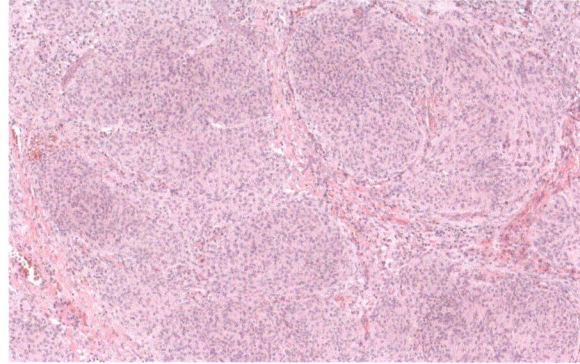

3.7   Familial Tumour Syndromes

Many genetic syndromes confer an increased risk of developing CNS tumours, including neurofibromatosis type 1 and 2, schwannomatosis, Von Hippel-Lindau disease, tuberous sclerosis, Li-Fraumeni syndrome, Cowden syndrome, Turcot syndrome, naevoid basal cell carcinoma syndrome and rhabdoid tumour predisposition syndrome. A specific follow-up of these patients is therefore warranted.

3.8   Metastatic Tumours

A considerable number of patients with systemic tumours (up to about 20%) develop secondary metastases to the CNS with a significant impact in terms of quality of life and overall prognosis. Lung, breast tumours and melanoma are the solid tumours that most commonly metastasize to the CNS. Metastatic lesions are usually multiple, preferentially located at the grey/white matter boundary, with variable dimensions and peripheral oedema. A specific kind of secondary CNS spread, which can occur both in patients with solid and haematological malignancies, is neoplastic meningitis which consists of leptomeningeal neoplastic involvement with circulation of neoplastic cell in the CSF. Identification of molecular markers associated with the risk of developing CNS metastases is warranted to optimize patients' management and follow-up.

3.9   Future Perspectives

The identification of novel diagnostic, prognostic and predictive markers for CNS tumours will help improve patients' care, which is also the ultimate aim of every tumour classification. Specific initiatives have therefore been proposed, like the cIMPACT-NOW Consortium, to facilitate the prompt introduction into clinical diagnosis and practice of the latest published research, even before WHO classification updates [34, 35]. The provided recommendations will hopefully help the medical community provide the most up-to-date diagnostic and therapeutic management to patients.

References

1. Ostrom QT, Gittleman H, Xu J, Kromer C, Wolinsky Y, Kruchko C, et al. CBTRUS statistical report: primary brain and other central nervous system tumors diagnosed in the United States in 2009–2013. Neuro-Oncology. 2016;18(Suppl_5):v1–v75. https://doi.org/10.1093/neuonc/now207.
2. Louis DN. International Agency for Research on Cancer. WHO classification of tumours of the central nervous system. Revised 4th ed. World Health Organization classification of tumours. Lyon: International Agency For Research On Cancer; 2016.

3. Reuss DE, Mamatjan Y, Schrimpf D, Capper D, Hovestadt V, Kratz A, et al. IDH mutant diffuse and anaplastic astrocytomas have similar age at presentation and little difference in survival: a grading problem for WHO. Acta Neuropathol. 2015;129(6):867–73. https://doi.org/10.1007/s00401-015-1438-8.

4. Hubner JM, Kool M, Pfister SM, Pajtler KW. Epidemiology, molecular classification and WHO grading of ependymoma. J Neurosurg Sci. 2017; https://doi.org/10.23736/S0390-5616.17.04152-2.

5. Waitkus MS, Diplas BH, Yan H. Isocitrate dehydrogenase mutations in gliomas. Neuro-Oncology. 2016;18(1):16–26. https://doi.org/10.1093/neuonc/nov136.

6. Walsh KM, Wiencke JK, Lachance DH, Wiemels JL, Molinaro AM, Eckel-Passow JE, et al. Telomere maintenance and the etiology of adult glioma. Neuro-Oncology. 2015;17(11):1445–52. https://doi.org/10.1093/neuonc/nov082.

7. Brennan CW, Verhaak RG, McKenna A, Campos B, Noushmehr H, Salama SR, et al. The somatic genomic landscape of glioblastoma. Cell. 2013;155(2):462–77. https://doi.org/10.1016/j.cell.2013.09.034.

8. LeBlanc VG, Marra MA. DNA methylation in adult diffuse gliomas. Brief Funct Genomics. 2016; https://doi.org/10.1093/bfgp/elw019.

9. Reuss DE, Kratz A, Sahm F, Capper D, Schrimpf D, Koelsche C, et al. Adult IDH wild type astrocytomas biologically and clinically resolve into other tumor entities. Acta Neuropathol. 2015;130(3):407–17. https://doi.org/10.1007/s00401-015-1454-8.

10. van den Bent MJ, Brandes AA, Taphoorn MJ, Kros JM, Kouwenhoven MC, Delattre JY, et al. Adjuvant procarbazine, lomustine, and vincristine chemotherapy in newly diagnosed anaplastic oligodendroglioma: long-term follow-up of EORTC brain tumor group study 26951. J Clin Oncol. 2013;31(3):344–50. https://doi.org/10.1200/JCO.2012.43.2229.

11. Cairncross G, Wang M, Shaw E, Jenkins R, Brachman D, Buckner J, et al. Phase III trial of chemoradiotherapy for anaplastic oligodendroglioma: long-term results of RTOG 9402. J Clin Oncol. 2013;31(3):337–43. https://doi.org/10.1200/JCO.2012.43.2674.

12. Stupp R, Hegi ME, Mason WP, van den Bent MJ, Taphoorn MJ, Janzer RC, et al. Effects of radiotherapy with concomitant and adjuvant temozolomide versus radiotherapy alone on survival in glioblastoma in a randomised phase III study: 5-year analysis of the EORTC-NCIC trial. Lancet Oncol. 2009;10(5):459–66. https://doi.org/10.1016/S1470-2045(09)70025-7.

13. Hartmann C, Hentschel B, Simon M, Westphal M, Schackert G, Tonn JC, et al. Long-term survival in primary glioblastoma with versus without isocitrate dehydrogenase mutations. Clin Cancer Res. 2013;19(18):5146–57. https://doi.org/10.1158/1078-0432.CCR-13-0017.

14. Rodriguez FJ, Scheithauer BW, Burger PC, Jenkins S, Giannini C. Anaplasia in pilocytic astrocytoma predicts aggressive behavior. Am J Surg Pathol. 2010;34(2):147–60. https://doi.org/10.1097/PAS.0b013e3181c75238.

15. Fernandez C, Figarella-Branger D, Girard N, Bouvier-Labit C, Gouvernet J, Paz Paredes A, et al. Pilocytic astrocytomas in children: prognostic factors--a retrospective study of 80 cases. Neurosurgery. 2003;53(3):544–53. discussion 54–5

16. Ida CM, Rodriguez FJ, Burger PC, Caron AA, Jenkins SM, Spears GM, et al. Pleomorphic Xanthoastrocytoma: natural history and long-term follow-up. Brain Pathol. 2015;25(5):575–86. https://doi.org/10.1111/bpa.12217.

17. de Ribaupierre S, Dorfmuller G, Bulteau C, Fohlen M, Pinard JM, Chiron C, et al. Subependymal giant-cell astrocytomas in pediatric tuberous sclerosis disease: when should we operate? Neurosurgery. 2007;60(1):83–9.; discussion 9–90. https://doi.org/10.1227/01.NEU.0000249216.19591.5D.

18. Pajtler KW, Witt H, Sill M, Jones DT, Hovestadt V, Kratochwil F, et al. Molecular classification of ependymal tumors across all CNS compartments, histopathological grades, and age groups. Cancer Cell. 2015;27(5):728–43. https://doi.org/10.1016/j.ccell.2015.04.002.

19. Parker M, Mohankumar KM, Punchihewa C, Weinlich R, Dalton JD, Li Y, et al. C11orf95-RELA fusions drive oncogenic NF-kappaB signalling in ependymoma. Nature. 2014;506(7489):451–5. https://doi.org/10.1038/nature13109.

20. Ellison DW, Kocak M, Figarella-Branger D, Felice G, Catherine G, Pietsch T, et al. Histopathological grading of pediatric ependymoma: reproducibility and clinical relevance in European trial cohorts. J Negat Results Biomed. 2011;10:7. https://doi.org/10.1186/1477-5751-10-7.
21. Chappe C, Padovani L, Scavarda D, Forest F, Nanni-Metellus I, Loundou A, et al. Dysembryoplastic neuroepithelial tumors share with pleomorphic xanthoastrocytomas and gangliogliomas BRAF(V600E) mutation and expression. Brain Pathol. 2013;23(5):574–83. https://doi.org/10.1111/bpa.12048.
22. Dougherty MJ, Santi M, Brose MS, Ma C, Resnick AC, Sievert AJ, et al. Activating mutations in BRAF characterize a spectrum of pediatric low-grade gliomas. Neuro-Oncology. 2010;12(7):621–30. https://doi.org/10.1093/neuonc/noq007.
23. Schindler G, Capper D, Meyer J, Janzarik W, Omran H, Herold-Mende C, et al. Analysis of BRAF V600E mutation in 1,320 nervous system tumors reveals high mutation frequencies in pleomorphic xanthoastrocytoma, ganglioglioma and extra-cerebellar pilocytic astrocytoma. Acta Neuropathol. 2011;121(3):397–405. https://doi.org/10.1007/s00401-011-0802-6.
24. Luyken C, Blumcke I, Fimmers R, Urbach H, Wiestler OD, Schramm J. Supratentorial gangliogliomas: histopathologic grading and tumor recurrence in 184 patients with a median follow-up of 8 years. Cancer. 2004;101(1):146–55. https://doi.org/10.1002/cncr.20332.
25. Majores M, von Lehe M, Fassunke J, Schramm J, Becker AJ, Simon M. Tumor recurrence and malignant progression of gangliogliomas. Cancer. 2008;113(12):3355–63. https://doi.org/10.1002/cncr.23965.
26. Karremann M, Pietsch T, Janssen G, Kramm CM, Wolff JE. Anaplastic ganglioglioma in children. J Neuro-Oncol. 2009;92(2):157–63. https://doi.org/10.1007/s11060-008-9747-6.
27. Kool M, Korshunov A, Remke M, Jones DT, Schlanstein M, Northcott PA, et al. Molecular subgroups of medulloblastoma: an international meta-analysis of transcriptome, genetic aberrations, and clinical data of WNT, SHH, group 3, and group 4 medulloblastomas. Acta Neuropathol. 2012;123(4):473–84. https://doi.org/10.1007/s00401-012-0958-8.
28. Zhukova N, Ramaswamy V, Remke M, Pfaff E, Shih DJ, Martin DC, et al. Subgroup-specific prognostic implications of TP53 mutation in medulloblastoma. J Clin Oncol. 2013;31(23):2927–35. https://doi.org/10.1200/JCO.2012.48.5052.
29. Ellison DW, Dalton J, Kocak M, Nicholson SL, Fraga C, Neale G, et al. Medulloblastoma: clinicopathological correlates of SHH, WNT, and non-SHH/WNT molecular subgroups. Acta Neuropathol. 2011;121(3):381–96. https://doi.org/10.1007/s00401-011-0800-8.
30. Korshunov A, Remke M, Gessi M, Ryzhova M, Hielscher T, Witt H, et al. Focal genomic amplification at 19q13.42 comprises a powerful diagnostic marker for embryonal tumors with ependymoblastic rosettes. Acta Neuropathol. 2010;120(2):253–60. https://doi.org/10.1007/s00401-010-0688-8.
31. Nobusawa S, Yokoo H, Hirato J, Kakita A, Takahashi H, Sugino T, et al. Analysis of chromosome 19q13.42 amplification in embryonal brain tumors with ependymoblastic multilayered rosettes. Brain Pathol. 2012;22(5):689–97. https://doi.org/10.1111/j.1750-3639.2012.00574.x.
32. Torchia J, Picard D, Lafay-Cousin L, Hawkins CE, Kim SK, Letourneau L, et al. Molecular subgroups of atypical teratoid rhabdoid tumours in children: an integrated genomic and clinicopathological analysis. Lancet Oncol. 2015;16(5):569–82. https://doi.org/10.1016/S1470-2045(15)70114-2.
33. Johann PD, Erkek S, Zapatka M, Kerl K, Buchhalter I, Hovestadt V, et al. Atypical teratoid/rhabdoid tumors are comprised of three epigenetic subgroups with distinct enhancer landscapes. Cancer Cell. 2016;29(3):379–93. https://doi.org/10.1016/j.ccell.2016.02.001.
34. Louis DN, Aldape K, Brat DJ, Capper D, Ellison DW, Hawkins C, et al. Announcing cIMPACT-NOW: the consortium to inform molecular and practical approaches to CNS tumor taxonomy. Acta Neuropathol. 2017;133(1):1–3. https://doi.org/10.1007/s00401-016-1646-x.
35. Louis DN, Aldape K, Brat DJ, Capper D, Ellison DW, Hawkins C, et al. cIMPACT-NOW (the consortium to inform molecular and practical approaches to CNS tumor taxonomy): a new initiative in advancing nervous system tumor classification. Brain Pathol. 2017;27(6):851–2. https://doi.org/10.1111/bpa.12457.

Clinical Concepts of Brain Tumors

Carlotta Chiavazza, Federica Franchino, and Roberta Rudà

Neurological symptoms and signs of brain tumors are not specifically tied to individual specific tumor types, but rather to location within the central nervous system (CNS). Tumor can damage neural tissue by infiltration or displace by compression, leading to focal symptoms. Direct invasion from a tumor typically occurs in gliomas, whereas meningiomas displace normal brain. The disruption of the blood–brain barrier by the tumor leads to vasogenic edema that is one of the main causes of neurological impairment: edema favors an increase of mass effect and thus a further compression of the surrounding brain [1].

Clinical symptoms of brain tumors can be divided into:

- Generalized symptoms (nausea, vomiting, and headache) related to increased intracranial pressure or hydrocephalus;
- Focal symptoms, related to the impaired function of the involved areas of the brain (focal seizures with or without secondary generalization, motor, sensitive and memory deficit, aphasia, ataxia, visual loss) [1].

Increased intracranial pressure leads to a syndrome that variably depends on the obstruction of the ventricular or venous system, the cerebrospinal fluid (CSF) flow impairment or the direct effect of the lesion and associated edema. As a matter of fact the skull contains three components, such as nervous tissue, cerebrospinal fluid, and blood. The increase of one of these components leads to the decrease of one of the others, and the intracranial pressure remains stable; however, this balance fails over time, so that even a little increase of brain, blood, or CSF volume leads to a rapid increase of intracranial pressure according to the Monro-Kellie hypothesis. Typical symptoms of increased intracranial pressure include headache, vomiting, papilledema, and impaired state of consciousness. An uncontrolled increase of the

C. Chiavazza · F. Franchino · R. Rudà (✉)
Department of Neuro-Oncology, University and City of Health and Science Hospital, Turin, Italy

© Springer Nature Switzerland AG 2019
M. Bartolo et al. (eds.), *Neurorehabilitation in Neuro-Oncology*,
https://doi.org/10.1007/978-3-319-95684-8_4

intracranial pressure will cause a herniation of specific cerebral structures, i.e., dislocation of cerebral tissue from one cerebral compartment to another. The most common herniations are:

- Temporal herniation through the tentorium: symptoms are due to the compression of brainstem structures, including III ipsilateral cranial nerve, contralateral pyramidal tracts, reticular formation, and autonomic brainstem centers. Neurological symptoms consist of ipsilateral III nerve palsy and pyramidal signs, blood pressure and breath alterations, impaired consciousness, and ultimately coma;
- Herniation of cingulus under the cerebral falx, with symptoms often related to local ischemic lesions;
- Herniation of cerebellar tonsils through the foramen magno, leading to bulbar compression and symptoms such as blood pressure and breath alterations, "cerebellar fits" and impaired consciousness, and coma [1, 2].

Hydrocephalus is an abnormal dilation of the ventricles of the brain. In brain tumors, hydrocephalus can be caused by obstruction of CSF circulation, occurring mainly in upper brainstem or infratentorial tumors, or by increased CSF production, e.g., in choroid plexus papillomas. By definition, these types of hydrocephalus lead to intracranial hypertension and related symptoms [3].

Moreover, meningeal symptoms (headache, vomiting, photophobia, cranial nerve impairment) and meningeal signs (rigor nucalis, Lasegue, Brudzinski, or Kernig signs) may be found in patients with leptomeningeal spread of tumor cells both in primary CNS and systemic tumors (e.g., breast cancer, lung cancer, melanoma, lymphomas, leukemias) [1].

4.1   Generalized Symptoms

4.1.1   Altered Mental Status and Behavior Changes

Symptoms such as confusion, disorientation, lethargy, and coma can be due to raised intracranial pressure, hydrocephalus, or involvement of deep seated structures (thalamus, corpus callosum, or reticular formation). Changes in personality, irritability, emotional lability, apathy, and slowed responses can be seen in about 16–34% of patients: these changes are related to the involvement of frontal and temporal lobes or the limbic system. Subtle symptoms of personality changes are often presenting symptoms of primary central nervous system lymphomas (PCNSL) [1, 4, 5].

4.1.2   Headache

Headache is rarely an isolated presenting symptom of a brain tumor, being usually associated with other symptoms. In patients presenting with headache, posterior fossa tumors (ependymomas or medulloblastomas) can often be found. In case of increased intracranial pressure, headache is typically associated with vomiting and is present on awakening, and persists during the day with variable characteristics (pulsating, dull, or diffuse pain, often with both frontal and nuchal localization) [1, 6, 7]. This type of headache worsens with Valsalva maneuver and has a poor response to analgesic treatments. Red flags that should raise the suspicion of a brain tumor include the association with neurological signs or a new headache, especially in an aged patient [8]. Headache can be found in case of leptomeningeal dissemination of a primary cerebral or extracerebral tumor due to meningeal irritation.

4.1.3   Nausea and Vomiting

Nausea and vomiting can be associated with increased intracranial pressure or hydrocephalus that leads to stimulation of the chemotactic trigger zone in the area postrema. Nausea and vomiting can also be due to the direct infiltration of the chemotactic trigger zone by posterior fossa tumors (e.g., in medulloblastomas or ependymomas of the fourth ventricle), or to the invasion of the nucleus solitarius in case of brainstem tumors [1]. In tumors involving the temporal lobe, nausea can also represent a manifestation of a seizure [9].

4.1.4   Papilledema

Papilledema, revealed by fundus oculi examination, is a sign of increased intracranial pressure, seen more often in children and young adults. Symptoms are usually bilateral, characterized by enlargement of blind spot or reduced visual acuity. Chronic condition, such as frontal lobe tumors or frontal-olfactory meningiomas, may rarely lead to the Foster Kennedy syndrome, characterized by optic atrophy on the side of the tumor and papilledema on the contralateral side due to increased intracranial pressure [1].

4.2   Focal Symptoms

4.2.1   Frontal Lobe Tumors

Prefrontal tumors produce changes in behavior and personality, including apathy, slowing of cognitive processes, attention and memory deficits, and disinhibition. If the tumor involves the olfactory cortex, the patients can complain of hyposmia. Lesions involving the pre-central cortex (Brodmann areas 4, 6, 8, and 44) cause contralateral hyposthenia (with variable combination of facial, brachial, or crural hyposthenia), skew deviation, motor or ideo-motor apraxia, or expressive aphasia (area 44). Moreover, frontal lesions cause focal frontal seizures with symptoms such as loss of consciousness with motor automatisms (prefrontal partial complex seizures), partial motor symptoms (areas 4, 6), sometimes with forced deviation of head and eyes (area 8), and aphasic symptoms (partial seizures involving area 44). Partial motor seizures are not rarely complicated by secondary generalization [1, 10].

4.2.2 Parietal Lobe Tumors

Lesions involving the post-central cortex cause contralateral hypoesthesia. Tumors in posterior parietal areas cause associative agnosia or specific syndromes related to the involvement of Brodmann areas 39 and 40: in the right hemisphere, the Anton Babinski syndrome (hemiasomatognosia with anosognosia); in the left hemisphere, the Gerstmann syndrome (left-right confusion, digital agnosia, agraphia, acalculia). Other symptoms of parietal lesions include constructional and ideational apraxia. Parietal lobe seizures present with contralateral paresthesias with craniocaudal or caudocranial spreading or with body perception illusions (the so-called Alice syndrome) [1, 10].

4.2.3 Temporal Lobe Tumors

Temporal lobe tumors frequently cause memory impairment due to the disruption of the Papez circuit: most patients complain of short-term or even anterograde memory deficits. Lesions involving Brodmann area 22 cause receptive aphasia, with difficulty or impossibility to understand words' meaning; lesions involving acoustic areas can cause contralateral hypoacusia. Seizures are very frequent in temporal tumors, due to the lower epileptogenic threshold of this part of the brain. Temporal partial complex seizures may include: olfactory hallucinations (usually disgusting smells); déjà-vu or déjà-vécu phenomena; psychic/emotional sensations ("forced thinking," depersonalization, unexplained joy, or sadness); loss of consciousness with oral, mimic, verbal, or walking automatisms [1, 10].

4.2.4 Occipital Lobe Tumors

Occipital lesions cause contralateral visual field defects (namely, contralateral homonymous hemianopsia) and optic agnosia. Occipital seizures can cause visual illusions or hallucinations, either simple (phosphenes) or complex, usually without emotional involvement [1, 10].

4.2.5 Corpus Callosum

Many brain tumors, especially gliomas or lymphomas, infiltrate corpus callosum. Symptoms are mainly cognitive, due to the disconnection of the cerebral hemispheres: in particular, the patient can present slowing of thinking, ideo-motor apraxia, tactile anomia, and visual anomia [1, 10].

4.2.6   Cerebellar Tumors

Tumors involving the vermis of the cerebellum cause ataxia, nystagmus, and dysarthria while hemispheric cerebellar lesions cause dysmetria, dizziness, and adyadococinesia [1, 10].

4.2.7   Brainstem Tumors

Symptoms are different, depending on the site of the lesion. One can find motor or sensitive deficits, cranial nerve palsies (in most cases diplopia or dysphagia), sphincteric dysfunctions, impaired consciousness, blood pressure variations, or respiratory changes [1, 10].

4.2.8   Sellar Tumors

Symptoms of tumors of the sella turcica include visual field defects (due to compression of optic chiasma), endocrinologic dysfunctions (pan or partial hypopituitarism), and symptoms of increased intracranial pressure [1, 10, 11].

4.3   Clinical Aspects of CNS Tumors Depending on Histology

Pilocytic astrocytomas are usually located in the chiasmatic/hypothalamic region or in the cerebellum. In the first case, patients show visual field defects or endocrinologic dysfunctions while in the second case ataxia, nystagmus, or dysmetria can be found. Grade II and III astrocytomas are typically located in the cerebral hemispheres, and seizures are symptoms at onset in a high percentage of patients. Astrocytomas are more frequent in the juvenile-adult age. On the contrary, glioblastomas (GBMs) are more frequent in the late-adult age and in the elderly: they are rapidly growing tumors, involving cerebral hemispheres with a tendency toward corpus callosum infiltration, subependymal diffusion, or multifocal spreading. Patients with glioblastoma show a wide range of symptoms, from loss of a specific area functions to seizures, headache, and vomiting (especially during tumor progression). In a late disease stage clinical signs of meningeal spread can be found. Oligodendrogliomas are adult-age tumors involving cerebral white matter and cortex: seizures are very frequent together with specific area-related dysfunctions. Gangliogliomas, gangliocytomas, and dysembryoplastic neuroepithelial tumors (DNET) involve the cerebral hemispheres, are typically located in the temporal lobe and associated to seizures, often pharmacoresistant, in the majority of cases. In patients with gliomatosis cerebri, which is a diffuse astrocytic or less frequently oligodendrocytic tumor, multiple signs and symptoms are found, given the frequent diffuse involvement of cerebral hemispheres, brainstem, and cerebellum. Cognitive symptoms are usually present. Also, primary CNS lymphomas often present with cognitive and psychic symptoms, due to the location in deep structures (corpus callosum, basal ganglia). Cerebellar tumors, such as medulloblastoma, hemangioblastomas, or IV ventricle ependymomas, show symptoms such as ataxia, dizziness, dysmetria, nystagmus, dysarthria, or symptoms of intracranial hypertension (sometimes with hydrocephalus). Papillomas of choroid plexus, central neurocytomas, colloid cysts, and meningiomas are brain tumors that can grow in the intraventricular space and produce hydrocephalus.

Grade I meningiomas have an extra-axial growth, with symptoms that emerge several years after the tumor birth, while grade II (atypical) or grade III (anaplastic) meningiomas have a more aggressive course characterized compression dislocation or infiltration of brain parenchyma. Falx meningiomas produce paraparesis, lower limbs numbness, and seizures; sellar meningiomas produce visual field loss, hypothalamic and hypophyseal dysfunctions; cavernous sinus meningiomas yield the "cavernous sinus syndrome," characterized by palsy of ipsilateral III, IV, VI, and ophthalmic branch of V cranial nerves; clivus meningiomas give dysfunctions of IX–XI cranial nerves. Tumors located in the pontocerebellar angle (neurinomas, meningiomas) produce peripheric palsy of the VII cranial nerve, deficit of V cranial nerve, dizziness, and ipsilateral dysmetria. In case of acoustic neuroma, the "brain" phase is preceded by otologic symptoms (hypoacusia, tinnitus, dizziness, and nystagmus due to the tumor growth inside the internal acoustic meatus) [1, 10].

Pineal gland tumors (pinealomas, pineoblastomas, germinomas) produce intracranial hypertension (due to aqueduct of Sylvius obstruction) and Parinaud syndrome (vertical gaze palsy); moreover, they can develop leptomeningeal spread with meningeal signs and symptoms.

Tumors of the sellar region include adenomas, craniopharyngioma, chordomas, and meningiomas. They produce multiple symptoms: visual field loss, due to optic chiasma involvement; endocrinological abnormalities, due to infiltration-compression of hypothalamus and hypophysis; and symptoms of intracranial hypertension [1, 10–12].

Brain metastases occur in 20–40% of patients with cancer and their frequency has increased over time. Lung, breast, and skin (melanoma) are the commonest sources of brain metastases, and in up to 15% of patients the primary site remains unknown [13]. Brain metastases can be asymptomatic in a number of patients. They are usually localized at the boundaries between cerebral (or cerebellar) grey and white matter; rarely, they are located in the brainstem or basal ganglia. Symptoms are typically subacute, with loss of specific brain functions or intracranial hypertension seizures can be found in 15–20% of cases. Intratumoral hemorrhage causes acute neurological symptoms and can be found in metastases from melanoma or renal cancer [13].

4.4   Brain Tumor-Related Epilepsy

Seizures occur in approximately one quarter to one half of patients with brain tumors and tumor-related seizures account for about 5% of new-onset seizures and more than 10% of lesional focal epilepsy [14, 15]. The prevalence rates of seizures vary depending on tumor type and grade and somewhat on age and tumor location. Generally, low-grade tumors with a longer disease duration appear to be slightly more epileptogenic than the more destructive high grade tumors. Recent data suggest rates of tumor-related epilepsy of 90% for low-grade glial tumors such as astrocytomas and oligodendrogliomas, compared with 30–50% for anaplastic astrocytomas or glioblastoma multiforme [16]. Seizures occur more commonly in patients with tumors located in cortical regions as opposed to subcortical areas, with a seizure frequency of 56% compared with 15%, respectively [17]. Frontal, temporal, insular, and centro-parietal regions are the most common cortical regions associated with symptomatic seizures. Incidence rates are higher for tumors located in eloquent cortical regions as opposed to functionally subtle or "clinically silent" areas.

Theories to explain tumor-related epilepsy have included architectural distortion of surrounding cortex, due to the tumor itself or peritumoral edema, vascular compression, and cerebral ischemia, or intracerebral hemorrhage creating mass effect or cortical irritation due to iron deposition. Additionally, based on intraoperative and extraoperative intracranial EEG recordings, cortical regions expressing high volume of interictal discharges are different from those invaded by the tumor. This means that the peritumoral tissue demonstrates greater irritability than tumor tissue. Other potential mechanisms of tumor-induced seizures are disturbances at the cellular level, such as alterations in synaptic and neuronal function and connectivity, free radical formation and excitotoxicity and alterations in the expression of specific genes and proteins relevant to intracellular communication, drug transport, drug resistance, and tumor growth. Among these mechanisms glutamate-induced excitotoxicity has gained popularity as a prolonged elevation of extracellular glutamate and imbalance in intracellular and extracellular glutamate levels have been shown to contribute to persistent neuronal network abnormalities that favor epileptogenesis [18–21]. In particular, studies have demonstrated a significant increase in glutamate concentrations in peritumoral tissue in brain tumor patients with seizures compared with those without seizures [22]. Other hypotheses for tumor-related epilepsy include mutation in specific genes, namely O6-methylguanine DNA-methyltransferases (MGMT), matrix metalloproteinases (MMPs), adenosine kinase (ADK), and isocitrate dehydrogenase (IDH). In particular, IDH1-2 mutations are more frequent in brain tumor patients with seizures, and this could be related to the similarity between 2-hydroxyglutarate (the product of the mutation) and glutamate [16].

Epilepsy in patients with brain tumors belongs to the type of partial epilepsy, either with or without secondary generalized seizures. For this type of seizures, the International League Against Epilepsy (ILAE) has updated the most appropriate AED choices, based on a meta-analysis of a large number of randomized controlled trials [23]. Levetiracetam (LEV), carbamazepine, phenytoin, and zonisamide have been classified as level A anticonvulsants, valproate (VPA) represents the only level B anticonvulsant, while gabapentin, lamotrigine, oxcarbazepine, phenobarbital, topiramate, and vigabatrin are level C. In neuro-oncology, consensus exists to avoid enzyme-inducing antiepileptic drugs (EIAEDs) due to interactions with antineoplastic drugs. Thus, older EIAED (e.g., phenobarbital, phenytoin, carbamazepine) should be avoided in favor of second and third generation AEDs (especially levetiracetam and lacosamide). Moreover, AED levels may be affected by some chemotherapeutic agents, such as methotrexate and cisplatin, that decrease the serum levels of valproic acid, carbamazepine, and phenytoin [19, 23, 24].

The most frequently used AED in patients with brain tumors is levetiracetam, based on a good efficacy versus toxicity profile, leading to a seizure reduction ≥50% and a seizure freedom in 65–100% and 20–77% of patients, respectively, when used in add/on, and seizure freedom in 76–91% of patients when used in monotherapy [25]. Valproic acid, sometimes used for a potential concomitant antineoplastic efficacy as well, yields a seizure freedom around 60% in add-on, and 30.4–77.8% in monotherapy [26]. Lacosamide is a new generation AED that yields a seizure reduction ≥50% in a great proportion of patients (up to 86%), and assures a good clinical response in case of status epilepticus [27, 28].

Common side effects of AEDs include irritability and depression (levetiracetam), thrombocytopenia (valproate, levetiracetam), weight gain (valproate), hyponatremia (carbamazepine, oxcarbazepine), rash (lamotrigine, phenytoin), and tremor (valproate) [28].

Tumor resection usually reduces seizure frequency in patients with tumor-related epilepsy, especially in case of gross total resection. Some authors suggest larger resections of margins to include peritumoral epileptogenic areas, identified by intraoperative awake mapping [29–31]. Patients whose seizures are well controlled by AEDs preoperatively and whose seizures are ≤1 year in duration usually achieve better seizure control post-surgery. Moreover, the presence of non-generalizing simple partial seizures has been associated with poorer outcome. No significant difference in epilepsy outcome exists between temporal and extratemporal tumors and between adults and children. In case of tumor progression, reoperation can be useful to improve seizure control [16, 19, 32, 33].

External radiotherapy has been reported to be effective in seizure control in 72–100% of patients with medically intractable epilepsy and lower grade gliomas (LGGs) [33, 34]. Patients may become seizure free (27–55%), and the median duration of seizure control is 12 months but can be as long as 8 years. In addition to a direct antitumor effect, one can speculate that ionizing radiation may decrease seizure activity by damaging epileptogenic neurons or inducing changes of the microenvironment in the peritumoral tissue. Concerning chemotherapy, seizure improvement in LGGs treated with alkylating agents (procarbazine + CCNU + vincristine, temozolomide) is usually obtained in 48–100% of patients, with 20–40% becoming seizure free [19, 32, 33]. Seizure reduction is more frequent than objective response on MRI and better correlated with decrease of uptake of methionine on PET.

As in LGGs seizure control can be achieved through different treatments (gross total resection, chemotherapy, or radiotherapy) seizures can be a surrogate marker for treatment response in patients with low-grade glioma and serve as an important secondary endpoint in clinical trials [35].

Seizure frequency may affect many aspects of a patient's life, including vocation and the ability to drive. In glioma patients with seizure freedom after successful antitumor therapy, the question is whether and until when AEDs should be continued. According to recent literature a safe withdrawal of AED medication is feasible, but overall, the benefit versus risks and timing of a withdrawal of AEDs in patients with gliomas are still unclear [19, 32, 33].

4.5 Clinical Complications of Treatments

4.5.1 Side Effects of Steroids

Brain tumors disrupt the blood–brain barrier by secreting factors, such as vascular endothelial growth factor (VEGF), that alter the permeability and lead to vasogenic edema. Edema spreads more prominently through white matter, and clinical effects depend on the location. Dexamethasone is the corticosteroid of choice because it has strong glucocorticoid but minimal mineralocorticoid activity, thereby exerting greater effects on the blood–brain barrier than on systemic fluid retention. It can reduce intracranial pressure and improve neurologic symptoms within 1–2 days. Short-term complications include hyperglycemia, insomnia, and mania. Long-term complications include the full range of Cushing syndrome. Steroid myopathy is particularly important for patients with preexisting weakness due to the brain tumor: it can persist as long as the patient receives dexamethasone, and recovery can be slow. Overall, for most patients, a 4-mg dose twice a day is sufficient and much better tolerated than higher doses. In the outpatient setting, the second dose should be administered in the afternoon to prevent insomnia [36–38].

4.5.2 Infectious Complications

Pneumocystis carinii pneumonia is a rare but potentially fatal infection seen in patients with brain tumors, and presents with fever, cough, and respiratory failure. Radiographic images demonstrate interstitial infiltrates, and diagnosis is made by demonstration of the microorganism. The key risk factor is lymphopenia caused by both temozolomide and glucocorticoids.

Immunosuppression from corticosteroids and chemotherapy also increases the risk for the development of Candida infection. This tends to be mild in patients with brain tumors, and primarily consists of an oropharyngeal candidiasis. This is often found incidentally on a routine throat examination, which should be part of each visit and include queries about dry mouth, poor taste, poor appetite, pain on swallowing, and nausea [36].

A cerebral abscess can mimic a brain tumor in both clinical presentation and imaging features. Patients with brain tumors are at risk of an abscess development as a complication of a neurosurgical intervention in the context of corticosteroid use. Chronic steroids further complicate the presentation because the patient's white blood cell count may already be elevated at baseline, and the ability to mount a fever can be impaired. Imaging typically reveals a ring-enhancing mass, which can be indistinguishable from a recurrent brain tumor on T1, T2/FLAIR, and gadolinium enhanced images. In a cerebral pyogenic abscess, diffusion-weighted imaging (DWI) demonstrates marked hyperintensity in the cavity with corresponding hypointensity on apparent diffusion coefficient (ADC) sequences, while recurrent tumor is hypointense in the necrotic core on DWI and hyperintense on an ADC map. Treatment consists of surgical aspiration and intravenous antibiotics [39, 40].

4.5.3 Vascular Complications

Venous thromboembolism is common in patients with brain tumors and is related to neurosurgical procedures, hemiparesis or decreased mobility, and hypercoagulability [41]. The most common time to develop venous thromboembolism is in the postoperative setting and the subsequent 6 months, but, in some patients with active malignancy, this risk can persist lifelong. Data for perioperative prophylaxis support the use of mechanical compression as well as chemical prophylaxis with low-molecular weight heparin that should start as early as 24–48 h after a craniotomy and continues as long as the patient is nonambulatory [42, 43]. Any patient with brain tumor, who presents with calf swelling, calf tenderness, shortness of breath, or tachycardia, should be urgently evaluated for evidence of venous thromboembolism with lower extremity ultrasound and helical CT chest with contrast. Studies in patients with cancer confirm that low-molecular weight heparin is superior to warfarin in preventing recurrent clots and is associated with low rates of intracranial hemorrhages [44]. Newer generation of oral anticoagulants do not require intensive monitoring or injections, but are expensive and have not been well studied in patients with either solid cancer or brain tumors. Thus far, these drugs lack data to support their use in lieu of low-molecular-weight heparin. The use of inferior vena cava filters should be limited to patients with recent or active intracranial hemorrhage or in patients with other medical contraindications to anticoagulation [45].

Although deep vein thrombosis and pulmonary embolism are the most common manifestations of venous thromboembolism, patients with malignant glioma can also develop cerebral venous sinus thrombosis. Presentation with headache, increased intracranial pressure, seizures, and focal neurologic symptoms are often attributed to the tumor itself, and the correct diagnosis can be missed. Despite a lack of evidence, standard management is to treat this complication with anticoagulants.

Clinically significant intracranial hemorrhage occurs in 1–2% of patients with glioblastoma. Bevacizumab, a monoclonal antibody to VEGF-A, is relatively contraindicated in patients with intracranial hemorrhage, but the risk of intracranial hemorrhage due to bevacizumab does not seem to be increased [46]. Stroke can also be a late effect of treatment, and is an important cause of morbidity in long-term survivors. Radiation-induced vasculopathy, due to accelerated atherosclerosis, can cause ischemic strokes 3–5 years after exposure to radiation [47]. Cerebral microbleeds can be a consequence of radiation therapy and are seen on gradient echo images: they can occur within 1–2 years of radiation therapy, are located within the field of radiation, have a direct relationship to radiation dose, may progress over time, and can be associated with cognitive dysfunctions [48, 49].

4.5.4 Hydrocephalus

The management of hydrocephalus associated with intracranial tumors is a growing concern in neurosurgery. A permanent CSF diversion procedure is indicated in patients prior to or after surgical resection of the tumor. Implantation of a ventriculoperitoneal (VP) shunt is the most widely used treatment for the management of hydrocephalus. Although CSF shunting reduces the morbidity and mortality of hydrocephalus, it is associated with potential complications that may require multiple surgical procedures, as well as shunt revisions during patient's lifetime. Causes for shunt complications or failures include obstruction, infection, mechanical disconnection, and overdrainage [3].

4.5.5 Endocrinological Complications

Diabetes mellitus is the most common endocrinologic comorbidity in patients with brain tumors, and may be induced or worsened by corticosteroid use. Tight control is important for quality of life, and may be associated with improved survival [50]. Increased intracranial pressure from a primary brain tumor can lead to the syndrome of inappropriate secretion of antidiuretic hormone (SIADH) and result in hyponatremia. As a consequence neurologic symptoms and seizures can worsen, and ultimately an encephalopathy can develop. In patients with tumors that infiltrate or exert mass effect on the posterior pituitary, an elevated sodium, excessive thirst, and excessive urination can result from diabetes insipidus or decreased production of antidiuretic hormone. Treatment requires supplementation with desmopressin or therapies that reduce the tumor's mass effect.

Cranial radiation therapy can impact pituitary function, and alterations in pituitary hormones can be either an early or late complication of therapy (especially after radiation of the sellar area) [36, 51]. Growth impairment and hypogonadism are common in childhood brain tumor survivors [52].

4.5.6 Mood and Cognitive Complications

A major depressive disorder is common in patients with brain tumors prior to diagnosis, at time of diagnosis, and during the course of the disease. Once a clinical diagnosis is made, an antidepressant drug can be considered, but no clear guidelines exist on which class of antidepressants to use or whether any of them are beneficial. Antidepressants are safe in patients with brain tumors, and, with the exception of bupropion, they do not meaningfully alter the seizure threshold. It is also important to minimize medications that can exacerbate depression and to consider nonpharmacologic therapies. Corticosteroids may have a profound impact on mood, but most commonly result in irritability, anxiety, insomnia, mania, and psychosis: in patients, who cannot taper corticosteroids, a concomitant antianxiety or antipsychotic medication may be indicated [36, 53].

A decline in cognitive function is experienced by many patients with primary brain tumors. This can be a direct result of the brain tumor that interferes with cognitive networks throughout the brain, but may be most pronounced in patients who have undergone radiation therapy. Patients have an impairment in multiple domains of cognition and imaging may reveal white matter damage and cortical atrophy. Cognitive dysfunctions from chemotherapy or radiation therapy within the first few years after therapy tend to be mild and manageable but, in some patients, can interfere with work and household activities. In most patients, symptoms are progressive, and in long-term survivors, symptoms gradually become more disabling with a negative impact on family relationships, job, and independence. No evidence exists to suggest that any pharmacologic intervention can be successful in preventing or treating memory dysfunctions from radiation therapy or chemotherapy, but the role of psychostimulants, cognitive-behavioral therapies, and cholinesterase inhibitors is being studied [54, 55].

4.6 Elderly Patients

Medical comorbidities and frailty in elderly patients are challenging to quantify, but likely play a role in survival and quality of life, especially in case of glioblastomas. Standard treatment options are often complicated by other medical considerations including comorbid disease, polypharmacy, and increased susceptibility to adverse events. Radiotherapy is less tolerated in elderly people, especially in case of tumors that did not receive resection (tumors located in deep structures or in eloquent areas) or in case of extensive post-surgical residual tumor. Fatigue is a frequent toxicity seen in the majority of patients receiving cranial radiation, and this may be more pronounced in the elderly. Cognitive decline is also a concern, particularly on a background of possible suboptimal cognitive baseline function or cognitive reserve. Chemotherapy can be less tolerated in terms of fatigue, nausea, or impaired blood examinations (in particular liver function) in patients with multiple comorbidities [56, 57].

Lastly, caregivers of elderly cancer patients are often elderly by themselves. This burden places both the patient and the caregiver at risk for health and psychosocial strain during the treatment process, and highlights the continuous need for nurse and physician assistance during the entire treatment journey.

References

1. Alentorn A, Hoang-Xuan K, Mikkelsen T. Presenting signs and symptoms in brain tumors. Handb Clin Neurol. 2016;134:19–26.
2. Posner JB, Saper CB, Schiff N, et al. Plum and Posner's diagnosis of stupor and coma. Oxford: Oxford University Press; 2007.
3. Reddy GK, Bollam P, Caldito G, Willis B, Guthikonda B, Nanda A. Ventriculoperitoneal shunt complications in hydrocephalus patients with intracranial tumors: an analysis of relevant risk factors. J Neurooncol. 2011;103(2):333–42.
4. Malamud N. Psychiatric disorder with intracranial tumors of limbic system. Arch Neurol. 1967;17(2):113–23.
5. Weitzner MA. Psychosocial and neuropsychiatric aspects of patients with primary brain tumors. Cancer Invest. 1999;17(4):285–91.
6. Forsyth PA, Posner JB. Headaches in patients with brain tumors: a study of 111 patients. Neurology. 1993;43(9):1678–83.
7. Vázquez-Barquero A, Ibáñez FJ, Herrera S, Izquierdo JM, Berciano J, Pascual J. Isolated headache as the presenting clinical manifestation of intracranial tumors: a prospective study. Cephalalgia. 1994;14(4):270–2.
8. Schaefer PW, Miller JC, Singhal AB, Thrall JH, Lee SI. Headache: when is neurologic imaging indicated? J Am Coll Radiol. 2007;4(8):566–9.
9. Chen C, Yen DJ, Yiu CH, Shih YH, Yu HY, Su MS. Ictal vomiting in partial seizures of temporal lobe origin. Eur Neurol. 1999;42(4):235–9.
10. Biller J, Brazis PW, Masdeu JC. Localization in clinical neurology. Philadelphia: Wolters Kluwer Health; 2011.
11. Raelson C, Chiang G. Chiasmatic-hypothalamic masses in adults: a case series and review of the literature. J Neuroimaging. 2015;25(3):361–4.
12. Sathananthan M, Sathananthan A, Scheithauer BW, Giannini C, Meyer FB, Atkinson JL, Erickson D. Sellar meningiomas: an endocrinologic perspective. Pituitary. 2013;16(2):182–8.
13. Soffietti R, Ducati A, Rudà R. Brain metastases. Handb Clin Neurol. 2012;105:747–55.
14. Politsky JM. Brain tumor-related epilepsy: a current review of the etiologic basis and diagnostic and treatment approaches. Curr Neurol Neurosci Rep. 2017;17(9):70.
15. Banerjee PN, Filippi D, Allen Hauser W. The descriptive epidemiology of epilepsy-a review. Epilepsy Res. 2009;85(1):31–45.
16. Rudà R, Bello L, Duffau H, Soffietti R. Seizures in low-grade gliomas: natural history, pathogenesis, and outcome after treatments. Neuro Oncol. 2012;14(Suppl 4):iv55–64.
17. Shady JA, Black PM, Kupsky WJ, Tarbell NJ, Scott RM, Leong T, Holmes G. Seizures in children with supratentorial astroglial neoplasms. Pediatr Neurosurg. 1994;21(1):23–30.
18. Shamji MF, Fric-Shamji EC, Benoit BG. Brain tumors and epilepsy: pathophysiology of peritumoral changes. Neurosurg Rev. 2009;32(3):275–84. discussion 284–6.
19. Rudà R, Soffietti R. What is new in the management of epilepsy in gliomas? Curr Treat Options Neurol. 2015;17(6):351.
20. Wolf H, Roos D, Blumcke I, Pietsch T, Wiestler O. Perilesional neurochemical changes in focal epilepsies. Acta Neuropathol. 1996;91:376–84.
21. Kohling R, Senner V, Paulus W, Speckmann E. Epileptiform activity preferentially arises outside tumor invasion zone in glioma xeno-transplants. Neurobiol Dis. 2006;22:64–75.
22. Yuen T, Morokoff A, Bjorksten A, D'Abaco G, Paradiso L, Finch S, et al. Glutamate is associated with a higher risk of seizures in patients with gliomas. Neurology. 2012;79:883–9.
23. Glauser T, Ben-Menachem E, Bourgeois B, Cnaan A, Guerreiro C, Kälviäinen R, ILAE Subcommission on AED Guidelines, et al. Updated ILAE evidence review of antiepileptic drug efficacy and effectiveness as initial monotherapy for epileptic seizures and syndromes. Epilepsia. 2013;54(3):551–63.
24. Kerrigan S, Grant R. Antiepileptic drugs for treating seizures in adults with brain tumours. Cochrane Database Syst Rev. 2011;8:CD008586.

25. Vecht CJ, Kerkhof M, Duran-Pena A. Seizure prognosis in brain tumors: new insights and evidence-based management. Oncologist. 2014;19:751–9.
26. Kerkhof M, Dielemans JC, van Breemen MS, et al. Effect of valproic acid on seizure control and on survival in patients with glioblastoma multiforme. Neuro-Oncology. 2013;15:961–7.
27. Rudà R, Pellerino A, Franchino F, Bertolotti C, Bruno F, Mo F, Migliore E, Ciccone G, Soffietti R. Lacosamide in patients with gliomas and uncontrolled seizures: results from an observational study. J Neuro-Oncol. 2018;136(1):105–14.
28. Lacy J, Saadati H, Yu JB. Complications of brain tumors and their treatment. Hematol Oncol Clin North Am. 2012;26(4):779–96.
29. Bourdillon P, Apra C, Guenot M, Duffau H. Similarity and differences in neuroplasticity mechanisms between brain gliomas and nonlesional epilepsy. Epilepsia. 2017;58(12):2038–47.
30. Duffau H. Brain mapping in tumors: intraoperative or extraoperative. Epilepsia. 2013;54(Suppl 9):79–83.
31. Duffau H. The challenge to remove diffuse low grade gliomas while preserving brain functions. Acta Neurochir. 2012;154:569–74.
32. Rudà R, Trevisan E, Soffietti R. Epilepsy and brain tumors. Curr Opin Oncol. 2010;22(6):611–20.
33. Roelcke U, Wyss MT, Nowosielski M, Rudà R, Roth P, Hofer S, Galldiks N, Crippa F, Weller M, Soffietti R. Amino acid positron emission tomography to monitor chemotherapy response and predict seizure control and progression-free survival in WHO grade II gliomas. Neuro Oncol. 2016;18(5):744–51.
34. Rudà R, Magliola U, Bertero L, Trevisan E, Bosa C, Mantovani C, Ricardi U, Castiglione A, Monagheddu C, Soffietti R. Seizure control following radiotherapy in patients with diffuse gliomas: a retrospective study. Neuro Oncol. 2013;15(12):1739–49.
35. Avila EK, Chamberlain M, Schiff D, Reijneveld JC, Armstrong TS, Ruda R, Wen PY, Weller M, Koekkoek JA, Mittal S, Arakawa Y, Choucair A, Gonzalez-Martinez J, MacDonald DR, Nishikawa R, Shah A, Vecht CJ, Warren P, van den Bent MJ, DeAngelis LM. Seizure control as a new metric in assessing efficacy of tumor treatment in low-grade glioma trials. Neuro Oncol. 2017;19(1):12–21.
36. Mohile NA. Medical complications of brain tumors. Continuum (Minneap Minn). 2017;23(6, Neuro-oncology):1635–52.
37. Machein MR, Kullmer J, Fiebich BL, et al. Vascular endothelial growth factor expression, vascular volume, and, capillary permeability in human brain tumors. Neurosurgery. 1999;44(4):732Y740. discussion 740Y741.
38. Gerstner ER, Duda DG, di Tomaso E, et al. VEGF inhibitors in the treatment of cerebral edema in patients with brain cancer. Nat Rev Clin Oncol. 2009;6(4):229Y236.
39. Schiff D. Pneumocystis pneumonia in brain tumor patients: risk factors and clinical features. J Neurooncol. 1996;27(3):235Y240.
40. Leuthardt EC, Wippold FJ 2nd, Oswood MC, Rich KM. Diffusion-weighted MR imaging in the preoperative assessment of brain abscesses. Surg Neurol. 2002;58(6):395–402.
41. Streiff MB, Ye X, Kickler TS, et al. A prospective multicenter study of venous thromboembolism in patients with newly-diagnosed high-grade glioma: hazard rate and risk factors. J Neurooncol. 2015;124(2):299–305.
42. Alshehri N, Cote DJ, Hulou MM, et al. Venous thromboembolism prophylaxis in brain tumor patients undergoing craniotomy: a meta-analysis. J Neurooncol. 2016;130(3):561–70.
43. Gerber DE, Grossman SA, Streiff MB. Management of venous thromboembolism in patients with primary and metastatic brain tumors. J Clin Oncol. 2006;24(8):1310–8.
44. Lee AY, Levine MN, Baker RI, et al. Low-molecular-weight heparin versus a coumarin for the prevention of recurrent venous thromboembolism in patients with cancer. N Engl J Med. 2003;349(2):146–53.
45. Levin JM, Schiff D, Loeffler JS, et al. Complications of therapy for venous thromboembolic disease in patients with brain tumors. Neurology. 1993;43(6):1111–4.
46. Gilbert MR, Dignam JJ, Armstrong TS, et al. A randomized trial of bevacizumab for newly diagnosed glioblastoma. N Engl J Med. 2014;370(8):699–708.

47. Kreisl TN, Toothaker T, Karimi S, DeAngelis LM. Ischemic stroke in patients with primary brain tumors. Neurology. 2008;70(24):2314–20.
48. Roongpiboonsopit D, Kuijf HJ, Charidimou A, et al. Evolution of cerebral microbleeds after cranial irradiation in medulloblastoma patients. Neurology. 2017;88(8):789–96.
49. Roddy E, Sear K, Felton E, et al. Presence of cerebral microbleeds is associated with worse executive function in pediatric brain tumor survivors. Neuro Oncol. 2016;18(11):1548–58.
50. McGirt MJ, Chaichana KL, Gathinji M, et al. Persistent outpatient hyperglycemia is independently associated with decreased survival after primary resection of malignant brain astrocytomas. Neurosurgery. 2008;63(2):286–91.
51. Sathyapalan T, Dixit S. Radiotherapy-induced hypopituitarism: a review. Expert Rev Anticancer Ther. 2012;12(5):669–83.
52. Pietilä S, Mäkipernaa A, Koivisto AM, Lenko HL. Growth impairment and gonadal axis abnormalities are common in survivors of paediatric brain tumours. Acta Paediatr. 2017;106(10):1684–93.
53. Rooney AG, Carson A, Grant R. Depression in cerebral glioma patients: a systematic review of observational studies. J Natl Cancer Inst. 2011;103(1):61–76.
54. Douw L, Klein M, Fagel SS, et al. Cognitive and radiological effects of radiotherapy in patients with low-grade glioma: long-term follow-up. Lancet Neurol. 2009;8(9):810–8.
55. Kaiser J, Bledowski C, Dietrich J. Neural correlates of chemotherapy-related cognitive impairment. Cortex. 2014;54:33–50.
56. Young JS, Chmura SJ, Wainwright DA, Yamini B, Peters KB, Lukas RV. Management of glioblastoma in elderly patients. J Neurol Sci. 2017;380:250–5.
57. de Moraes FY, Laperriere N. Glioblastoma in the elderly: initial management. Chin Clin Oncol. 2017;6(4):39.

Imaging in Neuro-Oncology

5

Giuseppe Minniti, Andrea Romano, Claudia Scaringi,
and Alessandro Bozzao

5.1 Introduction

The 2016 central nervous system (CNS) World Health Organization (WHO) classification of brain neoplasms has completely changed the way brain tumors are now classified, integrating both genotypic and phenotypic parameters, incorporated into the newly updated classification schema. This classification is based on a combination of histology and molecular patterns by direct evaluation of the mutated DNA or by immunohistochemistry, which evaluates the effects of the mutated genes on proteins (and this technique is more widely used also because of lower costs). Since histologic grading is still used in clinical practice, potential relevant inconsistency between the two might appear. The knowledge of this new classification is essential for radiologist as well as for all neuroscientists. The modern approach of imaging in the assessment of brain tumors aims to identify some morphological or metabolic patterns that may have an impact on their classification. This is synthesized in the term radiogenomics.

G. Minniti (✉)
Radiation Oncology Unit, University of Pittsburgh Medical Center, Hillman Cancer Center, San Pietro Hospital, Rome, Italy

IRCCS Neuromed, Pozzilli, IS, Italy
e-mail: minnitig@upmc.edu

A. Romano · A. Bozzao
Department of Neuroradiology, Sant' Andrea Hospital, University Sapienza, Rome, Italy

C. Scaringi
Radiation Oncology Unit, University of Pittsburgh Medical Center, Hillman Cancer Center, San Pietro Hospital, Rome, Italy

Radiation Oncology Unit, Sant' Andrea Hospital, University Sapienza, Rome, Italy

© Springer Nature Switzerland AG 2019
M. Bartolo et al. (eds.), *Neurorehabilitation in Neuro-Oncology*,
https://doi.org/10.1007/978-3-319-95684-8_5

5.2 Radiogenomics

The molecular stratification of brain tumors is quickly becoming an integral part of their diagnosis, prognosis, and clinical decision-making. Several studies over the past two decades provided insights into the genetic basis of tumorigenesis, explaining why tumors assigned to the same histopathological entity can have broadly different therapy responses and highly divergent clinical outcomes. The new 2016 WHO classification of CNS tumors uses, for the first time, molecular parameters in addition to histology to define many tumor entities [1, 2], thus clearly indicating the utmost significance of genome-wide biomarkers in the molecular era.

The molecular stratification is essential for estimating the individual prognosis [3–5]. The more relevant molecular biomarkers are isocitrate dehydrogenase (IDH) 1/2 mutation status and chromosome 1p/19q loss of heterozygosity (LOH). They are complemented by alpha-thalassemia/mental retardation syndrome X-linked (ATRX), which is predictive for associated IDH or H3F3A hotspot mutations [6]. The ATRX status itself confers a prognostic potential in diffuse gliomas [7]. The loss of ATRX expression is mostly induced by truncating ATRX mutations, resulting in an alternative lengthening of telomeres (ALT) phenotype [8, 9]. Moreover, O6-methylguanine DNA methyltransferase (MGMT) can be regarded as an independent prognostic factor in diffuse gliomas [10, 11], and the epidermal growth factor receptor (EGFR) amplification and EGFR variant III (EGFRvIII) mutation are related to neo-angiogenesis evaluation and representation.

Understanding how these molecular phenotypes are reflected on imaging is thus becoming increasingly important to define novel magnetic resonance imaging (MRI) biomarkers that can be used as surrogates for tissue-based molecular subtyping required to predict prognosis, to develop individualized patient therapies, and to follow up patients.

Radiogenomics is a new field of study aiming at determining the association between imaging features and molecular markers. Hence, more accurate approaches are recommended to identify the specific biological and microstructural characteristics of the underlying tumor tissue.

To this end, more sophisticated quantitative imaging approaches such as the analysis of texture features (i.e., pattern of local variations in image intensity) can be applied on anatomical MR images, seeking for correlations between tissue microstructure and thus tumor biology. Recent studies focused their attention on post-contrast T1-weighted and T2/FLAIR images searching for a link with molecular markers representing gene, protein, or metabolite expression, in order to create radiogenomics map to associate image features with biologic processes and molecular subgroups [12].

More recently, advanced imaging features derived from physiological imaging techniques, such as dMRI, PWI, and magnetic resonance spectroscopy (MRS), have shown to be promising to increase the accuracy of molecular subtyping by MRI.

5.3 Conventional Imaging

For many years computed tomography (CT) with contrast enhancement has been the gold standard for the diagnosis of brain tumors due to its ability to ascertain the presence of a brain lesion, to define its dimension and relation with surrounding brain structures, to assess perilesional edema, and to define the presence of multiple brain lesions. CT is superior to MRI for detecting calcifications, skull lesions, and hyper acute hemorrhage and helps direct differential diagnosis as well as immediate patient management [13, 14]. Continuous developments in MRI provide new insights into the diagnosis, classification, and understanding of the biology of brain tumors. MRI studies are characterized by higher contrast resolution associated with multiplanar views. MRI is characterized by high sensitivity for structural alterations caused by tumoral growth, which can be further enhanced by the use of paramagnetic contrast agents. Standard T1- and T2-weighted MRI acquisitions display high sensitivity for brain tumors and give information on the size and localization of the tumor [15]. A normal contrast-enhanced MRI scan essentially rules out the possibility of a brain tumor, but the role of neuroimaging is no longer simply to evaluate structural abnormality and to identify tumor-related complications. Functional, hemodynamic, metabolic, cellular, and cytoarchitectural alterations can be assessed by means of modern MRI. Thereby the current state of neuroimaging has evolved into a comprehensive diagnostic tool that allows the characterization of morphological as well as biological alterations, to diagnose and grade brain tumors, and to monitor and assess treatment response and patient prognosis [16]. Among advanced techniques, MR spectroscopy, diffusion-weighted imaging (DWI) and diffusion tensor imaging (DTI) with tractography, perfusion-weighted imaging, and functional MRI play a role in the transition of clinical MR imaging from a purely morphology-based discipline to one that combines structure with brain function.

Most IDH-mutant and non-mutant diffuse astrocytomas infiltrate the white matter (far behind the abnormal MR signal) sparing of the cortex with mild mass effect. They are typically hypointense on T1WI and hyperintense on T2/FLAIR, without enhancement following contrast administration (Fig. 5.1). Blooming T2* signal can be appreciated if calcifications are present. IDH-mutant anaplastic astrocytomas are hypointense on T1WI and hyperintense on T2/FLAIR as well. Contrast enhancement ranges from none to moderate, but 50–70% of lesions may show some degree of enhancement.

IDH-wild-type anaplastic astrocytoma shows a diffuse infiltrative pattern frequently involving more than three cerebral lobes. This feature was commonly described in the past as gliomatosis cerebri, a term that is no longer used in the pathologic report.

IDH-wild-type glioblastoma (GBM) shows T1WI hyposignal with poorly marginated margins; mixed signal indicating subacute hemorrhage can be seen. T2/FLAIR signal is heterogeneous as well with hyperintensity with indistinct tumor margins and vasogenic edema. Inside the neoplasm mixed signal can indicate necrosis, cysts, fluid and debris levels, and "flow voids" from neovascularization. Enhancement is strong and irregular and typically surrounds a central

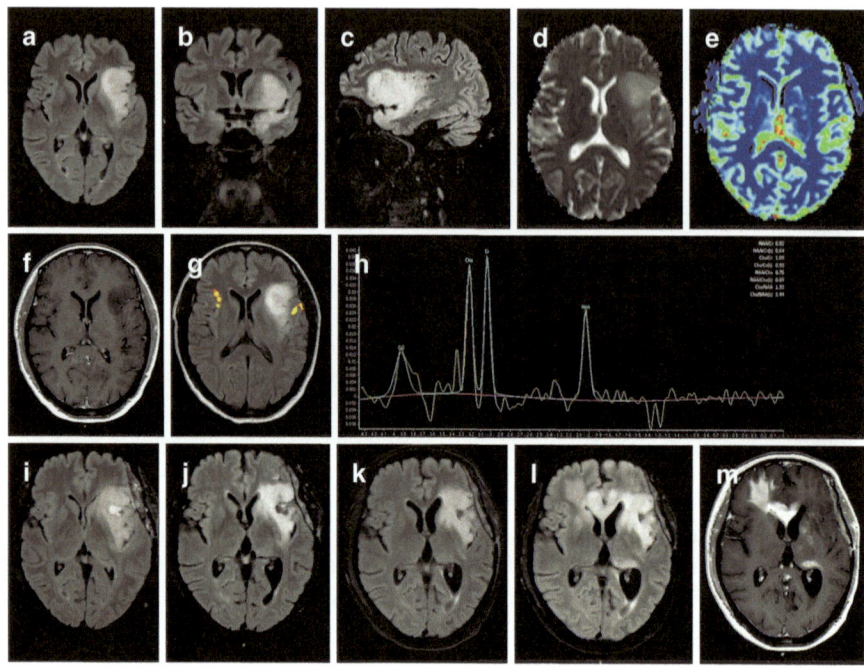

Fig. 5.1 A 52-year-old woman affected by recent epileptic episode. A hyperintense lesion on FLAIR images (**a–c**) is evident, with left fronto-temporal cortex involvement close to sylvian fissure. Low value of ADC (**d**) and relative CBV (**e**) with no enhancement after gadolinium injection (**f**) are visible. An area of BOLD signal changes close to the lesion after words recruitment task was interpreted as Broca's area (**g**). The spectroscopic evaluation reported a reduction of N-acetyl-aspartate into the lesion without significant increase of choline (**h**). After biopsy (**i**), a glioma was diagnosed, with lack of mutation of IDH1 (wild-type glioma) and methylation of MGMT. The follow-up examination (**j**, **k**) showed a stability of lesion extension. In the last follow-up (**l**, **m**) a significant progression of glioma with involvement of contralateral frontal lobe through genu of corpus callosum is appreciable with great enhancement after gadolinium injection. The patient died 13 months after diagnosis

non-enhancing core. Enhancement can be observed far from the central core of the neoplasm representing tumor extension into adjacent structures. This extension is microscopically evident even far from visible T2 signal alterations and areas of enhancement (Fig. 5.3).

IDH-mutant GBMs may appear non-enhancing, being somehow different from the classic large central necrotic core of IDH-wild-type GBMs.

Oligodendrogliomas (ODs) are glial neoplasms originated from oligodendrocytes that primarily affect supratentorial parenchyma (Fig. 5.2). Historically, co-deletion of whole chromosome arms 1p and 19q, namely 1p/19q co-deletion, has proved to be a diagnostic and prognostic biomarker of ODs. According to the 2016 WHO classification system, the "integrated diagnosis" of ODs requires histological classification, WHO grade, and molecular information (both IDH mutation and 1p/19q co-deletion). High-grade ODs are more prone to prominent edema and enhancement than low-grade ODs [17].

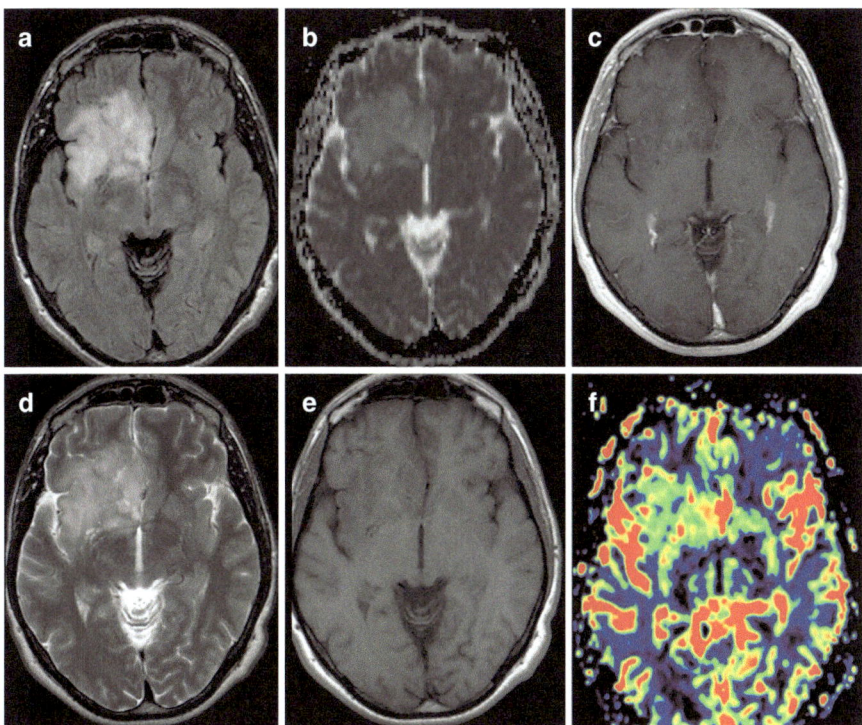

Fig. 5.2 Oligodendroglioma (both IDH1 mutation and 1p/19q co-deletion). Intra-axial lesion is evident in deep right fronto-basal region with T2-FLAIR hyperintensity (**a**, **d**), intermediate value of ADC (**b**), T1 iso-hypointensity (**e**), no enhancement after gadolinium injection (**c**), high values of CBV (**f**)

Some studies have tried to construct probabilistic radiographic atlases on anatomical magnetic resonance images of preoperative glioma locations, which may reflect the genetic profile of tumor precursor cells. IDH1 mutant tumors tended to be localized to the frontal lobe, whereas tumors with the methylation of the MGMT promoter occurred most frequently in the left temporal lobe, having a better prognosis than unmethylated tumors due to the higher sensitivity to chemotherapy [18].

A recent study assessed that tumor location was significantly different between MGMT promoter methylated and unmethylated groups, implying that the subventricular zone was more likely to be spared in patients with MGMT promoter methylation (Fig. 5.3). Besides, MGMT promoter methylation is prone to be associated with tumor necrosis. Other qualitative image features were not significantly different between these two groups, including multifocal, tumor cross midline, cyst, edema, enhancement, and side [19].

Some studies indicated that MGMT promoter methylation is poorly predicted with standard MRI features, such as T1-weighted images (T1WI), T2-weighted images (T2WI), and gadolinium (Gd)-enhanced T1WI.

Extracting additional information from medical imaging and relating it to a clinical variable of interest is broadly defined as radiomics. Radiomics is an emerging

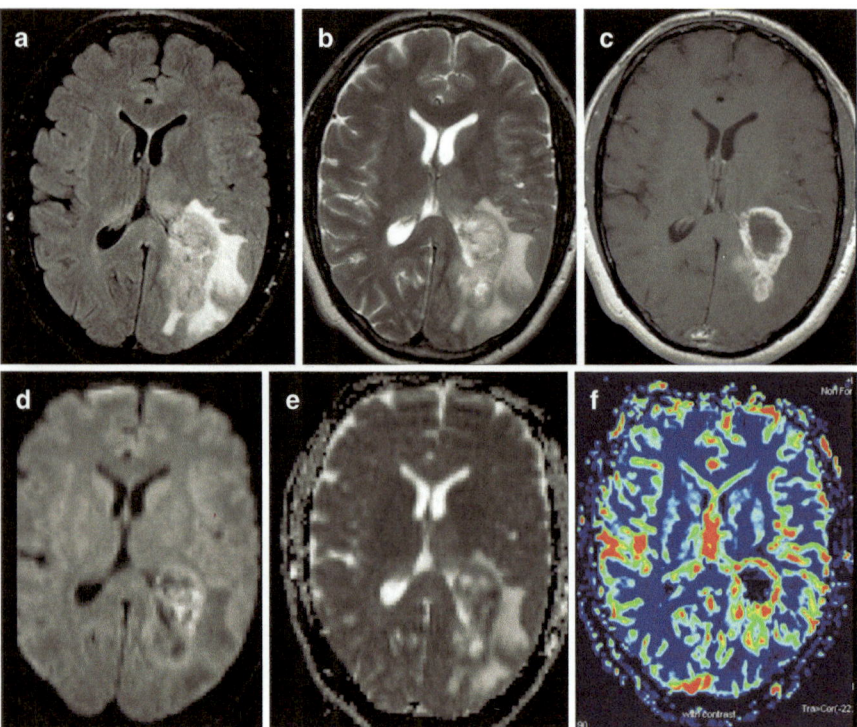

Fig. 5.3 Glioblastoma (wild-type glioma and unmethylated status). Left peritrigonal lesion characterized by un-homogeneous signal on FLAIR (**a**), T2 (**b**), peripheral enhancement after gadolinium (**c**), with restricted areas in DWI-ADC images (**d**, **e**), high values of CBV (**f**)

field that converts imaging data into a high-dimensional, mineable feature space using a large number of automatically extracted data characterization algorithms. Radiomics features include metrics such as spatial relationships, textural heterogeneity, and many other characteristics.

Radiomics features of GBM, especially the combination of enhanced T1W and T2W images, could reflect tumor molecular pathology indicators of MGMT methylation status. An association between imaging features and MGMT promoter methylation status in GBM could exist. MRI data could be applied to infer the molecular pathology of tumor target and may further guide clinical diagnosis and treatment [20].

Tumors with EGFR amplification and EGFRvIII mutation, which showed an increased angiogenesis, commonly occurred in the left temporal lobe anterior to the region identified by MGMT promoter methylation [2].

5.4 Advanced Techniques

5.4.1 Spectroscopy

The major clinical application of magnetic resonance spectroscopy for brain tumor patients has been its potential for non-invasive tumor grading [21–23]. These studies have predominantly used MR spectroscopy techniques that detect a signal spectrum from a small region of interest (single-voxel MR spectroscopy). Higher mean choline and lower mean NAA levels in higher-grade tumors have been reported. However, most of the studies found large standard deviations in metabolite ratios and substantial overlap in individual values, which may restrict the accuracy of the technique. Studies using sophisticated data analysis techniques have shown a higher degree of accuracy for in vitro and in vivo spectroscopy studies [24]. A significant improvement in accuracy was obtained using a two-dimensional MRS imaging technique [23]. The combination of improved spatial resolution and increased number of voxels provides much more data about tumor heterogeneity and contributes in exploring the tumor margin. As a result, it is possible to measure the metabolite content of different areas of neoplasms and surrounding normal tissue. This is very useful for better characterizing glial tumors, in which very often coexist areas with different grading, and for a more accurate monitoring of possible malignant degeneration of benign tumors. In a serial proton MRS imaging study it was clearly demonstrated that an increased choline signal is associated with malignant progression of cerebral gliomas and that serial MRS imaging effectively and accurately differentiates between stable and progressive disease [25]. Moreover, sampling of several voxels inside tumors is very important in guiding biopsies, surgery, and radiotherapy. Color choline maps are indeed helpful in guiding stereotactic biopsy, thus improving diagnostic accuracy with decreased sampling error. Multi-voxel MRS techniques provide important information about tumor heterogeneity and allow targeting the region for biopsy to that of maximum spectral abnormality, resulting in an improvement of the diagnosis [26]. It was recently described that 3T MRS may show an elevated 2-hydroxyglutarate peak (2-HG) resonating at 2.25 ppm in IDH-mutant diffuse astrocytomas. Mutations in IDH1/2 confer a gain-of-function neomorphic enzymatic activity, resulting in the aberrant production and subsequent accumulation of 2-HG, which has been suggested to be an oncometabolite for this genetic mutation [27]. Magnetic resonance spectroscopy (MRS) has been identified as a tool in the diagnosis of IDH-mutant gliomas via the non-invasive detection of 2-HG. Although 2-HG represents an attractive marker for diagnosis and monitoring of disease progression, unambiguous detection via MRS has proven difficult to establish. Complex spectral overlap by a number of metabolites, such as glutamate, glutamine, and gamma-aminobutyric acid (GABA), found in abundance within healthy brain tissue, often confound the identification and detection of 2-HG as well as compromise accurate quantification of metabolite concentration. Several methods for detection of 2-HG in vivo have been proposed to optimize MRS for this application [27–31]. These encompass a range of acquisition and post-processing protocols designed to eliminate the confounding spectral overlap, and reliably quantify the 2-HG concentration in patients with IDH-mutant gliomas. The feasibility of detection of 2-HG in vivo at clinical strengths (3 T), using a standard single-voxel double echo point-resolved spectroscopy (PRESS) sequence with a TE of 30 ms, has been reported [31, 32].

Spectroscopy studies are also very useful in the assessment of response to therapy. The sensitivity of this technique in fact exceeds that of conventional MRI, with useful information being provided in lesions treated with chemotherapy or radiation therapy. There is general agreement that within high-dose regions that correspond to the radiation target, treatment response is reflected in reduction in the levels of choline, creatine, and NAA 2–3 months after treatment. In regions that are not responsive to the radiation treatment, levels of choline may increase, corresponding to residual or recurrent tumor. This different behavior is of paramount importance in helping to differentiate between radio necrosis and recurrence, one of the most difficult topics in oncological neuroradiology. The possibility of monitoring the efficacy of new anti-tumoral compounds explains why MRS is included as a useful tool in many experimental protocols.

The high sensitivity of MRS is not matched by its specificity. Although several studies have reported that MRS makes possible the differentiation of diverse histological tumor types or abscesses or cystic lesions from neoplasms, the experience of routine daily practice has drawn attention to the risks related to the technique and warrants caution when considering differential diagnosis.

5.4.2   Diffusion Weighted Imaging and Diffusion Tensor Imaging

Diffusion-weighted MR has been widely used in the evaluation of brain tumors. With regard to extra-axial neoplasms, DWI can differentiate epidermoids from arachnoid cysts, both presenting similar signal intensity on T1- and T2-weighted images, while only epidermoids display very low ADC values [33, 34]. DWI has also been utilized in the differential diagnosis of malignant forms of meningiomas (grade WHO II–III) [35]. Primary cerebral lymphomas typically show signal hyperintensity in DWI with a low signal in the relative ADC maps, which is probably linked to the high cellularity of the tumor.

For intra-axial neoplasms it has been shown that pathological tissue has higher ADC values than healthy cerebral tissue and that the central necrotic component and the cystic component present greater diffusivity than the other components of neoplastic tissue [36]. Moreover, Brunberg et al. [37] demonstrated that edema and neoplastic tissue significantly differ in ADC values. Edema has a higher ADC value, which is probably linked to the preserved integrity of the myelin. Some studies have shown that water diffusibility is lower in high than in low-grade gliomas [38, 39], but a considerable overlap between ADCs has also been described [40]. DWI is commonly not restricted in IDH-mutant and non-mutant diffuse, anaplastic astrocytomas, and glioblastoma. ADC values obtained from standard clinical DWI are a highly significant predictor of non-enhancing glioma IDH status and may permit non-invasive molecular subtyping in accordance with the 2016 WHO classification. Low ADC values are associated with increased glioma cellularity and worse prognosis, supported by comparisons of diffusivity, histological specimens, and clinical data in multiple studies. Low diffusivity predicts poor astrocytoma survival independent from WHO grade and low ADC values are related to wild-type gliomas [41], as well as to high-grade ODs [17]. Older age, multifocality, brainstem involvement, lack of cystic change, and low ADC are independent predictors of IDH-wild-type grade II diffuse gliomas (DGs). Among these, ADC_{min} was most predictive with a threshold of $\leq 0.9 \times 10^{-3}$ mm^2/s conferring to it the greatest sensitivity (91%). Furthermore, while shorter progression free survival (PFS) and overall survival (OS) were seen in IDH-wild-type grade II DGs, combining IDH status and ADC_{min} better predicted PFS and OS than IDH status alone [42].

Some degree of DWI restriction is linked to other molecular characteristics of brain neoplasms such as MGMT methylation. MGMT promoter methylation is a strong predictor for response to alkylating agents and correlates with better survival. ADC was used as a potential surrogate biomarker for MGMT promoter methylation, however, with controversies [43–48]. In a study of Han et al. [19], the ADC value in GBMs with MGMT promoter methylation was higher than in those without MGMT promoter methylation. In accordance with several previous studies, ADC ratios or ADC minimum values are lower in tumors with unmethylated MGMT promoters than with methylated promoters [45, 46], and mean ADC had a positive relationship with the MGMT promoter methylation ratio [49] (Fig. 5.3). However, lower ADC value in MGMT promoter methylated GBMs was reported in a recent histogram analysis study [50]. Besides, no significant correlation between ADC values and MGMT promoter methylation status was also reported [48].

Diffusion tensor imaging is presently used to document the presence of white matter (WM) tracts and define their location with respect to the tumor (Fig. 5.4).

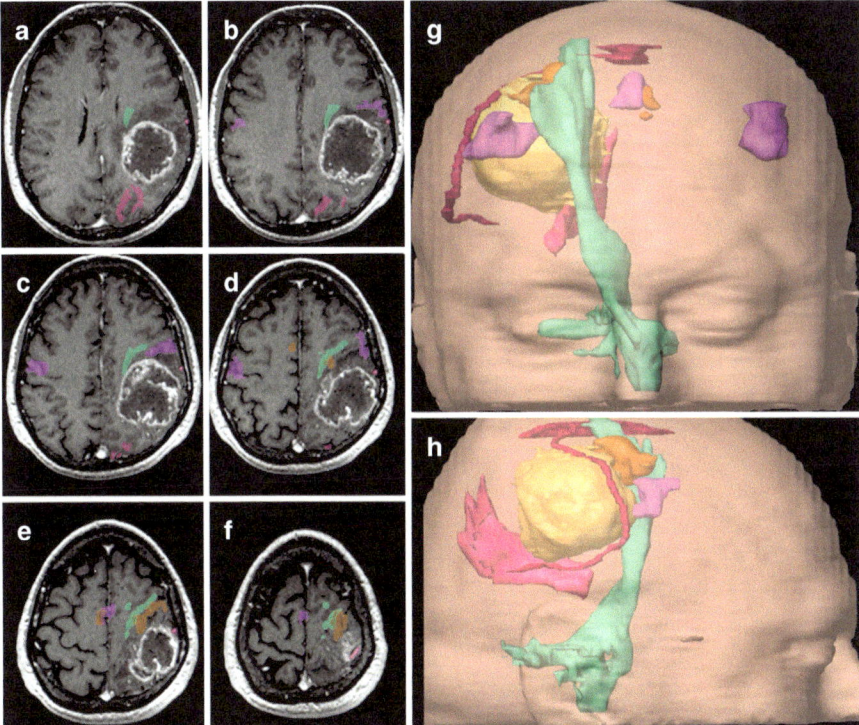

Fig. 5.4 Pre-surgical planning with tractographic reconstructions and motor area representation: axial (**a–f**) and volume rendering (**g, h**). Left fronto-parietal lesion (rolandic area) is evident (**a–f**). The lesion dislocated anteriorly the left cortico-spinal tract (green) (**a–f**), inferiorly the optic radiation (violet) (**g, h**). Motor areas of right hand (orange) (**d–f**) and right face (pink) (**b–d**) are dislocated anteriorly

Brain tumors may alter WM fibers in several ways: in particular, WM tracts may be displaced, infiltrated by tumor or edema, or destroyed [51]. Many studies have demonstrated that fractional anisotropy (FA), an index of fiber organization, decreases in the WM close to brain tumors [52, 53]. An increased ADC seems to play a major role in reducing the number of fibers, at least in symptomatic patients [54]. Diffusion tensor tractography (DTT), the main application of DTI, is the only imaging technique with the potential to generate realistic fiber-tract trajectories in the white matter (WM) of the brain in vivo [55]. DTI studies have demonstrated that edema, tissue compression, and degeneration may cause significant problems in the identification of trajectories compatible with WM tracts. Despite this, the combination of functional MRI (fMRI) and DTI is a useful tool for defining the seed region of interest for DTI-based tractography (DTT) and thus providing more comprehensive, functionally related, white matter mapping in preoperative assessment [56, 57]. Despite the high incidence of cases in which the lesion is responsible for changes that hinder the reconstruction of white matter tracts, the technique can change the surgical approach for corticotomy and define the extent of resection leading to change in the surgical procedure in 80% of cases [57, 58]. Combination of DTI-FT and intraoperative subcortical mapping makes possible the accurate identification of eloquent fiber tracts and enhances surgical performance and safety, while maintaining a high rate of functional preservation [58].

5.4.3 Perfusion Imaging

In the clinical setting, perfusion MRI has been proposed for tumor grading, identifying the best site for biopsy, for the differential diagnosis with non-neoplastic pathologies and to assess treatment response [59–61]. A cerebral blood volume ratio (rCBV) between the maximum value inside the tumor and the normal white matter higher than 1.75 was suggested as a threshold to distinguish between high- and low-grade gliomas [61].

In case of oligodendrogliomas (Fig. 5.2) these results are more debated since some studies demonstrated high rCBV even in low-grade tumors [62], whereas more recent studies demonstrated that perfusion MR is helpful in differentiating low-grade from anaplastic oligodendrogliomas [63]. In transforming low-grade gliomas, MR perfusion imaging demonstrated significant increases in rCBV up to 12 months before contrast enhancement was apparent on T1-weighted MR images, thus indicating the potential role of the technique in predicting malignant transformation [64]. As in high-grade gliomas, metastatic lesions show elevated rCBV. Lower rCBV values outside the enhancing component of the lesion might differentiate secondary from primary neoplasms, with a lower value in metastatic disease [65].

Moreover, $rCBV_{max}$ values are significantly associated with the IDH mutational status. Recent research showed that IDH mutation leads to 2HG accumulation, resulting in decreased hypoxia-inducible-factor 1-activation and downstream inhibition of angiogenesis-related signaling [66]. As demonstrated by Kickingereder et al. [67], IDH-mutant and wild-type tumors were both associated with distinct imaging phenotypes and were predictable with rCBV imaging in a clinical setting (i.e., IDH-mutant tumors represented considerably lower rCBV). In a recent study, the $rCBV_{max}$ values in IDH-mutant tumors were significantly lower than in wild types [66]. Similar results are reported in a study of Lin et al. [17] on ODs, showing that rCBV values can differentiate low- and high-grade types.

The MGMT can be regarded as an independent prognostic factor in patients with primary GBM as MGMT promoter methylation increases responsiveness to temozolomide chemotherapy. The association between MGMT methylation and CBV results is debated. Ryoo et al. [68] found significantly higher rCBV values in GBMs with an unmethylated MGMT promoter than in those with a methylated MGMT; however, they did not take the IDH1/2 mutation status into account and analyzed only a small cohort of 25 patients. Conversely, in a study of Hempel et al. [3], rCBV values were significantly higher in IDH-wild-type GBMs with a methylated MGMT than in those with an unmethylated MGMT. These findings support the hypotheses of Chahal et al. [69], who found that MGMT-positive cells displayed higher levels of vascular endothelial growth factor receptor 1 (VEGFR-1) compared with MGMT unmethylated U87/EV cells leading to higher vascularization of GBM.

Perfusion MRI might help in the differential diagnosis with non-neoplastic disease. In demyelinating lesions and abscess rCBV is lower than in high-grade neoplasm and in cases of demyelinating disease even lower than in normal brain tissue [70].

The size of an enhancing lesion is commonly used as a feature of tumor behavior after therapy. Despite this, it has been demonstrated that rCBV and permeability (Ktrans) assessed with perfusion MR may decrease after therapy indicating success even without changes in tumor size. Consensus panels have published recommendations concerning the use of perfusion MR in monitoring the efficacy of therapy in intra-axial tumors [71].

Lastly, recurrent high-grade neoplasms are typically characterized by high rCBV, whereas tumor necrosis is generally associated with lack of rCBV elevation [72].

5.4.4 Functional MRI

In brain tumor patients, the aim of neurosurgery is to remove as much pathologic tissue as possible, thereby increasing survival time, while simultaneously minimizing the risk of postoperative neurological deficits [73]. Functional MR imaging is increasingly being used as part of the routine preoperative work-up of patients to establish the relationship of the lesion to eloquent areas, such as language or motor areas, and to evaluate hemispheric dominance. Identifying these areas purely on an anatomical basis is inexact, owing to considerable interindividual anatomical and functional variability, especially for language representation. Moreover, in the presence of a lesion, functional areas may be displaced due to mass effect, or function may have shifted to other areas in the brain due to plasticity [74] (Fig. 5.4). A preoperative functional MR imaging study of the main brain functions provides information on the feasibility of surgery and allows adequate assessment of the risk of postoperative neurologic deficits.

For optimal results, the relationship between the tumor margins and the functionally important brain areas needs to be established as accurately as possible [75].

The correlation between functional areas, as established with functional MR imaging versus intraoperative electrocortical stimulation, has been studied for both motor and, to a lesser extent, language representation brain areas. A high correlation has been shown for motor representation areas, but results from language representation studies are conflicting and disappointing.

Bizzi et al. [76] showed that the diagnostic performance of functional MR imaging may change according to the grade of the glioma: sensitivity is higher and specificity is lower in grade II and III gliomas than in glioblastoma multiforme, particularly for functional MR imaging of language. In patients with Rolando area tumors, the sensitivity and specificity of functional MR imaging are higher (88% and 87%, respectively) than in patients with a mass near language cortical areas (80% and 78%, respectively).

In conclusion, although functional MR imaging cannot yet replace intraoperative electrocortical stimulation in patients undergoing neurosurgery, it may be useful for guiding surgical planning and mapping, thereby reducing the extent and duration of craniotomy [77]. Moreover the combination of functional MRI and DTI-based tractography provides more complete preoperative cortical and subcortical mapping.

References

1. Louis DN, Perry A, Reifenberger G, von Deimling A, Figarella-Branger D, Cavenee WK, et al. The 2016 World Health Organization classification of tumors of the central nervous system: a summary. Acta Neuropathol. 2016;131:803–20.
2. Castellano A, Falini A. Progress in neuro-imaging of brain tumors. Curr Opin Oncol. 2016;28:484–93.
3. Hempel JM, Schittenhelm J, Klose U, Bender B, Bier G, Skardelly M, et al. In vivo molecular profiling of human glioma: cross-sectional observational study using dynamic susceptibility contrast magnetic resonance perfusion imaging. Clin Neuroradiol. 2018:21.
4. Reuss DE, Kratz A, Sahm F, Capper D, Schrimpf D, Koelsche C, et al. Adult IDH wild type astrocytomas biologically and clinically resolve into other tumor entities. Acta Neuropathol. 2015;130:407–17.
5. Reuss DE, Mamatjan Y, Schrimpf D, Capper D, Hovestadt V, Kratz A, et al. IDH mutant diffuse and anaplastic astrocytomas have similar age at presentation and little difference in survival: a grading problem for WHO. Acta Neuropathol. 2015;129:867–73.
6. Ebrahimi A, Skardelly M, Bonzheim I, Ott I, Mühleisen H, Eckert F, et al. ATRX immunostaining predicts IDH and H3F3A status in gliomas. Acta Neuropathol Commun. 2016;4:60.
7. Pekmezci M, Rice T, Molinaro AM, Walsh KM, Decker PA, Hansen H, et al. Adult infiltrating gliomas with WHO 2016 integrated diagnosis: additional prognostic roles of ATRX and TERT. Acta Neuropathol. 2017;133:1001–16.
8. Abedalthagafi M, Phillips JJ, Kim GE, Mueller S, Haas-Kogen DA, Marshall RE, et al. The alternative lengthening of telomere phenotype is significantly associated with loss of ATRX expression in high-grade pediatric and adult astrocytomas: a multi-institutional study of 214 astrocytomas. Mod Pathol. 2013;26:1425–32.
9. Hegi ME, Diserens AC, Gorlia T, Hamou MF, de Tribolet N, Weller M, et al. MGMT gene silencing and benefit from temozolomide in glioblastoma. N Engl J Med. 2005;352:997–1003.

10. Stupp R, Mason WP, van den Bent MJ, Weller M, Fisher B, Taphoorn MJ, et al. Radiotherapy plus concomitant and adjuvant temozolomide for glioblastoma. N Engl J Med. 2005;352:987–96.
11. van den Bent MJ, Baumert B, Erridge SC, Vogelbaum MA, Nowak AK, Sanson M, et al. Interim results from the CATNON trial (EORTC study 26053-22054) of treatment with concurrent and adjuvant temozolomide for 1p/19q non-co-deleted anaplastic glioma: a phase 3, randomised, open-label intergroup study. Lancet. 2017;390:1645–53.
12. Gevaert O, Mitchell LA, Achrol AS, Xu J, Echegaray S, Steinberg GK, et al. Glioblastoma multiforme: exploratory radiogenomic analysis by using quantitative image features. Radiology. 2015;276:313.
13. Falini A, Romano A, Bozzao A. Tumours. Neurol Sci. 2008;29:S327–32.
14. Del Sole A, Falini A, Ravasi L, Ottobrini L, De Marchis D, Bombardieri E, et al. Anatomical and biochemical investigation of primary brain tumours. Eur J Nucl Med. 2001;28:1851–72.
15. Jacobs AH, Kracht LW, Gossmann A, Rüger MA, Thomas AV, Thiel A, et al. Imaging in neurooncology. NeuroRx. 2005;2:333–47.
16. Cha S. Update on brain tumor imaging: from anatomy to physiology. AJNR Am J Neuroradiol. 2006;27:475–87.
17. Lin Y, Xing Z, She D, Yang X, Zheng Y, Xiao Z, et al. IDH mutant and 1p/19q co-deleted oligodendrogliomas: tumor grade stratification using diffusion-, susceptibility-, and perfusion-weighted MRI. Neuroradiology. 2017;59:555–62.
18. Ellingson BM, Lai A, Harris RJ, Selfridge JM, Yong WH, Das K, et al. Probabilistic radiographic atlas of glioblastoma phenotypes. AJNR Am J Neuroradiol. 2013;34:533–40.
19. Han Y, Yan LF, Wang XB, Sun YZ, Zhang X, Liu ZC, et al. Structural and advanced imaging in predicting MGMT promoter methylation of primary glioblastoma: a region of interest based analysis. BMC Cancer. 2018;18:215.
20. Xi YB, Guo F, Xu ZL, Li C, Wei W, Tian P, et al. Radiomics signature: a potential biomarker for the prediction of MGMT promoter methylation in glioblastoma. J Magn Reson Imaging. 2018;47:1380–7.
21. Demaerel P, Johannik K, Van Hecke P, Van Ongeval C, Verellen S, Marchal G, et al. Localized 1H NMR spectroscopy in fifty cases of newly diagnosed intracranial tumors. J Comput Assist Tomogr. 1991;15:67–76.
22. Negendank WG, Sauter R, Brown TR, Evelhoch JL, Falini A, Gotsis ED, et al. Proton magnetic resonance spectroscopy in patients with glial tumors: a multicenter study. J Neurosurg. 1996;84:449–58.
23. Preul MC, Caramanos Z, Collins DL, Villemure JG, Leblanc R, Olivier A, et al. Accurate, non-invasive diagnosis of human brain tumors by using proton magnetic resonance spectroscopy. Nat Med. 1996;2:323–5.
24. Somorjai RL, Dolenko B, Nikulin AK, Pizzi N, Scarth G, Zhilkin P, et al. Classification of 1H MR spectra of human brain neoplasms: the influence of preprocessing and computerized consensus diagnosis on classification accuracy. J Magn Reson Imaging. 1996;6:437–44.
25. Tedeschi G, Lundbom N, Raman R, Bonavita S, Duyn JH, Alger JR, et al. Increased choline signal coinciding with malignant degeneration of cerebral gliomas: a serial proton magnetic resonance spectroscopy imaging study. J Neurosurg. 1997;87:516–24.
26. Dowling C, Bollen AW, Noworolski SM, McDermott MW, Barbaro NM, Day MR, et al. Preoperative proton MR spectroscopic imaging of brain tumors: correlation with histopathologic analysis of resection specimens. AJNR Am J Neuroradiol. 2001;22:604–12.
27. Dang L, White DW, Gross S, Bennett BD, Bittinger MA, Driggers EM, et al. Cancer-associated IDH1 mutations produce 2-hydroxyglutarate. Nature. 2009;462:739–44.
28. Choi C, Ganji SK, DeBerardinis RJ, Hatanpaa KJ, Rakheja D, Kovacs Z, et al. 2-Hydroxyglutarate detection by magnetic resonance spectroscopy in IDH-mutated patients with gliomas. Nat Med. 2012;18:624–9.
29. Andronesi OC, Kim G, Gerstner E, Batchelor T, Tzika AA, Fantin VR, et al. Detection of 2-hydoxyglutarate in IDH-mutated glioma patients by spectral-editing and 2D correlation magnetic resonance spectroscopy. Sci Transl Med. 2012;4:116ra4.

30. Emir UE, Larkin SJ, De Pennington N, Voets N, Plaha P, Stacey R, et al. Noninvasive quantification of 2-hydroxyglutarate in human gliomas with IDH1 and IDH2 mutations. Cancer Res. 2016;76:43–9.
31. Pope WB, Prins RM, Thomas MA, Nagarajan R, Yen KE, Bittinger MA, et al. Non-invasive detection of 2-hydroxyglutarate and other metabolites in IDH1 mutant glioma patients using magnetic resonance spectroscopy. J Neurooncol. 2012;107:197–205.
32. Leather T, Jenkinson MD, Das K, Poptani H. Magnetic resonance spectroscopy for detection of 2-hydroxyglutarate as a biomarker for IDH mutation in gliomas. Metabolites. 2017;7:29.
33. Tsuruda J, Chew W, Moseley M, Norman D. Diffusion-weighted MR imaging of the brain: value of differentiating between extra-axial cysts and epidermoid tumors. AJNR Am J Neuroradiol. 1990;11:925–31.
34. Maeda M, Kawamura Y, Tamagawa Y, Matsuda T, Itoh S, Kimura H, et al. Intravoxel incoherent motion (IVIM) MRI in intracranial, extra-axial tumors and cysts. J Comput Assist Tomogr. 1992;16:514–8.
35. Filippi CG, Edgar MA, Ulug A, Prowda JC, Heier LA, Zimmerman RD. Appearance of meningiomas on diffusion- weighted images: correlating diffusion constants with histopathologic findings. AJNR Am J Neuroradiol. 2001;22:65–72.
36. Tien R, Felsberg G, Friedman H, Brown M, MacFall J. MR imaging of high grade cerebral gliomas: value of diffusion-weighted echoplanar pulse sequences. AJR Am J Roentgenol. 1994;162:671–7.
37. Brunberg J, Chenevert T, Mckeever P, Ross DA, Junck LR, Muraszko KM, et al. In vivo MR determination of water diffusion coefficients and diffusion anisotropy: correlation with structural alteration in gliomas of the cerebral hemisphere. AJNR Am J Neuroradiol. 1995;16:361–7.
38. Yang D, Korogi Y, Sugahara T, Kitajima M, Shigematsu Y, Liang L, et al. Cerebral gliomas: prospective comparison of multivoxel 2D chemical-shift imaging proton MR spectroscopy, echoplanar perfusion and diffusion weighted MRI. Neuroradiology. 2002;44:656–66.
39. Bulakbasi N, Kocaoglu M, Ors F, Tayfun C, Uçöz T. Combination of single-voxel proton MR spectroscopy and apparent diffusion coefficient calculation in the evaluation of common brain tumors. AJNR Am J Neuroradiol. 2003;24:225–33.
40. Kono K, Inoue Y, Nakayama K, Shakudo M, Morino M, Ohata K, et al. The role of diffusion weighted imaging in patients with brain tumors. AJNR Am J Neuroradiol. 2001;22:1081–8.
41. Thust SC, Hassanein S, Bisdas S, Rees JH, Hyare H, Maynard JA, et al. Apparent diffusion coefficient for molecular subtyping of non-gadolinium-enhancing WHO grade II/III glioma: volumetric segmentation versus two-dimensional region of interest analysis. Eur Radiol. 2018;28:3779–88.
42. Villanueva-Meyer JE, Wood MD, Choi BS, Mabray MC, Butowski NA, Tihan T, et al. MRI features and IDH mutational status of grade II diffuse gliomas: impact on diagnosis and prognosis. AJR Am J Roentgenol. 2018;210:621–8.
43. Ahn SS, Shin NY, Chang JH, Kim SH, Kim EH, Kim DW, et al. Prediction of methylguanine methyltransferase promoter methylation in glioblastoma using dynamic contrast-enhanced magnetic resonance and diffusion tensor imaging. J Neurosurg. 2014;121:367–73.
44. Gupta A, Omuro AM, Shah AD, Graber JJ, Shi W, Zhang Z, et al. Continuing the search for MR imaging biomarkers for MGMT promoter methylation status: conventional and perfusion MRI revisited. Neuroradiology. 2012;54:641–3.
45. Moon WJ, Choi JW, Roh HG, Lim SD, Koh YC. Imaging parameters of high grade gliomas in relation to the MGMT promoter methylation status: the CT, diffusion tensor imaging, and perfusion MR imaging. Neuroradiology. 2012;54:555–63.
46. Romano A, Calabria LF, Tavanti F, Minniti G, Rossi-Espagnet MC, Coppola V, et al. Apparent diffusion coefficient obtained by magnetic resonance imaging as a prognostic marker in glioblastomas: correlation with MGMT promoter methylation status. Eur Radiol. 2013;23:513–20.
47. Rundle-Thiele D, Day B, Stringer B, Fay M, Martin J, Jeffree RL, et al. Using the apparent diffusion coefficient to identifying MGMT promoter methylation status early in glioblastoma: importance of analytical method. J Med Radiat Sci. 2015;62:92–8.

48. Choi YS, Ahn SS, Kim DW, Chang JH, Kang SG, Kim EH, et al. Incremental prognostic value of ADC histogram analysis over MGMT promoter methylation status in patients with glioblastoma. Radiology. 2016;281:175–84.
49. Sunwoo L, Choi SH, Park CK, Kim JW, Yi KS, Lee WJ, et al. Correlation of apparent diffusion coefficient values measured by diffusion MRI and MGMT promoter methylation semiquantitatively analyzed with MS-MLPA in patients with glioblastoma multiforme. J Magn Reson Imaging. 2013;37:351–8.
50. Pope WB, Lai A, Mehta R, Kim HJ, Qiao J, Young JR, et al. Apparent diffusion coefficient histogram analysis stratifies progression-free survival in newly diagnosed bevacizumab-treated glioblastoma. AJNR Am J Neuroradiol. 2011;32:882–9.
51. Laundre BJ, Jellison BJ, Badie B, Alexander AL, Field AS. Diffusion tensor imaging of corticospinal tract before and after mass resection as correlated with clinical motor findings: preliminary data. AJNR Am J Neuroradiol. 2005;26:791–6.
52. Field AS, Alexander AL, Wu YC, Hasan KM, Witwer B, Badie B. Diffusion tensor eigenvector directional color imaging patterns in the evaluation of cerebral white matter tracts altered by tumor. J Magn Reson Imaging. 2004;20:555–62.
53. Price SJ, Burnet NG, Donovan T, Green HA, Peña A, Antoun NM, et al. Diffusion tensor imaging of brain tumors at 3T: a potential tool for assessing white matter tract invasion? Clin Radiol. 2003;58:455–62.
54. Romano A, Fasoli F, Ferrante M. Fiber density index, fractional anisotropy, ADC and clinical motor findings in the white matter of patients with glioblastoma. Eur Radiol. 2008;18:331–6.
55. Dong Q, Welsh RC, Chenevert TL, Carlos RC, Maly-Sundgren P, Gomez-Hassan DM, et al. Clinical application of diffusion tensor imaging. J Magn Reson Imaging. 2004;19:6–18.
56. Arfanakis K, Gui M, Lazar M. Optimization of white matter tractography for pre-surgical planning and image-guided surgery. Oncol Rep. 2006;15:1061–4.
57. Romano A, Ferrante M, Cipriani V. Role of magnetic resonance tractography in the preoperative planning and intraoperative assessment of patients with intra-axial brain tumours. Radiol Med. 2007;112:906–20.
58. Bello L, Gambini A, Castellano A, Carrabba G, Acerbi F, Fava E, et al. Motor and language DTI Fiber tracking combined with intraoperative subcortical mapping for surgical removal of gliomas. NeuroImage. 2008;39:369–82.
59. Law M, Yang S, Wang H, Babb JS, Johnson G, Cha S, et al. Glioma grading: sensitivity, specificity, and predictive values of perfusion MR imaging and proton MR spectroscopic imaging compared with conventional MR imaging. AJNR Am J Neuroradiol. 2003;24:1989–98.
60. Aronen HJ, Pardo FS, Kennedy DN, Belliveau JW, Packard SD, Hsu DW, et al. High microvascular blood volume is associated with high glucose uptake and tumor angiogenesis in human gliomas. Clin Cancer Res. 2000;6:2189–200.
61. Knopp EA, Cha S, Johnson G, Mazumdar A, Golfinos JG, Zagzag D, et al. Glial neoplasms: dynamic contrast-enhanced T2*-weighted MR imaging. Radiology. 1999;211:791–8.
62. Lev MH, Ozsunar Y, Henson JW, Rasheed AA, Barest GD, Harsh GR 4th, et al. Glial tumor grading and outcome prediction using dynamic spin-echo MR susceptibility mapping compared with conventional contrast-enhanced MR: confounding effect of elevated rCBV of oligodendrogliomas. AJNR Am J Neuroradiol. 2004;25:214–21.
63. Spampinato MV, Smith JK, Kwock L, Ewend M, Grimme JD, Camacho DL, et al. Cerebral blood volume measurements and proton MR spectroscopy in grading of oligodendroglial tumors. AJR Am J Roentgenol. 2007;188:204–12.
64. Danchaivijitr N, Waldman AD, Tozer DJ, Benton CE, Brasil Caseiras G, et al. Low-grade gliomas: do changes in rCBV measurements at longitudinal perfusion- weighted MR imaging predict malignant transformation. Radiology. 2008;247:170–8.
65. Cha S, Lupo JM, Chen MH, Lamborn KR, McDermott MW, Berger MS, et al. Differentiation of glioblastoma multiforme and single brain metastasis by peak height and percentage of signal intensity recovery derived from dynamic susceptibility-weighted contrast-enhanced perfusion MR imaging. AJNR Am J Neuroradiol. 2007;28:1078–84.

66. Xing Z, Yang X, She D, Lin Y, Zhang Y, Cao D. Noninvasive assessment of IDH mutational status in World Health Organization grade II and III astrocytomas using DWI and DSC-PWI combined with conventional MR imaging. AJNR Am J Neuroradiol. 2017;38:1138–44.
67. Kickingereder P, Sahm F, Radbruch A, Wick W, Heiland S, Deimling AV, et al. IDH mutation status is associated with a distinct hypoxia/angiogenesis transcriptome signature which is noninvasively predictable with rCBV imaging in human glioma. Sci Rep. 2015;5:16238.
68. Ryoo I, Choi SH, Kim JH, Sohn CH, Kim SC, Shin HS, et al. Cerebral blood volume calculated by dynamic susceptibility contrast-enhanced perfusion MR imaging: preliminary correlation study with glioblastoma genetic profiles. PLoS One. 2013;19:8.
69. Chahal M, Xu Y, Lesniak D, Graham K, Famulski K, Christensen JG, et al. MGMT modulates glioblastoma angiogenesis and response to the tyrosine kinase inhibitor sunitinib. Neuro-Oncology. 2010;12:822–33.
70. Bernarding J, Braun J, Koennecke HC. Diffusion and perfusion-weighted MR imaging in a patient with acute demyelinating encephalomyelitis (ADEM). J Magn Reson Imaging. 2002;15:96–100.
71. Leach MO, Brindle KM, Evelhoch JL, et al. Assessment of anti-angiogenic and anti-vascular therapeutics using magnetic resonance imaging: recommendations for appropriate methodology for clinical trials. In: Proceedings of the Eleventh Meeting of the International Society for Magnetic Resonance in Medicine. Berkeley: International Society for Magnetic Resonance in Medicine; 2003. p. 1268.
72. Wenz F, Rempp K, Hess T, Debus J, Brix G, Engenhart R, et al. Effect of radiation on blood volume in low-grade astrocytomas and normal brain tissue: quantification with dynamic susceptibility contrast MR imaging. AJR Am J Roentgenol. 1996;166:187–93.
73. Duffau H. Lessons from brain mapping in surgery for low-grade glioma: insights into associations between tumour and brain plasticity. Lancet Neurol. 2005;4:476–86.
74. Sunaert S, Yousry TA. Clinical applications of functional magnetic resonance imaging. Neuroimaging Clin N Am. 2001;11:221–36.
75. Oritz C, Haughton V. Functional MR imaging: paradigms for clinical preoperative mapping. Magn Reson Imaging Clin N Am. 2003;11:529–42.
76. Bizzi A, Blasi V, Falini A, Ferroli P, Cadioli M, Danesi U, et al. Presurgical functional MR imaging of language and motor functions: validation with intraoperative electrocortical mapping. Radiology. 2008;248:579–89.
77. Smits M, Visch-Brink E, Schraa-Tam CK, Koudstaal PJ, van der Lugt A. Functional MR imaging of language processing: an overview of easy-to implement paradigms for patient care and clinical research. Radiographics. 2006;26(Suppl 1):S145–58.

Tumors of the Central Nervous System: Therapeutic Approaches

Alessia Pellerino and Riccardo Soffietti

6.1 Introduction

Brain tumors include both primary and secondary tumor subtypes with different therapeutic approaches according to the histology and the molecular profile. In this regard, the World Health Organization (WHO) 2016 classification of CNS tumors has integrated the histological and molecular factors in order to identify patients with different outcomes in terms of prognosis and to personalize treatments [1, 2]. Furthermore, some clinical factors must be also considered to choose the most adequate therapy. Among high-grade gliomas (HGGs) significant prognostic factors are age (<50 years or ≥50 years), Karnofsky performance status (KPS < or ≥ 70), mental alteration (yes or no), neurological function (work or not), extent of resection (biopsy versus partial/gross total), radiation dose (< or ≥ 54.4 Gy) [3], isocitrate dehydrogenase status (IDH 1–2 mutation), and methylation of the *O6-methylguanine-DNA methyltransferase* (MGMT) promoter [4], while in brain metastasis (BM) the primary tumor histology and molecular subtype, the number of brain metastasis, and the presence of extracranial tumor activity may play a significant role to determine the survival [5].

In the last years, some driver mutations involved in the tumor growth have been identified and may be druggable by different compounds. Encouraging data have been provided in BM from large international clinical trials with increasing disease control rate, progression-free survival (PFS), and overall survival (OS) compared with traditional therapies, while in HGGs disappointing results from antiangiogenic therapy and immunotherapy have been reported thus far.

Considering the WHO 2016 classification and the most recent data from clinical trials, here we report general considerations regarding the treatment of brain

A. Pellerino (✉) · R. Soffietti
Department of Neuro-Oncology, University and City of Health and Science Hospital,
Turin, Italy
e-mail: alessia.pellerino@unito.it; riccardo.soffietti@unito.it

© Springer Nature Switzerland AG 2019
M. Bartolo et al. (eds.), *Neurorehabilitation in Neuro-Oncology*,
https://doi.org/10.1007/978-3-319-95684-8_6

tumors, including low grade (LGGs) and HGGs, ependymomas, medulloblastomas, meningiomas, and BM.

6.2 Surgery in Gliomas

Surgery is the first step in the management of brain gliomas. Biopsy or resection is
mandatory to obtain tissue for diagnostic confirmation, typing, grading, and molecular characterization and relieves symptoms from intracranial hypertension or spinal compression. Moreover, surgery has shown to improve seizure control, especially
in LGGs [6, 7]. The extent of resection is significantly correlated with the overall
survival and quality of life (QoL) [8]. Lacroix and coworkers reported a significant
survival advantage in glioblastoma (GBM) with resection more than 98% of the
tumor volume (median OS 13 months, 95% CI 11.4–14.6 months) compared with a
median OS of 8.8 months (95% CI 7.4–10.2 months) for resection of less than 98%
[9]. In another study, Laws and coworkers described a survival benefit for both
grade III and IV gliomas (58% and 11% at 24 months, respectively) [10]. Some
recent data suggest that a supramaximal resection beyond FLAIR altered area could
represent a promising strategy to improve outcome in either LGGs [11] or GBM
patients [12] with limited postoperative complications, even in eloquent areas.
Several techniques have been employed to maximize the effect of the surgery and
facilitate the impact of adjuvant therapy. In particular, intraoperative mapping,
aggressive microsurgical resection, intraoperative magnetic resonance imaging,
intraoperative ultrasonography, and fluorescence-guided surgery can be valuable
tools to safely reduce the tumor burden of LGGs and HGGs [13]. Similarly, gross-
total resection can be achieved in BM with lower morbidity [14] and may be also
considered for patients with two to three surgically accessible brain metastases in
good neurological condition and controlled systemic disease.

6.3 Glioblastomas (Grade IV)

6.3.1 Standard Treatment in Newly Diagnosed GBM

The current standard of care (SOC) in GBM is represented by a maximal safe resection followed by radiotherapy (60 Gy/30 fractions) with concomitant and adjuvant
temozolomide (TMZ) for six cycles (Stupp regimen) [15]. The MGMT methylation
is a strong predictive factor of response to alkylating agents (mOS 23.4 months in
MGMT methylated patients versus 12.6 months in MGMT unmethylated patients)
[16]. In 10–30% of GBM a progressive enhancing MRI lesion may appear shortly
following radiotherapy, and is considered as a pseudoprogression. Pseudoprogression
may be accompanied by clinical signs and symptoms, but more often remains
asymptomatic. This treatment-related effect has implications for patient management and may result in premature discontinuation of an effective adjuvant therapy
and erroneous inclusion into clinical trials for recurrent gliomas.

In many countries, the Stupp regimen is prolonged up to 12 cycles of TMZ with the expectation to delay recurrences. However, continuing TMZ beyond 6 cycles has not shown to increase the OS in newly GBM [17], as well as the use of intensified TMZ schedule, regardless the MGMT methylation status [18, 19].

A new SOC has been defined for the population of elderly patients with GBM, which is increasing overtime. Patients with tumors lacking MGMT promoter methylation could receive hypofractionated radiotherapy alone, while those with methylated MGMT GBM could be treated with TMZ alone (treatment for 5 of every 28 days until progression or for 12 months), according to the findings from the NOA-08 and Nordic trials. Recently, Perry and coworkers have established a new SOC in elderly GBM, which consists in a short course radiation (40 Gy/15 fractions) associated with concomitant and adjuvant TMZ by reporting a median OS longer with radiotherapy plus TMZ than with radiotherapy alone (9.3 months vs. 7.6 months) as well as a prolonged median PFS (5.3 months vs. 3.9 months) [20]. However, this new SOC can be applied to fit patients only.

The locoregional use of alternating electric fields to treat tumors, called TTF, represents a novel treatment modality. Low-intensity (1–3 V/cm), intermediate-frequency (200 kHz) fields may selectively disrupt the microtubule assembly and interfere with mitotic spindle formation, causing apoptosis of rapidly dividing malignant cells. TTF is administered via transducer arrays, which are applied to the patient's shaved scalp for 18 h/day. The EF-14 trial has investigated the efficacy and tolerability of TTF in patients with GBM, who had already completed temozolomide chemoradiotherapy. The primary endpoint was either PFS, which improved from a median of 4.0–7.1 months or OS from a median of 16.6–19.6 months [21]. Some limitations are present in the study: patients and investigators were not blind and patients randomized to TTF received additional training and support necessary for the use of the TTF device. Together, these factors may have conferred a placebo benefit. Moreover, TTF is very expensive, and this represents a major obstacle for an extensive application of the device in a large population.

6.3.2   Treatment of Recurrent GBM

The three strategies of medical treatment for GBM, recurrent following the Stupp regimen, that are most often used in Europe, include alternative dosing regimens of TMZ, nitrosourea-based regimens, and bevacizumab [22]. Different phase II trials (RESCUE, NCT00657267, and BR12) suggested that there is no rationale for the use of dose-intensified TMZ in recurrent GBM, while some activity of lomustine has been confirmed in the control groups of different randomized trials [23, 24] with PFS at 6 months of 20%. Fotemustine is a third-generation nitrosourea showing some efficacy in GBM; the dosage may range from 60 to 100 mg/m^2 every 2 weeks (induction phase) or 4 weeks (maintenance phase) achieving a median PFS of 3–6 months [25–27].

Bevacizumab, a humanized monoclonal antibody which binds VEGF-A, is the most studied antiangiogenic agent for GBM. The results from the BRAIN trial have led to the approval by the US FDA of bevacizumab for the first recurrence of GBM [28]. In Europe, the BELOB trial [29] has shown encouraging results for the combination of bevacizumab and lomustine versus either agent alone. However, the subsequent phase III trial, which has compared the combination of lomustine and bevacizumab with lomustine alone, did not report advantages in OS [30]. Similarly, bevacizumab has been investigated in the setting of newly diagnosed GBM in two independent randomized phase III trials (AVAGlio and RTOG-0825) [31, 32]: PFS was prolonged in both trials in the bevacizumab arms (median 10.7 vs 7.3 months in RTOG0825; 10.6 vs 6.2 months in AvAGlio); however, this did not translate into prolongation of OS. Moreover, the median OS of 16 months of AVAGlio and RTOG trials is not substantially longer than the OS in prior TMZ-containing trials (EORTC-NCIC trial). QoL appears to be improved due to the delayed progression in the experimental arm in AVAGlio, while RTOG patients have shown cognitive deterioration (especially in executive and speed processing functions) during PFS in BEV-treated patients. In general, the clinical indication for bevacizumab includes progressive tumors with a great amount of enhancement and edema. The proneural variant of GBM has been suggested to be more sensitive to the bevacizumab [33], but this evidence would need to be prospectively validated.

6.3.3 Immunotherapy in GBM

The success of immune-based therapies in cancers, such as melanoma and NSCLC, has led to investigate the potential efficacy of immunotherapies in GBM. In this regard, several clinical trials using these agents, including antitumor vaccines, autologous cell-based therapies, and immune checkpoint inhibitors, are ongoing.

When using peptide-based vaccination, patients are directly inoculated with one or more tumor-associated antigens in order to stimulate an immune response against tumor cells. The most extensively evaluated vaccine-based therapy for glioma is rindopepimut, which consists of the amino acid sequence of EGFR variant III (EGFRvIII) conjugated to keyhole limpet hemocyanin. The ACT trials have investigated the role of rindopepimut in newly diagnosed GBM harboring the EGFRvIII mutation. The phase II trial reported a median PFS and OS of 9.2 and 21.8 months, respectively, which were significantly longer than matched controls [34]. However, the phase III trial did not confirm the survival benefit [35]. Notably, the EGFRvIII mutation has been found as lost following reoperation for tumor progression, thus it is unknown whether this represents a development of a secondary resistance or the natural evolution of the disease. In patients with recurrent GBM, the phase II ReACT trial showed significant OS improvement from 8.8 to 12.0 months with rindopepimut plus bevacizumab versus bevacizumab alone [36].

When using cell-based vaccination, the autologous antigen-presenting cells (APCs) (i.e., dendritic cells) are exposed to a lysate of the patient's own tumor cells in order to stimulate the specific T-cell activation and create a personalized vaccine. Although this therapeutic approach is a highly personalized therapy with a limited toxicity due to the specificity of the targeted antigens, these agents are expensive to produce. In fact, the enrollment in the phase III trial ICT-107-301 (educated dendritic cells against six different tumor-associated antigens) was prematurely closed by the company due to inability to ensure sufficient financial resources. To date, there are no other reported phase III trials of cell-based therapies, so the clinical utility of these agents remains to be determined.

Immune check point inhibitors have been tested in recurrent GBM with unsatisfactory results. In particular, the phase III trial CheckMate 143 in patients with recurrent GBM showed no benefit for nivolumab over bevacizumab [37]. The activity of nivolumab in GBM seems to be modest, probably due to a low mutational burden of HGG and an immunosuppressive cellular environment. Despite these poor results, two different phase III trials are now evaluating the efficacy of nivolumab in newly diagnosed GBM (CheckMate 498 for MGMT unmethylated patients and CheckMate 548 for MGMT methylated patients, respectively) and the preliminary results are awaited.

6.3.4 Targeted Therapies in GBM

The EGF receptor (EGFR) is overexpressed in about 50% of GBM and represents a potential druggable target. Several EGFR inhibitors have been evaluated in GBM trials, including the small molecule inhibitors such as gefitinib, erlotinib, and afatinib or the monoclonal antibodies such as cetuximab, mAb 425, and nimotuzumab. Unfortunately, the results have shown a limited activity in GBM, even among those with EGF receptor amplification.

A new therapeutic option is represented by the depatuxizumab mafodotin (ABT-414) in GBM with EGFR amplification. The antibody component of ABT-414 binds to mutant/amplified EGFR with consistent diffusion to the blood brain barrier (BBB), then delivers the cytotoxic drug component (monomethyl auristatin F—MMAF) into the tumor cell. In recurrent GBM, van den Bent and coworkers have reported a prolonged PFS at 6 months (28.8%, a median PFS of 1.7 months), an OS at 6 months of 72.5%, and a median OS of 9.3 months compared with control [38]: these results are encouraging and warrant further investigations in phase III trials (NCT02573324, NCT02343406).

Early evidence showed cilengitide (an integrin inhibitor) as a promising therapeutic option, especially in GBM with MGMT promoter methylation, but a large randomized phase III trial (CENTRIC) has not demonstrated any survival benefit [39], as well as other compounds, including panobinostat (histone deacetylase inhibitor), galunisertib (TGF-β receptor-1 inhibitor), and selinexor (exportin-1 inhibitor).

Overall, the greatest limitation for target therapies is that a consistent driver mutation in GBM is still unknown so far, thus limiting their impact on the disease.

6.4 Anaplastic Gliomas (Grade III)

Treatment recommendations in anaplastic diffuse gliomas are based on the long-term results of four phase III trials and on the first results of the CATNON trial. The RTOG 9402 and the EORTC 26951 trials have demonstrated that

1p/19q-codeleted anaplastic oligodendrogliomas benefit from the addition of PCV (procarbazine, CCNU, and vincristine) chemotherapy to radiotherapy. It is still unknown whether PCV chemotherapy may be replaced by TMZ and is currently under investigation by the CODEL trial comparing radiotherapy and PCV versus radiotherapy and concomitant and adjuvant TMZ. A critical point of chemoradiation is the risk of cognitive dysfunctions in long-term survivors due to radiotherapy neurotoxicity. Some data suggest that PCV chemotherapy alone as an up-front treatment may prolong OS with limited cognitive dysfunctions. This issue is currently being investigated in the POLCA trial which is comparing initial treatment with radiotherapy and PCV vs. PCV alone (radiotherapy being postponed at the time of progression) in 1p/19q codeleted-anaplastic oligodendrogliomas (NCT02444000).

Conversely, in 1p/19-intact anaplastic gliomas the OS was similar with either radiotherapy alone or radiotherapy plus PCV in both RTOG 9402 and EORTC 26951 trials.

Recently, the EORTC 26053 CATNON trial on anaplastic gliomas has reported that the combination of radiotherapy and adjuvant temozolomide was associated with both longer PFS and OS compared with radiotherapy alone in 1p/19q non codeleted patients. Further follow-up is needed to evaluate the impact of concomitant TMZ and the predictive value of IDH mutation and MGMT methylation status.

Treatment for recurrent anaplastic gliomas is poorly codified and relies on a second surgery, when it is feasible, reirradiation, and second-line chemotherapy with alkylating agents.

The eflornithine, an irreversible inhibitor of ornithine decarboxylase (ODC), is being investigated in a phase III trial in association with lomustine compared with lomustine alone in anaplastic astrocytomas recurrent following radiation and TMZ (NCT02796261). The mechanism of action is based on decrease of the intracellular polyamine accumulation. A phase II trial has demonstrated that in patients receiving up to 12 months of eflornithine-PCV, m-PFS improved of 2.8 years as well as mOS improved of 2.5 years.

Targeting the oncogenic IDH mutation is an attractive approach: different drugs are being tested, such as inhibitors of IDH 1/2 mutant enzymes, mutation-specific vaccination, and glutaminase inhibitors.

6.5   Low-Grade Gliomas (Grade II)

The optimal management of LGGs is still controversial regarding the timing and sequence of radiotherapy and chemotherapy.

One issue is whether patients with maximal resection need additional treatment or may be observed. Considering that more than 50% of patients recur within 5 years following gross-total resection [40], an initial observation with MRI is a reasonable postoperative option in low-risk patients (age < 40 years, gross-total resection, the absence of seizures, or other neurological impairment).

High-risk LGGs are characterized by either an incomplete resection with or without seizures or a progression following initial observation with MRI. The EORTC 22033-26033 trial has enrolled patients with high-risk LGGs to either TMZ or standard radiation therapy. For IDH mutated and 1p19q codeleted LGGs (mainly oligodendrogliomas), the OS was similar with TMZ and radiotherapy (55.0 versus 61.6 months), while in IDH mutated but 1p/19 non-codeleted (mainly astrocytomas) patients PFS was inferior with TMZ (36.0 versus 55.4 months). Overall, survival data from this trial are not yet mature.

In 1998, a phase III trial in LGGs on radiotherapy with or without adjuvant PCV was launched by RTOG. The first publication in 2012 did not report an OS advantage with the addition of chemotherapy [41], despite an improvement of PFS. With longer follow-up, a statistically significant benefit for OS in radiotherapy plus PCV arm as compared with radiotherapy alone was significant (13.3 versus 7.8 years, respectively) [42].

Similar to anaplastic gliomas, open questions are whether an increased survival from chemoradiation is balanced by the risk of late cognitive defects, and how to treat the heterogeneous group of the IDH wild-type LGGs. Most of IDH wild-type LGGs have a clinical course similar to HGGs and tend to be treated with chemoradiation. Recently, some molecular alterations (trisomy of chromosome 7, loss of chromosome 10, and TERT mutation) have been suggested as prognostic factors in IDH wild-type LGGs leading to the identification of different molecular risk groups [43].

6.6 Meningiomas

Although meningiomas are the most common non-glial brain tumors (12–20% of primary intracranial tumors), the level of evidence to provide recommendations for the treatment is low compared with other tumors. In this regard, the European Association of Neuro-Oncology (EANO) has provided guidelines for clinicians, [44] suggesting that therapy for patients with meningiomas needs to be personalized.

Asymptomatic, incidentally discovered meningiomas can be managed by observation alone, while for patients with symptomatic meningiomas, surgery represents the first therapeutic option in order to relieve neurological symptoms and obtain a histological diagnosis, grading, and hopefully molecular profiling. Grade I meningiomas are usually treated by surgery and complete resection (Simpson grade I) is the primary goal. Stereotactic radiosurgery (SRS) or fractionated radiotherapy (SFRT) as an adjuvant treatment may be considered in tumors not accessible for surgery, or after an incomplete resection, or in grade II and III meningiomas. In particular, for grade III meningiomas adjuvant radiation improves long-term control and OS. Conversely, there is conflicting evidence on the value of radiotherapy in grade II meningiomas. In this regard, the ROAM/EORTC 1308 trial is evaluating the impact of adjuvant radiotherapy in terms of delay of recurrence in incompletely resected grade II meningiomas.

To date, there are no FDA and EMA approved chemotherapeutic agents for treatment of refractory meningioma, as they have very limited efficacy. Small retrospective series and case reports have reported some activity of drugs, such as hydroxyurea, doxorubicin, temozolomide, bevacizumab, IFNα, and octreotide agonists.

Trabectedin, a compound with activity in sarcomas, failed to demonstrate an efficacy in the EORTC 1320 phase II trial and displayed severe side effects. Currently, two different trials are being evaluating the efficacy of the Novo-TTF (NCT01892397) and the combination of everolimus and octreotide (CEVOREM): the results are awaited in 2018.

New oncogenic mutations have been described in meningiomas, such as NF2 mutation (24–36%), AKT1 mutation (8–13%), and SMO mutation (4–5%). Interestingly, these mutations may be druggable by specific compounds, such as vismodegib (SMO inhibitor), AZD5363 (AKT inhibitor), and GSK2256098 (NF2-FAK inhibitor) which are investigated in the phase II Alliance/NCI trial (A071401).

6.7 Ependymal Tumors

Ependymomas are the most common intramedullary spinal cord tumors in adults, especially the myxopapillary type in the filum terminale or conus. Conversely, intracranial ependymomas are most common in children: 60% are infratentorial, 40% are supratentorial, and up to 30% are anaplastic (WHO grade III). Recently, Pajtler et al. [45] have identified nine major molecular subgroups of ependymomas, with three in each compartment of the CNS, namely spine, posterior fossa, and supratentorial. Guidelines for management of ependymomas have been recently drawn by the EANO [46]. Surgery is the mainstay of treatment, and a total resection should be performed whenever feasible. Radiotherapy is employed in case of an incomplete resection of grade II ependymomas. A postoperative conformal radiotherapy with doses up to 60 Gy is recommended for patients with WHO grade III ependymomas regardless the extent of resection, while doses of 54–55 Gy are used for grade II ependymomas. A craniospinal radiotherapy of 36 Gy is recommended only in case of CSF dissemination with a boost up to 45–54 Gy on focal lesions.

The role of chemotherapy for treatment of recurrent ependymoma in adults remains unclear and is considered only when local treatment options (surgery and radiotherapy) have been exhausted. TMZ has shown some efficacy for the treatment of adult patients, as well as platinum-based regimens and bevacizumab.

A postoperative staging with MRI of whole CNS and examination are mandatory and because of the risk of asymptomatic and/or late relapses, patients should be followed long term with enhanced craniospinal MRI.

6.8 Medulloblastomas

Medulloblastomas are aggressive embryonal tumors representing the most frequent primary malignant brain cancer in children and more often is located in the cerebellum vermis. Maximal safe resection, craniospinal irradiation (CSI), and chemotherapy remain the mainstays of first-line treatment. Medulloblastomas tend to metastasize to the cranial and spinal cord leptomeninges, thus this justifies the irradiation of the entire CNS and not just the primary tumor bed.

Currently, medulloblastomas in children between 3 and 5 years are stratified in low-risk and high-risk groups. High-risk patients are defined by the presence of a residual disease >1.5 cm^2 and/or metastatic spread, while low-risk patients are characterized by gross-total resection and the absence of CSF spread. High-risk patients are treated with craniospinal irradiation of 36–39 Gy, with a boost to 55 Gy to the posterior fossa–tumor bed, followed by cisplatin and cyclophosphamide-based chemotherapy, while low-risk patients receive 23.4 Gy of craniospinal irradiation, with a boost to 55 Gy to the posterior fossa–tumor bed, followed by adjuvant chemotherapy. Low-risk patients achieve an OS of 80% at 5 years, while high-risk medulloblastomas have a shorter outcome (36% of OS at 5 years).

The irradiation of the entire CNS increases the risk of severe neurocognitive dysfunctions in long-term medulloblastoma survivors. Considering these long-term sequelae, patients younger than 3 years are treated with radiation-sparing approaches and more intensive chemotherapy achieving similar results in terms of OS compared with patients treated with radiotherapy and better neurocognitive outcomes.

Medulloblastomas in young and adult patients are more located in the cerebellar hemisphere and relatively less aggressive than tumors in children. Total resection is feasible in many patients and in this instance only whole CNS radiotherapy is performed, while chemotherapy is added in high-risk patients.

The 2016 WHO classification of the CNS tumors divides medulloblastomas into wingless (WNT)-activated, sonic hedgehog (SHH)-activated-TP53 wild-type, SHH-activated-TP53 mutant, and non-WNT-SHH (group 3 and group 4 medulloblastomas).

WNT patients have a favorable outcome in terms of OS (95% at 5 years) and current clinical trials are focused on the de-escalation of therapy (NCT02066220, NCT01878617, and NCT02724579).

Outcomes of SHH tumors are age specific. Infants have an excellent outcome, while in childhood TP53-mutant SHH tumors have a dismal prognosis. To date, SHH pathway antagonists, such as SMO inhibitors (LDE225/Sonidegib and GDC-0449/Vismodegib) are currently being evaluated in clinical trials. Conversely, targeted therapies for group 3 and 4 medulloblastomas are still missing [47].

6.9 Brain Metastasis

The EANO has recently drawn guidelines for the management of brain metastasis [48]. Surgical resection and stereotactic radiosurgery (SRS) yield similar outcomes in terms of survival for patients with oligometastases. The choice between surgery and SRS should be made considering factors, such as number, location, and size of BM, neurologic symptoms, patient preference, and physician expertise. In case of a measurable tumor following surgery, postoperative SRS improves local control with good cognitive outcomes, preservation of quality of life, and functional independence as demonstrated by the phase III N107C/CEC·3 trial [49]. SRS allows to deliver high radiation doses on a well-defined and limited target volume (3.0–3.5 cm diameter). A high single radiation dose to large tumors is associated with neurotoxicity (especially brain edema), thus hypofractionated regimens (SFRT) may be considered in order to achieve adequate local control. Patients with a single BM, KPS > 70, and controlled extracranial disease achieve longer survival, including cases of radioresistant tumors, such as melanoma and renal cell carcinoma, as well as patients with a limited number of BM (1–3). Yamamoto and coworkers have reported that patients with a high number of BM (up to 10) have similar OS (10.8 months) and treatment-related toxicity compared with those with 2–4 BM [50], but these data need to be validated in randomized trials. The risk of adverse radiation effects following SRS/SFRT increases with the increase of radiation dose and the size of lesion. The early adverse events (AEs) tend to appear within 2 weeks after the start of treatment. Typical symptoms are headache, nausea and vomiting, worsening of neurological deficits, seizures, and are reversible with steroids. The late AEs tend to appear later with pseudoprogression (months) and radionecrosis (months to years) and consist in an increase of contrast enhancement, necrosis, and edema. Treatment with steroids or bevacizumab may be effective to control neurological symptoms and mass effect.

Since the 1950s WBRT has been the most widely used treatment for patients with brain metastasis, given its effectiveness in palliation, widespread availability, and ease of delivery. A neurological improvement and radiological response following WBRT as an up-front treatment have been reported in up to 60% of patients with multiple BM (10–15% alive at 1 year). However, a phase III trial (QUARTZ), comparing WBRT versus supportive care in non-small cell lung cancer (NSCLC) patients with BM, has reported no differences in terms of OS and QoL. Typical acute adverse effects of WBRT include temporary alopecia, mild dermatitis, mild fatigue, and less commonly otitis media or externa. Infrequently, worsening of cognitive and neurologic deficits may develop during treatment due to a transient edema, which usually responds to corticosteroids.

The role of WBRT following surgery or SRS is limited. Three large phase III trials have demonstrated that the omission of WBRT in patients with limited number of BM after either complete surgery or SRS results in worse local and distant control, but do not affect the overall survival (OS). Other two trials have reported a higher incidence of cognitive deficit (in particular memory deficits) in patients receiving SRS plus WBRT versus SRS alone [51, 52]. Moreover, a negative impact of WBRT on quality of life, resulting in a transient lower physical and cognitive functioning score in health-related quality of life (HRQOL) tests, has been reported [53]. Considering all these limitations, the American Society for Radiation Oncology (ASTRO) evidence-based guidelines [54] and the EANO guidelines [48] recommend WBRT alone as a palliative treatment only in patients with multiple BM and/or progressive systemic disease. The use of memantine (noncompetitive NMDA antagonist receptor with neuroprotective effect in preclinical models) and the intensity-modulated radiotherapy (IMRT) that allows a major sparing of the cognitive hippocampal areas are being investigated.

In general, the response rates to chemotherapeutic agents of brain metastases reflect the sensitivity of primary solid tumor (30–80% in SCLC, 30–50% in breast cancer, 10–30% in NSCLC, 10–15% in melanoma). The association of RT and chemotherapy may improve response rate compared with RT alone, but not survival. Targeted agents are able to induce higher response rate than those observed following cytotoxic chemotherapy in specific molecular subgroups. Moreover, the activity of targeted therapies is higher in patients with small, asymptomatic, and radiotherapy-naïve patients.

Melanoma, lung, and breast cancer represent the major sources of brain/leptomeningeal metastases. Alkylating agents, such as temozolomide and fotemustine, either as single agent or in combination, have some activity against BM from melanomas. Selective inhibitors of the kinases BRAF and MEK are efficacious as single agents as well as in combination regimens in BRAF-V600-mutated melanoma. Similarly, selective blockers of cytotoxic T-lymphocyte-associated antigen-4 (CTLA-4) and programmed-death-1 (PD-1), known as checkpoint inhibitors (ICIs), are effective in metastatic melanoma as single agents and in combination.

The association of SRS to BRAF/MEK inhibitors may increase intracranial disease control and OS; however, some studies report higher CNS toxicity, requiring caution in clinical use. The association between SRS and anti-PD1 appears safe and active in terms of intracranial disease control and OS, but needs further investigations. The combination of SRS and anti-CTLA-4 is promising and shows improvement over anti-CTLA-4 alone or SRS alone.

Regarding NSCLC, platinum compounds (cisplatin, carboplatin) and pemetrexed, alone or in association (etoposide, vinorelbine, radiotherapy), are the most commonly used chemotherapeutics.

Thirty-three percent of BM from NSCLC has the expression of the mutant epidermal growth factor receptor (EGFR) and other 5–10% has the anaplastic lymphoma kinase (ALK) rearrangement, which are druggable by EGFR tyrosine kinase inhibitors (EGFR TKIs) and ALK inhibitors, respectively.

The first (erlotinib, gefitinib) and second (afatinib) generation of EGFR TKIs have a limited BBB penetration. Up to 60% of NSCLC patients develop resistance to first and second-generation EGFR TKIs due to the presence of new mutation (T790M). In this regard, two different drugs (osimertinib and AZD3759) targeting the resistance mutation and with higher CSF concentration are being investigated with preliminary interesting results. Different studies have investigated whether the association of EGFR TKIs (erlotinib and gefitinib) and radiotherapy (SRS or WBRT) may increase the response rate. Patients with ALK rearrangement respond well to the ALK inhibitors (crizotinib in first line, ceritinib and alectinib as second line). Brigatinib and lorlatinib that represent a third generation of ALK inhibitors with better activity and CSF penetration are now being investigated. ICIs (nivolumab and pembrolizumab) are investigated in patients without EGFR mutations or ALK rearrangements, and hopefully could in the future represent an option for patients with asymptomatic brain metastases.

Regarding breast cancer, chemotherapy regimens that combine cyclophosphamide, 5-fluorouracil, methotrexate, vincristine, cisplatin, and etoposide are active in patients with BM. In HER2-positive breast cancer targeted therapies are widely used (trastuzumab, trastuzumab emtansine, pertuzumab). The dual HER-2 and EGFR tyrosine kinase inhibitor lapatinib has shown activity in HER2-positive BM (CNS objective responses to lapatinib in 6% of patients). Finally, new more potent HER2+ inhibitors (neratinib) are being investigated in order to improve CNS concentration and local control rate.

Acknowledgments Founding: None.
Conflict of interest: None declared from the authors.

References

1. Louis DN, Perry A, Reifenberger G, et al. The 2016 World Health Organization classification of tumors of the central nervous system: a summary. Acta Neuropathol. 2016;131(6): 803–20.
2. van den Bent MJ, Weller M, Wen PY, et al. A clinical perspective on the 2016 WHO brain tumor classification and routine molecular diagnostics. Neuro-Oncology. 2017;19(5): 614–24.
3. Li J, Wang M, Won M, et al. Validation and simplification of the Radiation Therapy Oncology Group recursive partitioning analysis classification for glioblastoma. Int J Radiat Oncol Biol Phys. 2011;81(3):623–30.
4. Wee CW, Kim E, Kim N, et al. Novel recursive partitioning analysis classification for newly diagnosed glioblastoma: a multi-institutional study highlighting the MGMT promoter methylation and IDH1 gene mutation status. Radiother Oncol. 2017;123(1):106–11.
5. Sperduto PW, Chao ST, Sneed PK, et al. Diagnosis-specific prognostic factors, indexes, and treatment outcomes for patients with newly diagnosed brain metastases: a multi-institutional analysis of 4,259 patients. Int J Radiat Oncol Biol Phys. 2010;77(3):655–61.
6. Chang EF, Potts MB, Keles GE, et al. Seizure characteristics and control following resection in 332 patients with low-grade gliomas. J Neurosurg. 2008;108(2):227–35.
7. Avila EK, Chamberlain M, Schiff D, et al. Seizure control as a new metric in assessing efficacy of tumor treatment in low-grade glioma trials. Neuro-Oncology. 2017;19(1):12–21.
8. Brown PD, Maurer MJ, Rummans TA, et al. A prospective study of quality of life in adults with newly diagnosed high-grade gliomas: the impact of the extent of resection on quality of life and survival. Neurosurgery. 2005;57(3):495–504.
9. Lacroix M, Abi-Said D, Fourney DR, et al. A multivariate analysis of 416 patients with glioblastoma multiforme: prognosis, extent of resection, and survival. J Neurosurg. 2001;95(2): 190–8.
10. Laws ER, Parney IF, Huang W, et al. Survival following surgery and prognostic factors for recently diagnosed malignant glioma: data from the Glioma Outcomes Project. J Neurosurg. 2003;99(3):467–73.
11. Duffau H. Long-term outcomes after supratotal resection of diffuse low-grade gliomas: a consecutive series with 11-year follow-up. Acta Neurochir. 2016;158(1):51–8.
12. Pessina F, Navarria P, Cozzi L, et al. Maximize surgical resection beyond contrast-enhancing boundaries in newly diagnosed glioblastoma multiforme: is it useful and safe? A single institution retrospective experience. J Neuro-Oncol. 2017;135(1):129–39.
13. Watts C, Sanai N. Surgical approaches for the gliomas. Handb Clin Neurol. 2016;134: 51–69.
14. Patel AJ, Suki D, Hatiboglu MA, et al. Impact of surgical methodology on the complication rate and functional outcome of patients with a single brain metastasis. J Neurosurg. 2015;122(5):1132–43.

15. Stupp R, Mason WP, Van Den Bent MJ, et al. Radiotherapy plus concomitant and adjuvant temozolomide for glioblastoma. N Engl J Med. 2005;352(10):987–96.
16. Stupp R, Hegi ME, Mason WP, et al. Effects of radiotherapy with concomitant and adjuvant temozolomide versus radiotherapy alone on survival in glioblastoma in a randomised phase III study: 5-year analysis of the EORTC-NCIC trial. Lancet Oncol. 2009;10(5):459–66.
17. Blumenthal DT, Gorlia T, Gilbert MR, et al. Is more better? The impact of extended adjuvant temozolomide in newly diagnosed glioblastoma: a secondary analysis of EORTC and NRG oncology/RTOG. Neuro-Oncology. 2017;19(8):1119–26.
18. Gilbert MR, Wang M, Aldape KD, et al. Dose-dense temozolomide for newly diagnosed glioblastoma: a randomized phase III clinical trial. J Clin Oncol. 2013;31(32):4085–91.
19. Perry JR, Bélanger K, Mason WP, et al. Phase II trial of continuous dose-intense temozolomide in recurrent malignant glioma: RESCUE study. J Clin Oncol. 2010;28(12):2051–7.
20. Perry JR, Laperriere N, O'Callaghan CJ, et al. Short-course radiation plus temozolomide in elderly patients with glioblastoma. N Engl J Med. 2017;376(11):1027–37.
21. Stupp R, Taillibert S, Kanner AA, et al. Maintenance therapy with tumor-treating fields plus temozolomide vs temozolomide alone for glioblastoma: a randomized clinical trial. JAMA. 2015;314(23):2535–43.
22. Weller M, van den Bent M, Hopkins K, et al. EANO guideline for the diagnosis and treatment of anaplastic gliomas and glioblastoma. Lancet Oncol. 2014;15(9):e395–403.
23. Wick W, Puduvalli VK, Chamberlain MC, et al. Phase III study of enzastaurin compared with lomustine in the treatment of recurrent intracranial glioblastoma. J Clin Oncol. 2010;28:1168–74.
24. Batchelor TT, Mulholland P, Neyns B, et al. Phase III randomized trial comparing the efficacy of cediranib as monotherapy, and in combination with lomustine, versus lomustine alone in patients with recurrent glioblastoma. J Clin Oncol. 2013;31:3212–8.
25. Brandes AA, Tosoni A, Franceschi E, et al. Fotemustine as second-line treatment for recurrent or progressive glioblastoma after concomitant and/or adjuvant temozolomide: a phase II trial of Gruppo Italiano Cooperativo di Neuro-Oncologia (GICNO). Cancer Chemother Pharmacol. 2009;64(4):769–75.
26. Addeo R, Caraglia M, de Santi MS, et al. A new schedule of fotemustine in temozolomide-pretreated patients with relapsing glioblastoma. J Neuro-Oncol. 2011;102(3):417–24.
27. Santoni M, Scoccianti S, Lolli I, et al. Efficacy and safety of second-line fotemustine in elderly patients with recurrent glioblastoma. J Neuro-Oncol. 2013;113(3):397–401.
28. Cohen MH, Shen YL, Keegan P, et al. FDA drug approval summary: bevacizumab (Avastin) as treatment of recurrent glioblastoma multiforme. Oncologist. 2009;14(11):1131–8.
29. Taal W, Oosterkamp HM, Walenkamp AM, et al. Single-agent bevacizumab or lomustine versus a combination of bevacizumab plus lomustine in patients with recurrent glioblastoma (BELOB trial): a randomised controlled phase 2 trial. Lancet Oncol. 2014;15(9):943–53.
30. Wick W, Brandes AA, Gorlia T, et al. EORTC 26101 phase III trial exploring the combination of bevacizumab and lomustine in patients with first progression of a glioblastoma. J Clin Oncol. 2016;34(15 Suppl):2001.
31. Chinot OL, Wick W, Mason W, et al. Bevacizumab plus radiotherapy-temozolomide for newly diagnosed glioblastoma. N Engl J Med. 2014;370(8):709–22.
32. Gilbert MR, Dignam JJ, Armstrong TS, et al. A randomized trial of bevacizumab for newly diagnosed glioblastoma. N Engl J Med. 2014;370(8):699–708.
33. Sandmann T, Bourgon R, Garcia J, et al. Patients with proneural glioblastoma may derive overall survival benefit from the addition of bevacizumab to first-line radiotherapy and temozolomide: retrospective analysis of the AVAglio trial. J Clin Oncol. 2015;33(25):2735–44.
34. Schuster J, Lai RK, Recht LD, et al. A phase II, multicenter trial of rindopepimut (CDX-110) in newly diagnosed glioblastoma: the ACT III study. Neuro-Oncology. 2015;17(6):854–61.

35. Weller M, Butowski N, Tran DD, et al. Rindopepimut with temozolomide for patients with newly diagnosed, EGFRvIII-expressing glioblastoma (ACT IV): a randomised, double-blind, international phase 3 trial. Lancet Oncol. 2017;18(10):1373–85.
36. Reardon DA, Schuster J, Tran DD, et al. ReACT: overall survival from a randomized phase II study of rindopepimut (CDX-110) plus bevacizumab in relapsed glioblastoma. J Clin Oncol. 2015;33(15 Suppl):2009.
37. Reardon DA, Omuro A, Brandes AA, et al. Randomized phase 3 study evaluating the efficacy and safety of nivolumab vs bevacizumab in patients with recurrent glioblastoma: CheckMate 143. Neuro Oncol. 2017;19(Suppl. 3):iii21.
38. van den Bent M, Gan HK, Lassman AB, et al. Efficacy of depatuxizumab mafodotin (ABT-414) monotherapy in patients with EGFR-amplified, recurrent glioblastoma: results from a multi-center, international study. Cancer Chemother Pharmacol. 2017;80(6):1209–17.
39. Stupp R, Hegi ME, Gorlia T, et al. Cilengitide combined with standard treatment for patients with newly diagnosed glioblastoma with methylated MGMT promoter (CENTRIC EORTC 26071–22072 study): a multicentre, randomised, open-label, phase 3 trial. Lancet Oncol. 2014;15(10):1100–8.
40. Shaw EG, Berkey B, Coons SW, et al. Recurrence following neurosurgeon-determined gross-total resection of adult supratentorial low-grade glioma: results of a prospective clinical trial. J Neurosurg. 2008;109(5):835–41.
41. Shaw EG, Wang M, Coons SW, et al. Randomized trial of radiation therapy plus procarbazine, lomustine, and vincristine chemotherapy for supratentorial adult low-grade glioma: initial results of RTOG 9802. J Clin Oncol. 2012;30(25):3065–70.
42. Buckner JC, Shaw EG, Pugh SL, et al. Radiation plus procarbazine, CCNU, and vincristine in low-grade glioma. N Engl J Med. 2016;374(14):1344–55.
43. Wijnenga MMJ, Dubbink HJ, French PJ, et al. Molecular and clinical heterogeneity of adult diffuse low-grade IDH wild-type gliomas: assessment of TERT promoter mutation and chromosome 7 and 10 copy number status allows superior prognostic stratification. Acta Neuropathol. 2017;134(6):957–9.
44. Goldbrunner R, Minniti G, Preusser M, et al. EANO guidelines for the diagnosis and treatment of meningiomas. Lancet Oncol. 2016;17(9):383–91.
45. Pajtler KW, Mack SC, Ramaswamy V, et al. The current consensus on the clinical management of intracranial ependymoma and its distinct molecular variants. Acta Neuropathol. 2017;133(1):5–12.
46. Rudà R, Reifenberger G, Frappaz D, et al. EANO guidelines for the diagnosis and treatment of ependymal tumors. Neuro Oncol. 2018;20(4):445–56.
47. Khatua S, Song A, Sridhar DC, et al. Childhood medulloblastoma: current therapies, emerging molecular landscape and newer therapeutic insights. Curr Neuropharmacol. 2018;16(7):1045–58.
48. Soffietti R, Abacioglu U, Baumert B, et al. Diagnosis and treatment of brain metastases from solid tumors: guidelines from the European Association of Neuro-Oncology (EANO). Neuro-Oncology. 2017;19(2):162–74.
49. Brown PD, Ballman KV, Cerhan JH, et al. Postoperative stereotactic radiosurgery compared with whole brain radiotherapy for resected metastatic brain disease (NCCTG N107C/CEC·3): a multicentre, randomised, controlled, phase 3 trial. Lancet Oncol. 2017;18(8):1049–60.
50. Yamamoto M, Serizawa T, Shuto T, et al. Stereotactic radiosurgery for patients with multiple brain metastases (JLGK0901): a multi-institutional prospective observational study. Lancet Oncol. 2014;15(4):387–95.
51. Brown PD, Jaeckle K, Ballman KV, et al. Effect of radiosurgery alone vs radiosurgery with whole brain radiation therapy on cognitive function in patients with 1 to 3 brain metastases: a randomized clinical trial. JAMA. 2016;316(4):401–9.
52. Chang EL, Wefel JS, Hess KR, Allen PK, Lang FF, Kornguth DG, et al. Neurocognition in patients with brain metastases treated with radiosurgery or radiosurgery plus whole-brain irradiation: a randomised controlled trial. Lancet Oncol. 2009;10(11):1037–44.

53. Soffietti R, Kocher M, Abacioglu UM, et al. A European Organisation for Research and Treatment of Cancer phase III trial of adjuvant whole-brain radiotherapy versus observation in patients with one to three brain metastases from solid tumors after surgical resection or radiosurgery: quality-of-life results. J Clin Oncol. 2013;31(1):65–72.
54. ASTRO releases second list of five radiation oncology treatments to question, as part of national Choosing Wisely® campaign. 2014. www.choosingwisely.org/astro-releases-second-list. Accessed 1 July 2016.

Side Effects of Therapies for Brain Tumours

7

Robin Grant

7.1 Introduction

The brain is the most complex organ in the body and although there are some areas of the brain that are more "eloquent" (e.g., the speech centre, motor and sensory strips, dominant temporal lobe and optic radiations) than others (frontal lobes, non-dominant temporal lobe), all are important. Where tests are not sophisticated enough to show a problem, this does not mean that the person will be free from problems affecting day-to-day abilities.

Focal therapies such as surgery, focal radiotherapy or intra-tumoural chemotherapy and local gene therapy may produce either immediate, sub-acute or late side effects in many patients, some of which will be evident and others which will go unnoticed, if not checked for systematically.

Systemic therapies aimed at symptomatic control of oedema (e.g., dexamethasone), the effect of the tumour on cortical neurones (anti-epileptic drugs [AEDs]) or the tumour (e.g., systemic chemotherapy; immunotherapy), will largely produce similar multi-system allergic or toxic side effects profiles. There may be some specific organs or structures that are more susceptible to toxicity. Largely, side effects will fall into the categories of early allergic or dose-dependent toxicity – which will be reversible by drug withdrawal or dose reduction – or late cumulative toxicity, which largely will be irreversible and may even progress despite drug withdrawal, e.g., nitrosourea-related pulmonary fibrosis and cisplatin-related neuropathy.

R. Grant (✉)
Edinburgh Centre for Neuro-Oncology, Western General Hospital, Edinburgh, UK
e-mail: robin.grant@nhslothian.scot.nhs.uk

© Springer Nature Switzerland AG 2019
M. Bartolo et al. (eds.), *Neurorehabilitation in Neuro-Oncology*,
https://doi.org/10.1007/978-3-319-95684-8_7

85

7.2   Symptomatic Medication Complications

Avoidance of side effects starts with consideration of whether a therapy is really required. Symptomatic management with dexamethasone in the perioperative period is only required where there is headache suggestive of raised intracranial pressure or where there is a focal neurological deficit that is causing distress. The dose of dexamethsone should be in line with the severity of the symptoms and requirement for a fast symptomatic response. Dexamethasone is not required for tumour-associated epilepsy. Similarly, the prescription of AEDs in patients who have never had a seizure is increasing and is now often included in perioperative protocols in some centres, without acknowledgement that there is inadequate evidence for the efficacy of prophylactic AEDs and in the certain knowledge that 10–15% of patients are likely to experience side effects. These may be difficult to distinguish from the effect of the tumour or surgery, e.g., fatigue and neurocognitive, personality and mood-related effects. Prophylactic proton pump inhibitors (PPIs) or H2 receptor antagonists are inadvertently continued in >6% of hospital discharges without any evidence of a requirement to be on these drugs, when dexamethasone is discontinued [1].

(a) *Dexamethasone*

Dexamethasone is the most common steroid used. The benefit of steroids, when used at the appropriate doses and timings, are obvious and almost always outweigh the risk of side effects. However, dexamethasone should be used cautiously in the elderly, especially if there is heart, liver or renal failure; diabetes; hypertension; glaucoma or a past history of severe psychosis. Early side effects include sleep disturbance, emotional lability and psychiatric, gastrointestinal and endocrine symptoms. Insomnia is very common, particularly if the drug is prescribed after 12 midday. Neuropsychiatric effects, such as euphoria, anxiety, acute confusion and psychosis, usually occur early and are dose related. Gastrointestinal symptoms include dyspepsia, abdominal distension and, rarely, gastrointestinal ulceration or acute pancreatitis. Gastrointestinal side effects can be minimised by keeping the steroid dose as low as possible and giving an H2 receptor antagonist or a PPI (e.g., omeprazole, lansoprazole). Endocrine effects of dexamethasone, such as increased appetite, unmasked diabetes, and increased susceptibility to infection, e.g., candida, occur early, within the first few weeks, while weight gain is a late effect as a result of the increased appetite, reduced mobility and the effect of dexamethasone on metabolism and body deposition of fat. Ankle oedema, skin atrophy, bruising, striae, and acne can occur after a few weeks at high dosage (e.g., 4 mg twice daily). Rarely, an acute myopathy can come on within a week of a patient starting high-dose corticosteroids, but more commonly, a proximal myopathy starts after a few weeks; this is painless and mainly affects the proximal lower limb muscles and proximal upper limbs to a lesser extent. It is twice as common in women than in men. Recovery after withdrawal can take weeks or months. With long-term usage, elevation in blood sugar occurs in 47–72% of patients, peripheral oedema in 11%, anxiety or psychiatric disorders in 10%, oro-pharyngeal candidiasis in 6–8%, Cushing's syndrome in 15% and muscular weakness in 60%. Osteoporosis with vertebral fractures, avascular necrosis of the hip and tendon rupture are the result of long-term high-dose usage, as is psychological dependence and fatigue associated with adrenal suppression. Ophthalmological complications such as worsening of glaucoma are a rare, but serious, early complication, while cataract and scleral thinning occur commonly with prolonged use.

Withdrawal of dexamethasone after usage for some months should be done slowly. It may be associated with changes in mood, the development of myalgia/muscle cramps, arthropathy, or headaches. Dexamethasone withdrawal headache is non-specific and may lead to the reinstatement of higher doses due to concerns of raised intracranial pressure. Imaging evidence of reduced tumour mass effect and patient re-assurance and education that dexamethasone withdrawal can cause headache, may aid eventual withdrawal and limit psychological dependence. Dexamethasone-induced adrenal insufficiency from long-term dexamethasone may persist for 6–12 months after the withdrawal of dexamethasone.

(b) *Anti-epileptic drugs (AEDs)*

Early allergic responses that necessitate the withdrawal of AEDs include hypersensitivity syndrome, which is characterized by multi-system involvement, fever, lymphadenopathy, rash, abnormal liver function and eosinophilia. More commonly, a less severe rash occurs in 5–10% of patients within the first 2 months of taking enzyme-inducing AEDs (phenytoin, phenobarbital, carbamazepine) or lamotrigine. There is cross-reactivity between these AEDs. Accompanying steroids may lessen or delay the appearance of allergic rash, which might only subsequently appear on steroid withdrawal. Levetiracetam, valproate, topiramate, or tiagabine are moderately safe alternative choices of AEDs with a lower risk of rash. All AEDs (especially valproate) can cause serious hepatic toxicity and liver failure. Although this is rare, it is advisable to monitor liver function during the introduction of AEDs and for the following 6 months. The incidence of haematological toxicity is low, but valproate may cause dose-dependent thrombocytopenia (Table 7.1). Carbamazepine can cause a mild neutropenia and hyponatraemia that may influence the later use of chemotherapy. Valproate is often associated with weight gain, especially if the patient is also taking dexamethasone. Valproate can also inhibit platelet aggregation and the coagulation cascade, which may lead to a higher tendency to haemorrhage when used with heparins, warfarin or non-steroidal anti-inflammatory drugs. Valproate can also cause fine tremor, which is often more noticeable in the hemiparetic limb. Toxicity from any of the AEDs may lead to dysarthria, diplopia, ataxia with nystagmus, lethargy and weakness, and can be easily mistaken for tumour progression, although the presence of nystagmus and intermittent diplopia and the absence of papilloedema or focal neurological deficits are helpful pointers to the likely diagnosis of AED toxicity. Idiosyncratic side effects of AEDs include headache; cognitive, speech or

Table 7.1 Cautions, toxicity and side effects of anti-epileptic drugs commonly used in tumour-associated epilepsy

Carbamazepine	Cautions	Hepatic, renal, cardiac disease. Glaucoma
	Toxicity	Diplopia, dizziness; confusion, ataxia, tremor
	Side effects	Early severe blood disorders and leucopenia. Rash, hypersensitivity reaction, agitation; jaundice, renal failure, depression, psychosis, alopecia, hyponatraemia, oedema, osteomalacia
Lamotrigine	Cautions	Hepatic, renal disease
	Toxicity	Diplopia, dizziness; confusion and ataxia
	Side effects	Early severe blood disorders and aplastic anaemia and leucopenia. Rash, hypersensitivity reaction, flu-like illness, worsening seizures; dizziness, drowsiness, insomnia, headache, agitation
Levetiracetam	Cautions	Hepatic, renal disease
	Toxicity	Drowsiness, tiredness and dizziness
	Side effects	Drowsiness, tiredness and dizziness. Rarely, amnesia, psychiatric symptoms (e.g., aggression), insomnia, headache, rash, anaemia (folate deficiency)
Phenytoin	Cautions	Hepatic disease
	Toxicity	Diplopia, dizziness; confusion, ataxia, tremor
	Side effects	Early severe blood disorders and leucopenia. Rash, agitation, jaundice, systemic lupus erythematosus, hypersensitivity reaction, depression, psychosis, gum hypertrophy, peripheral neuropathy, megaloblastic anaemia, osteomalacia
Topiramate	Cautions	Hepatic and renal disease. May cause secondary acute angle closure glaucoma in myopes in first month
	Toxicity	Diplopia, dizziness; confusion, ataxia, tremor
	Side effects	Rash, agitation; leucopenia, jaundice, weight loss, paraesthesia, memory problems, fatigue, speech problems, depression, psychosis
Valproate	Cautions	Hepatic disease, clotting disorders. Pancreatitis
	Toxicity	Tremor. Diplopia, dizziness; confusion, ataxia
	Side effects	Leucopenia, alopecia, weight gain, gastrointestinal side effects, memory problems, dementia, gynaecomastia

memory problems; or psychiatric symptoms. Patients with cognitive problems may be best suited to using agents, e.g., levetiracetam, lamotrigine, tiagabine or oxcarbazepine by extrapolation from studies in people with non-tumour-associated epilepsy. Obese patients may benefit from topiramate or zonisamide, as these have a tendency to produce weight loss, but topiramate may cause memory, concentration and speech problems and acute angle closure glaucoma. These phenomena reverse when the drug is withdrawn. Levetiracetam, commonly used as a first-line AED in brain tumour patients, can cause fatigue, or personality change with anger and irritability or low mood in 10–15% of cases and causation may be difficult to separate from the effect of radiotherapy or tumour or psychiatric issues related to the diagnosis.

(c) *Gastric acid suppressants* (H2 receptor antagonists and proton pump inhibitors)

These agents should only be prescribed if patients are symptomatic or at risk (e.g., on anti-inflammatory drugs or dexamethasone). They can cause headache, dizziness, rash and tiredness and, rarely, confusion, depression and hallucinations. Leucopenia, thrombocytopenia, rash and disturbance of hepatic enzymes are possible. It may be difficult to distinguish the side effects of these agents from those related to AEDs or chemotherapy. Omeprazole and lansoprazole can, rarely, be associated with hyponatraemia, confusion and agitation.

7.3   Surgical Complications

Patients with tumours present with: *progressive focal neurological deficits,* e.g., unilateral motor or sensory symptoms, dysphasia, and visual field defect; *progressive cognitive changes*, e.g., subacute confusion or memory loss; *headache alone or associated with change in personality, mood and memory or associated with papilloedema* and lastly with *late-onset seizures.* Twenty-five percent of an unselected series of people with a brain tumour lacked capacity to give informed consent for surgery when more formally assessed [2]. This is the background from which to determine the side effects profile of surgical procedures.

Specific risks of brain tumour surgery include: seizures, weakness, balance and coordination difficulties, memory and cognitive problems, spinal fluid leakage, meningitis, brain swelling and stroke. General risks include infection, bleeding, blood clots, pneumonia and blood pressure instability. The overall major complication rate is between 27 and 36%, with neurological complications being the most frequently encountered. Infra-tentorial tumour location, age over 60 years, eloquent area, severe pre-operative deficit and severe concomitant disease were risk factors for systemic complications [3]. Previous radiotherapy and re-operations are factors strongly related to the incidence of complications. While most surgical complications are obvious immediately after surgery, some – such as posterior fossa syndrome/cerebellar mutism and supplementary motor area syndrome – may only appear hours or days after surgery and can appear devastating, although both improve significantly in 4–6 weeks [4, 5].

7.4   Radiotherapy Complications

The side effects of radiotherapy are related to demographic, radiation and tumour factors. Age; past medical history (e.g., vascular disease/hypertension); pre-existing brain heath (e.g., stroke, dementia); tumour size and grade; and radiation volume, total dose and fraction size should all be taken into account when considering the likelihood of developing complications from radiotherapy.

1. *Acute reaction*

   If the tumour has not been adequately resected, or steroids are not continued in an appropriately high dose, there is a risk of developing an acute radiation reaction during radiotherapy, with worsening of focal signs or headache and somnolence. This may require an increase in dexamethasone dosage or even consideration of a further debulking. Somnolence usually improves by 6–8 weeks. Hair loss, nausea, anorexia and fatigue can occur within the first 4–6 weeks of treatment.

2. *Early delayed reaction*

   In about one-third of patients, "early delayed" radiation reaction/"pseudo-progression" will occur in the first 3 months after completion of radiation. This presents as tiredness, subtle difficulty in thinking clearly and with memory loss and sometimes confusion or worsening of focal symptoms, possibly with headaches. There may be a need to restart or increase steroids for a few weeks to manage symptoms. Magnetic resonance imaging (MRI) might suggest tumour progression. "Pseudo-progression" is related to demyelination/inflammation and will settle down. Pseudoprogression is more common in glioblastoma with high levels of methylguanine methyl transferase (MGMT) promotor methylation.

   Fatigue is the most common symptom post-treatment. The prevalence of fatigue ranges between 25% and 90% and occurs at all stages of care. The fatigue may be related to primary causes affecting the brain (tumour, irradiation, injury), secondary causes (psychological; sleep disturbance; pain; comorbid conditions [underactive pituitary, infection, malnutrition]), or medication [6]. Medications to treat epilepsy, pain, nausea may contribute to fatigue. Endocrine dysfunction may also contribute to fatigue. Management of fatigue should include the removal of drugs that may be associated with fatigue; advice about sleep and healthy living, diet, and physical exercise; and, if anxiety or depression is present, the management of these through talking therapies, cognitive behavioural therapy, mindfulness, or antidepressants. A Cochrane review of studies on the management of fatigue in adult brain tumour patients [7] found only one randomised controlled trial [8] that included solely patients with high levels of fatigue. The other studies were looking at prevention of fatigue and recruited patients who may or may not have had fatigue at entry. Fatigue is complex and the evidence that a specific drug will significantly help fatigue in everyone is lacking.

3. *Late effects*

   Late effects of radiotherapy are usually degenerative or vascular in nature [9]. The target tissue may be brain, pituitary gland, cranial nerve/end organ and second tumours.

   In the brain, white matter damage, leuco-encephalopathy with ex-vacuo hydrocephalus (Fig. 7.1), is associated with a slow continuous subtle drop-off in memory, attention and executive function. This is particularly the case when the radiotherapy includes the hippocampus. The effect on the developing brain is more pronounced than the effect in adults. Damage to oligodendrocyte 0-2A progenitor cells may result in failure to replace myelin, and damage to astrocytes

Fig. 7.1 T2-weighted image showing brain atrophy and radiation-related leucoencephalopathic changes

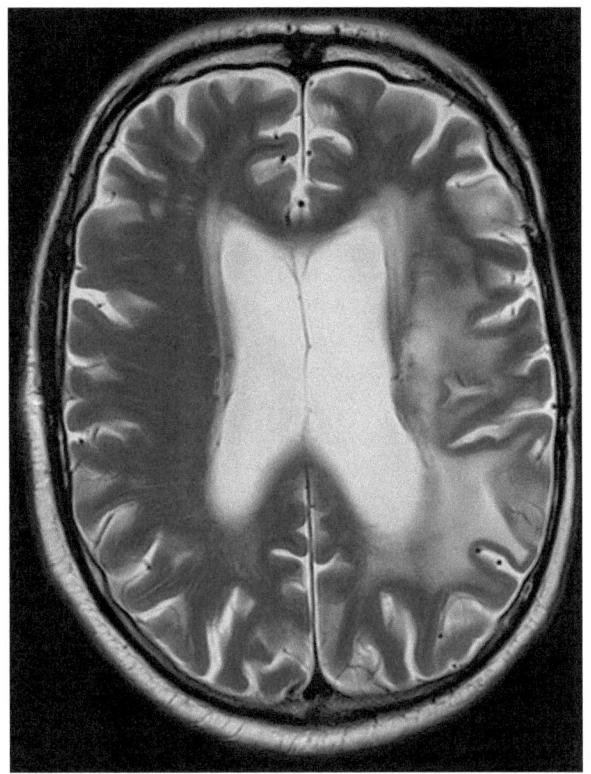

may influence growth factors, with the development of "reactive" astrocytes that express glial fibrillary acidic protein, which releases pro-inflammatory cytokines [10]. Activated microglia may also produce cytokines that mediate a chronic inflammation within the brain [11]. The neuro-pathological correlates show vascular abnormalities, e.g., endothelial cell nuclei damage, capillary loss, and vascular thickening and dilatation [12], breakdown of the blood brain barrier and radiation necrosis with blockage of small blood vessels. These changes are dose and volume related.

(a) *Radiation-induced dementia*

Some identifiable radiation-induced cognitive impairment can be found on neurocognitive testing in up to 90% of adult brain tumour patients who survive for >6 months post-irradiation [13]. Cognitive areas affected early are verbal memory, spatial memory, attention, and problem-solving ability. This is often associated with fatigue and changes in mood. By 2 years about 50% of patients will be aware of cognitive decline and by 5 years after radiotherapy this has increased to between 70–80% [14]. With time either a solely profound memory and cognitive disturbance is found or sometimes a "normal pressure hydrocephalus" like clinical picture will develop with progressive gait apraxia, subcortical dementia and urinary incontinence.

(b) *Radionecrosis*

Radionecrosis is a delayed effect of the radiotherapy that occurs in patients who have survived radiotherapy or radiosurgery. It can occur from 6 months to several years after the radiation treatment, but it usually occurs within the first 1 to 2 years [15]. Clinically it produces subacute progressive focal neurological problems that are difficult to distinguish from tumour recurrence in the irradiated brain. MRI perfusion studies can sometimes be helpful, or MR spectroscopy, which typically shows low choline and creatine and N-acetylaspartate (NAA) in radiation necrosis, whereas with tumour recurrence choline, lipids and lactates are increased. Pathologically, radiation necrosis primarily affects the smaller arterioles and arteries, causing coagulative, fibrinoid necrosis of the vascular walls with endothelial thickening and infiltration of lymphocytes and macrophages, resulting in occlusion and infarction. A randomised trial in 200 adult patients with low-grade glioma who received either 50.4 Gy or 64.8 Gy at 1.8 Gy per fraction demonstrated that the 5-year incidence of radiation necrosis was 10% in patients receiving 64.8 Gy versus 5% for those given 50.4 Gy [16].

(c) *Vascular disorders.*

Stroke-like migraine after radiotherapy (SMART)

Stroke-like migraine after radiotherapy (SMART) is a late complication [17]. SMART attacks are more common in patients treated for brain tumours in childhood or in patients living with low-grade glioma. The symptoms come on over minutes or hours with a spread of "negative" phenomena (e.g., numbness, weakness, dysphasia or visual aura) which may help distinguish from stroke which presents with sudden onset, or seizures which produce "positive" phenomena (jerking, tingling) that spreads over seconds. Cases generally also have headache with migrainous features. Occasionally, seizures do occur during an attack and then the differential diagnosis of SMART attack will have to include seizures with prolonged Todd's paresis. Symptoms may take several days or weeks to recover. Diagnosis is based on medical history, clinical characteristics, and radiological investigations. Attacks can start as early as 1 year after treatment or as late as 35 years, but most frequently occur between 1 and 5 years after treatment. Attacks are more frequent in males. Diagnosis requires: (a) a history of cranial irradiation without evidence of recurrent neoplasm and (b) prolonged, reversible signs and symptoms referable to a unilateral cortical region. These may include: "negative" phenomena, such as visuo-spatial deficits, confusion, hemisensory deficits, hemiparesis, and aphasia, or "positive" phenomena, such as seizures. There is often an antecedent migraine headache, with or without aura. Imaging shows transient, diffuse, unilateral cortical gadolinium enhancement of the cerebral gyri, sparing the white matter, within the previous radiation field. Lastly, the condition must not be attributed to tumour recurrence or another identifiable disorder, e.g. posterior reversible encephalopathy syndrome (PRES) related to immunosuppressant drugs or hypertension, where neuroradiological changes involve both hemispheres, usually in the occipital lobes and the MR changes involve the white matter. The MRI abnormalities in SMART demonstrate cortical enhancement on T1-weighted images and T2-weighted images are suggestive of parenchymal hyperperfusion in the underlying brain. These changes settle. Fluorodeoxyglucose positron emission tomography (FDG PET) has demonstrated hypermetabolism in the involved areas. Electroencephalograms (EEGs) may show slowing over the affected area and a few may demonstrate seizures [18], but epileptiform activity should not put one off the clinical diagnosis of SMART where seizures do not explain the clinical and radiological features.

Stroke

Late ischaemic complications, including transient ischaemic attacks (TIAs) or established ischaemic stroke, can occur as a late effect of cranial radiation on cerebral vessels many years after radiotherapy. TIAs are focal, sudden-onset phenomena with unilateral weakness, numbness, dysphasia, homonymous visual field loss or visual loss in one eye, lasting less than 24 h, whereas stroke will persist and be accompanied by MRI changes to support infarction. Management is as with any new stroke—correction of any risk factors, e.g., smoking, hypercholesterolaemia and hypertension and secondary prevention with anti-platelets, a statin and anti-hypertensives.

Cavernomas and microhaemorrhages

Cavernomas are thin-walled dilated capillary spaces within the brain, found in up to one in 200 people. Cavernomas are thought to be congenital but can be acquired after radiotherapy (Fig. 7.2a, b). Cavernomas have been hypothesized to result from a proliferative vasculopathy that begins with the development of capillary telangiectasias triggered by radiation injury to the cerebral microcirculation [19]. An alternative explanation is that radiation may cause direct DNA damage, which leads to the formation of cavernomas. Cavernomas have been correlated with radiation dose. At doses >30 Gy, there is a shorter latency to the development of cavernomas [20]. Cavernomas can sometimes be misdiagnosed as tumour progression, especially if they are associated with symptomatic haemorrhage or seizures. Intervention is not usually required, as these are low-pressure bleeds from the capillary structures. Multiple micro-haemorrhages may also be found on scans and are often asymptomatic (Fig. 7.2c, d).

(d) *Hypopituitarism*

Disturbances in pituitary hormone secretion are common following radiotherapy to the hypothalamicpituitary axis. Hormonal deficiencies may affect body image, growth, sexual function, skeletal health and quality of life. It is important that cancer survivors are tested regularly, e.g., annually, to screen for pituitary insufficiency and timely treatment with hormone replacement is offered. The severity and frequency of pituitary disturbance correlates with the total radiation dose and length of follow-up. It is possible that concomitant chemotherapy may potentiate the action of radiotherapy. Children are most seriously at risk, as the first hormone to be affected is growth hormone (GH) resulting in slow growth, poor bone development, increased subcutaneous fat and fatigue. Loss of GH in adults is not such a serious matter although has been associated with fatigue. Isolated GH deficiency can occur after doses as low as 18 Gy. GH deficiency occurs within 5 years in 30% of patients given <30 Gy and within 3–5 years in 50–100% of patients treated with 30–50 Gy. Multiple hormonal deficiencies occur by 10 years of follow-up in patients given doses >30 Gy of

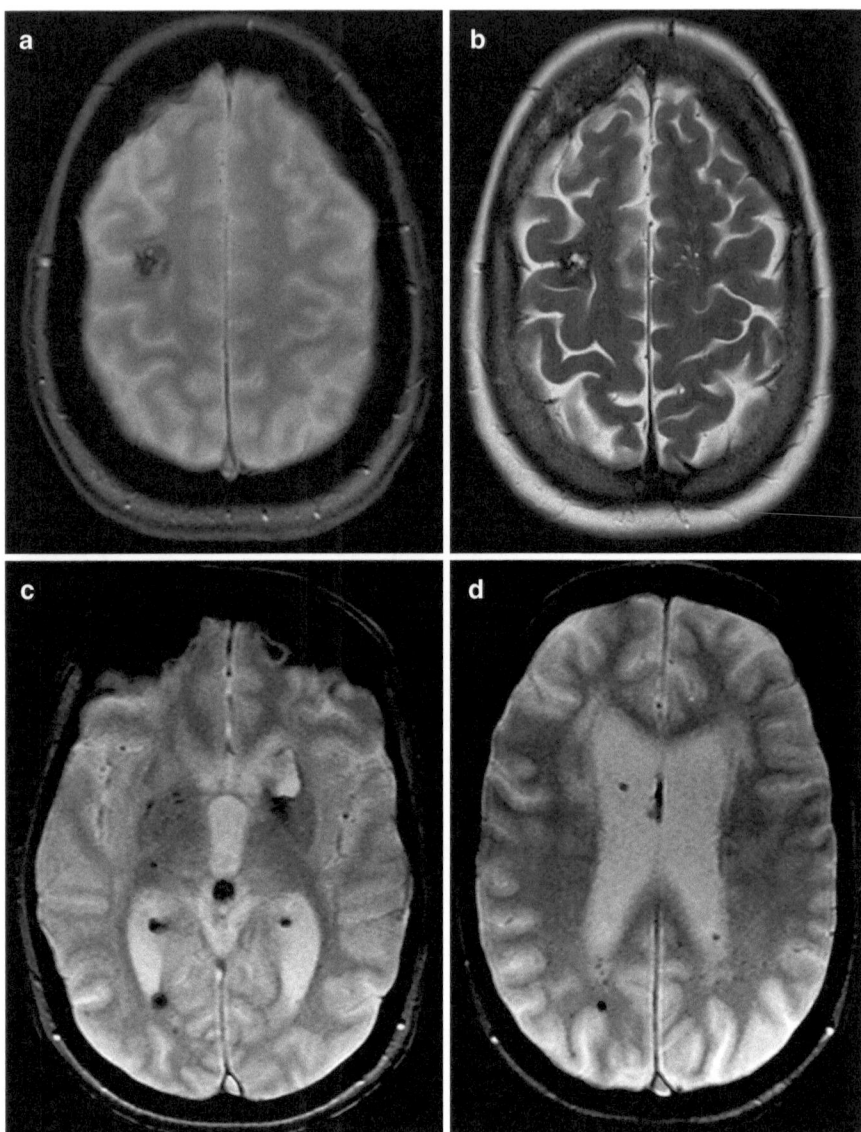

Fig. 7.2 (**a**, **b**) Radiation-induced right frontal cavernoma. (**c**, **d**) Radiation-induced multiple microhaemorrhages

radiation include deficiencies in GH (30–60%), sex hormone (20–30%), thyroid-stimulating hormone (TSH; 3–9%) and adrenocorticotropic hormone (ACTH; 3–6%) [21].

In children, injection of GH-releasing hormone (GHRH) analog therapy (e.g., Genotropin [somatotropin, Pfizer Inc. New York, New York) helps. Replacement can be associated with injection-site reactions, such as pain, redness/swelling, inflammation, bleeding, scarring, lumps, or rash.

Gonadotropin deficiency will affect secondary sex characteristics, fertility and bone and muscle mass. Diagnosis is confirmed by normal or low normal basal luteinizing hormone (LH)/follicle-stimulating hormone (FSH) with low circulating sex hormone concentrations in the blood. In children, because of the influence on bone age, treatment with sex steroids is required to aid the development of secondary sex characteristics. In adults, amenorrhoea, sweating and flushes may occur in women and in men there may be reduced libido, erectile dysfunction, reduced shaving frequency, fatigue and mood changes. Sex steroid replacement improves quality of life generally.

Hyperprolactinaemia predominantly occurs in young women; it is usually subclinical, but can affect 20–50% of women who have had cranial irradiation. Prolactin levels can be assessed using blood tests. If hyperprolactinaemia is high enough to impair gonadotropin release it can cause galactorrhoea and ovarian dysfunction in females or affect libido and cause impotence in males. If symptomatic, hyperprolactinaemia can be treated with dopamine agonists such as cabergoline. Low serum testosterone can be replaced.

TSH deficiency usually requires radiation doses of >40 Gy to be associated with a high risk of involvement. Hypothyroidism will cause hair loss, dry skin, weight gain, cold intolerance, bowel change, fatigue and memory problems, and muscle weakness and is easily treated with thyroxine replacement.

Cortisol deficiency secondary to ACTH deficiency, similarly, is seen at higher treatment doses. IIt causes fatigue and memory problems, muscle weakness, nausea, and dizziness, but with weight loss and hypoglycemia. Both cortisol defiiency and thyroid hormone deficiencies are more commonly seen in children treated for central nervous system (CNS) malignancies, where the pituitary is within the radiation field, but these features can occur years after the treatment of brain tumours adjacent to the pituitary gland where the pituitary is within the treatment field. Cortisol deficiency is treated with oral hydrocortisone twice daily.

(e) *Cranial nerve/end organ radiation damage*
    Cranial and peripheral nerves are generally considered to be radio-resistant; however, radiation also commonly damages end organs, e.g., the cochlea – leading to sensorineural hearing loss – or it damages the lens, retina and optic nerve – leading to multifactorial visual loss.

    Deafness is very common in survivors of medulloblastoma, ependymoma or astrocytoma within the posterior fossa. The rate of deafness appears to increase with age >50 years. The mean total dose to the cochlea during fractionated radiotherapy appears to be an important factor in predicting deafness in those treated in childhood. The effect of dose per fraction ($\leq$ or > 2.0 Gy) is probably also relevant. Chemotherapy combined with radiotherapy may have a synergistic effect, especially if the chemotherapy is ototoxic in its own right.

    The optic nerve and eye are generally shielded where possible when treating intracranial tumours. However, where it is not possible to shield the eye, a variety of complications are possible, from an early increase in intraocular pressure during treatment, to the development of late complications of cataract, dry eye from lacrimal gland damage, and retinopathy or optic neuropathy.

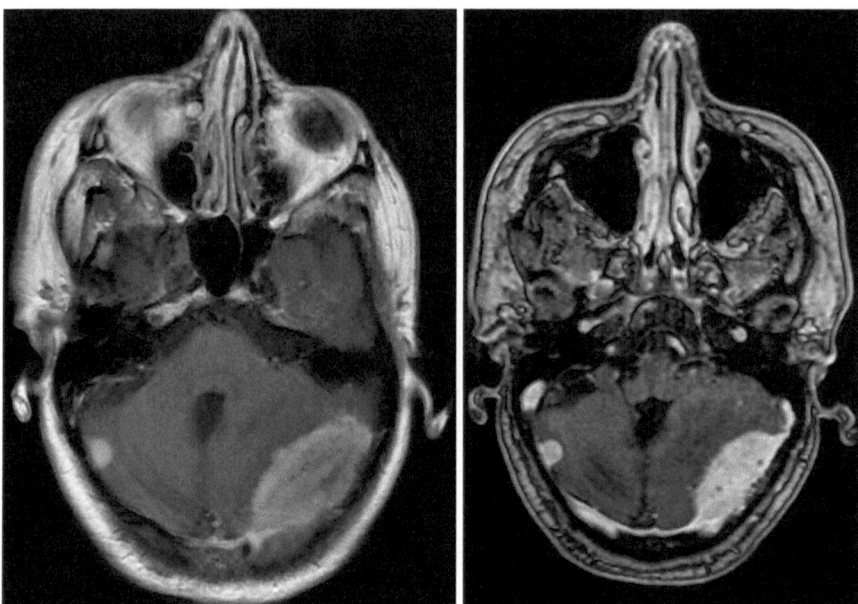

Fig. 7.3 T1-weighted gadolinium enhanced magnetic resonance image showing radiation-induced meningiomas 15 years after treatment of medulloblastoma

(f) *Second tumours*

Radiation to the central nervous system may be required for different tumour types e.g. acute lymphoblastic leukaemia (ALL), childhood medulloblastoma, ependymoma or astrocytoma, head and neck soft tissue sarcoma, and retinoblastoma. A late complication is development of a different tumour type within the radiation field. Second neoplasms are infrequent but with higher doses of radiation used for brain tumours, and where survival from the primary tumour is excellent, there is an increased risk for meningiomas (Fig. 7.3) and glial tumours [22].

7.5   Chemotherapy Complications

Chemotherapy that crosses the blood brain barrier is most likely to be effective. Drugs such as alkylating agents (temozolomide, procarbazine,) and nitrosoureas (e.g., 1-(2-chloroethyl)-cyclo-hexyl-1-nitrosourea—CCNU [lomustine]) are most commonly used, alone or in combination (e.g., procarbazine, CCNU, vincristine [PCV]).

Patients being prescribed chemotherapy should avoid aspirin and not receive immunisation or vaccination, nor should they become pregnant and they should therefore use barrier contraception. Nursing mothers should not breastfeed. Patients should avoid sun exposure and keep well hydrated, eat in small amounts and frequently and get plenty of rest. Avoid things that may worsen the symptoms of nausea, such as heavy or greasy/fatty, spicy or acidic foods (lemons, tomatoes, oranges). Brush teeth with a soft bristle toothbrush.

Patients should report signs of infection, e.g., fever, to their GP early and will get regular blood tests between treatments. Hair may appear thin and brittle and fall out 2–3 weeks after the starting of many chemotherapy drugs.

7.5.1   Temozolomide

Temozolomide is an alkylating agent and the first-line chemotherapy for patients with glioblastoma. It is most commonly given along with radiotherapy (concomitantly) and after completion of radiotherapy for 5 days every 4 weeks, for six courses. Temozolomide causes haematological toxicity (lymphopenia, neutropenia, thrombocytopenia) in >10% of patients. Elderly patients and women have a higher risk of developing haematological toxicities or myelodysplastic syndrome. Pneumocystis pneumonia (PCP) is a risk, especially in patients requiring high-dose steroids or those who have lymphocyte counts <500 cells/μm. PCP prophylaxis is required for "high-risk" patients who are receiving concomitant temozolomide and radiotherapy. All patients, particularly those receiving steroids, should be observed closely for the development of lymphopenia and PCP. Care should be given when treating patients with severe renal or hepatic impairment. Severe hepatotoxicity can be fatal. Temozolomide may interact with valproate, an anti-epileptic drug (AED), to reduce the excretion of temozolomide, other AEDs, steroids and sulpha drugs. Forty-nine percent of patients treated with temozolomide report one or more severe reactions, most commonly fatigue (13%), convulsions (6%), headache (5%) or thrombocytopenia (5%). The common side effects (>10%) are: gastrointestinal (e.g., nausea and vomiting – clinical toxicity criteria (CTC) grade 3/4 in 6–10%), anorexia, constipation or diarrhoea; muco-cutaneous (rash, mouth ulcers); neurological (headache, dizziness, abnormal taste); or generalized, e.g., sleep disturbance, fatigue (16%). To reduce nausea and vomiting, temozolomide should be given on an empty stomach and an anti-emetic may be advised before treatment. Immunosuppression can be associated with new infections or the reactivation of infections e.g. cytomegalovirus (CMV); hepatitis B infections and herpes simplex encephalitis, including cases with fatal outcomes. Sixty to seventy percent of patients with glioblastoma (grade 4) derive no survival benefit and for the recurrent anaplastic gliomas (grade 3), more than 50% of patients have tumour progression at 6 months [23]. Selection of patients for treatment is important with those who have highly methylated MGMT obtaining more benefit from chemotherapy.

7.5.2   Procarbazine

Procarbazine is usually given in conjunction with CCNU and vincristine as PCV. It is the first-line combination for patients with oligodendroglioma and is also commonly given after the failure of temozolomide. Procarbazine is an alkylating agent.

Patients taking procarbazine should avoid several food types that are high in tyramine, including: avocados, bananas, figs, papaya, raisins, and sauerkraut; beef or chicken liver; meats prepared with tenderizer; bologna, pepperoni, summer sausage, game meat, and meat extracts; pickled or smoked fish, anchovies, dried fish, herring, caviar, and shrimp paste; beer (alcoholic and nonalcoholic); wine (especially red wine), champagne, sherry, vermouth, and other distilled spirits; caffeine (including coffee, tea, cola), ginseng; cheese; chocolate; yogurt; soy sauce, miso soup, and bean curd; and fava beans.

As with all chemotherapy, haematological side effects are dose-limiting and recovery may be delayed. Leukopenia, anaemia, and thrombocytopenia have been reported frequently. Pancytopenia, eosinophilia, hemolytic anaemia, and bleeding tendencies, including petechiae, purpura, epistaxis, hematuria and hemoptysis, have also been reported. Gastrointestinal side effects, including nausea and vomiting, are the most commonly reported. Hepatic dysfunction, jaundice, stomatitis, hematemesis, melena, diarrhoea, dysphagia, anorexia, abdominal pain, constipation, and dry mouth are also reported. Peripheral neuropathy with paraesthesia of the extremities and depressed deep tendon reflexes have been reported to occur in 17% of patients, but usually when procarbazine is given in combination with vincristine. Nervous system side effects, including leucoencephalopathy, coma, convulsions, neuropathy, ataxia, paraesthesia, nystagmus, diminished reflexes, falling, foot drop, headache, dizziness, chills, weakness, fatigue, hallucinations and unsteadiness have also been reported. Psychiatric side effects, including hallucinations, depression, apprehension, agitation, psychosis, nervousness, confusion, mania and nightmares can occur. Hypotension, tachycardia, and syncope also occur, as can pneumonitis, pleural effusion, retinal haemorrhage, papilloedema, photophobia and diplopia.

7.5.3 CCNU

1-(2-Chloroethyl)-cyclo-hexyl-1-nitrosourea (CCNU, lomustine) is an alkylating agent given by mouth in capsule form. It is often given in combination with procarbazine and vincristine. Other alkylating agents such as 1,3-bis-(2-chloroethyl)-1-nitrosourea (BCNU, carmustine) are frequently given intravenously. As with all chemotherapy there is a range of side effects that can affect all systems. Haematological toxicity increases with the number of courses, with a nadir in platelet count at 4–5 weeks with recovery at 5–6 weeks and white cell count nadir at 5–6 weeks and recovery by 6–8 weeks.

Poor appetite and nausea occur within 5–6 h after taking the medication and can be helped by taking prophylactic anti-nauseant agents, while neurocutaneous symptoms such as hair loss and mouth ulcers occur in >10% of patients. Pulmonary and renal toxicity is cumulative with dosage and may be delayed for years after diagnosis. Pulmonary infiltrates and fibrosis can occur.

7.5.4 Vincristine

Vincristine is a plant vinca alkaloid that is given intravenously. It is a vesicant and care must be given when it is given intravenously. Partial or complete hair loss is common and the nadir in blood count occurs at 7–10 days, with recovery by 21 days.

Side effects include gastrointestinal symptoms and peripheral neuropathy, generally with paraesthesia and numbness in the feet and, less commonly, the hands.

7.6 Targeted and Immunotherapy Agent Complications

Targeted and immunotherapy agents have been used alone, in combination, or along with other types of therapy. Targeted therapies aimed at growth factor receptors, e.g., *epidermal growth factor receptor* (EGFR), e.g., cetuximab, gefitinib; *vascular endothelial growth factor receptor* (VEGFR), e.g., bevacizumab, cediranib; *platelet-derived growth factor receptor* (PDGFR), e.g., temsirolimus, have all been tried in brain tumours with very limited success. Complications are similar between agents and bevacuzimab and ipilimumab will be used as examples.

Immunotherapy has a different mechanistic approach compared with that of chemotherapy, radiation and surgery. Most of the current immunologic treatments are antibody-based therapies, but some, more recently, have been cell-based therapies and there are several tumour vaccine strategies. Immunotherapy can be passive or active. In passive immunotherapy, a patient is given immune cells or antibodies that target the tumour cell and this does not require activation of the patient's own immune system. Active immunotherapy boosts the patient's own immune system. Passive immunotherapy can be divided into three types: therapies in which there is direct injection of monoclonal antibodies, e.g., bevacizumab, a humanized IgG1 monoclonal antibody that binds to and neutralizes VEGF; therapies in which there is cytokine stimulation, e.g., interleukin 2 (IL2); and therapies in which there are stimulated immune effector cells (adoptive or cell-based immunotherapy), e.g., lymphocyte-activated killer cells (LAKs) and cytotoxic T-lymphocytes (CTLs). Active immunotherapy boosts the patient's immune system by priming it with antigen exposure. There is a relatively high frequency of immune-related adverse effects from immunotherapies, ranging from endocrine, hepatic, gastrointestinal, and dermatological toxicities. The side effects are due to the aberrant infiltration of stimulated $CD4^+$ and $CD8^+$ T-cells into normal tissues, along with elevated levels of pro-inflammatory cytokines [24]. The stimulated immune response can overshoot its target and attack healthy tissues and organs, similarly to an autoimmune disorder.

7.6.1 Bevacizumab

Bevacizumab is the most commonly used targeted agent. It is given by infusion once every 2 weeks. It can lead to improvements on scanning by its influence on the blood brain barrier and can reduce the need for dexamethasone. The most common side effects are high blood pressure (18%), proteinuria (7%), infusion reactions (3%), bleeding (nose/rectum), back pain, headache, taste disturbance, diarrhoea and loss of appetite or skin problems (dryness or inflammation), watery eyes or jaw pain, and swelling or numbness. The most serious side effects may be gastrointestinal perforation, poor wound healing and serious bleeding. Bevacizumab should not be used for 28 days before or after surgery and until surgical wounds are fully healed; it should not be used before or during pregnancy or breastfeeding. It is often given with chemotherapy, where it amplifies the risk of toxicities.

7.6.2 Ipilimumab

Ipilimumab (CTLA-4 checkpoint inhibitor) may be associated with pneumonitis, colitis, bowel perforation, hepatitis, pancreatitis, skin rash and mouth ulcers. It may also cause neurological complications including paralysis (acute inflammatory demyelinating neuropathy; Guillain-Barre); chronic inflammatory demyelinating polyneuropathy (CIDP); transverse myelitis; myositis; myasthenia gravis. Hormonal upset of thyroid, pituitary and adrenal glands and eye problems with blurred vision and eye pain and redness may occur. Side effects are best managed by steroids and antihistamines.

7.7 Conclusion

Early side effects of brain tumour treatment usually resolve with steroids to treat brain oedema, demyelination or immunotherapy reactions. Drug withdrawal or dose reduction may be necessary to manage acute toxic effects of chemotherapy or targeted immunotherapy. Late effects are becoming an increasing problem as survival improves and depend on factors that are often not reversible – e.g., radiotherapy dose and volume. There is no good evidence that there are effective treatments to prevent, delay or reverse late cognitive effects, stroke like complications and fatigue, but more high quality clinical research is required. Prevention of late effects by increasing fractionation schemes, reducing dose per fraction or total dose of radiation and hippocampal sparing techniques are a balance between effectively treating the tumour and preventing long-term brain injury. It seems likely that technologies such as proton beam treatments may play an increasing role by more selectively targeting the tumour, although their value has yet to be proven in good randomised clinical trials or long-term prognostic studies. As aggressive primary brain tumours are often highly resistant to chemotherapy and targeted and immunotherapy, care must be taken to choose those most likely to respond to these potentially toxic treatments and advise against active treatment where they may just accentuate acute toxicities for no discernible benefit. Supportive and palliative care should be advocated in parallel, rather than leaving such care until it is too late to be helpful.

References

1. Scales DC, Fischer HD, Li P, et al. Unintentional continuation of medications intended for acute illness after hospital discharge: a population-based cohort study. J Gen Intern Med. 2016;31:196.
2. Kerrigan S, Erridge SE, Liaquat I, et al. Mental incapacity in patients undergoing neuro-oncologic treatment: a cross-sectional study. Neurology. 2014;83(6):537–41.
3. Brell M, Ibanez J, Caral L, Ferrer E. Factors influencing surgical complications of intra-axial brain tumours. Acta Neurochir (Wein). 2000;142:739–50.

4. Gudrunardottir T, Sehested A, Juhler M, Schmiegelow K. Cerebellar mutism: review of the literature. Childs Nerv Syst. 2011;27(3):355–63.
5. Potgieser ARE, de Jong BM, Wagemakers M, Hoving EW, Groen RJM. Insights from the supplementary motor area syndrome in balancing movement initiation and inhibition. Front Hum Neurosci. 2014;8:960.
6. Armstrong TS, Cron SG, Bolanos EV, et al. Risk factors for fatigue severity in primary brain tumor patients. Cancer. 2010;116(11):2707–15.
7. Day J, Yust-Katz S, Cachia D, et al. Interventions for the management of fatigue in adults with a primary brain tumour. Cochrane Database Syst Rev. 2016;(4):CD011376. https://doi.org/10.1002/14651858.CD011376.pub2.
8. Boele FW, Douw L, de Groot M, et al. The effect of modafinil on fatigue, cognitive functioning, and mood in primary brain tumor patients: a multicenter randomized controlled trial. Neuro-Oncology. 2013;15(10):1420–8.
9. Robbins ME, Zhao W. Chronic oxidative stress and radiation-induced late normal tissue injury: a review. Int J Radiat Biol. 2004;80:251–9.
10. Wilson CM, Gaber MW, Sabek OM, Zawaski JA, Merchant TE. Radiation-induced astrogliosis and blood–brain barrier damage can be abrogated using anti-TNF treatment. Int J Radiat Oncol Biol Phys. 2009;74:934–41.
11. Lee WH, Sonntag WE, Mitschelen M, Yan H, Lee YW. Irradiation induces regionally specific alterations in pro-inflammatory environments in rat brain. Int J Radiat Biol. 2010;86:132–44.
12. Brown WR, Blair RM, Moody DM, Thore CR, Ahmed S, Robbins ME, Wheeler KT. Capillary loss precedes the cognitive impairment induced by fractionated whole-brain irradiation: a potential rat model of vascular dementia. J Neurol Sci. 2007;257:67–71.
13. Meyers CA, Brown PD. Role and relevance of neurocognitive assessment in clinical trials of patients with CNS tumors. J Clin Oncol. 2006;24:1305–9.
14. Nieder C, Leicht A, Motaref B, Nestle U, Niewald M, Schnabel K. Late radiation toxicity after whole brain radiotherapy: the influence of antiepileptic drugs. Am J Clin Oncol. 1999;22:573–9.
15. Chung C, Brown PD. Interventions for the treatment of brain radionecrosis after radiotherapy or radiosurgery. Cochrane Database Syst Rev. 2015;(1):CD011492. https://doi.org/10.1002/14651858.CD011492.
16. Shaw E, Arusell R, Scheithauer B, et al. A prospective randomized trial of low- versus high-dose radiation therapy in adults with supratentorial low-grade glioma: initial report of a NCCTG-RTOG-ECOG Study. J Clin Oncol. 2002;20:2267–76.
17. Kerklaan JP, Lycklama A Nijeholt GJ, Wiggenraad RG, Berghuis B, Postma TJ, Taphoorn MJ. SMART syndrome: a late reversible complication after radiation therapy for brain tumours. J Neurol. 2011;258(6):1098–104.
18. Bradshaw J, Chen L, Saling M, Fitt G, Hughes A, Dowd A. Neurocognitive recovery in SMART syndrome: a case report. Cephalalgia. 2011;31:372–6.
19. Larson JJ, Ball WS, Bove KE, et al. Formation of intracerebral cavernous malformations after radiation treatment for central nervous system neoplasia in children. J Neurosurg. 1998;88:51–6.
20. Heckl S, Aschoff A, Kunze S. Radiation-induced cavernous hemangiomas of the brain: a late effect predominantly in children. Cancer. 2002;94:3285–91.
21. Darzy KH, Shalet SM. Hypopituitarism following radiotherapy revisited. Endocr Dev. 2009;15:1–24.
22. Pui CH, Cheng C, Leung W, et al. Extended follow-up of long-term survivors of childhood acute lymphoblastic leukemia. N Engl J Med. 2003;349:640–9.
23. Chamberlain M. Temozolomide: therapeutic limitations in the treatment of adult high grade gliomas. Expert Rev Neurother. 2010;10(10):1537–44.
24. Kaehler KC, Piel S, Livingstone E, Schilling B, Hauschild A, Schadendorf D. Update on immunologic therapy with anti-CTLA-4 antibodies in melanoma: identification of clinical and biological response patterns, immune-related adverse events, and their management. Semin Oncol. 2010;37(5):485–98.

Neurorehabilitation in Neuro-Oncology

8

Michelangelo Bartolo and Isabella Springhetti

8.1   Introduction

Brain tumours (BT) represent a diverse spectrum of highly morbid neoplasms arising from different cells both from within central nervous system and from systemic tumours that have metastasized to the brain [1]. Intracranial metastases from systemic cancers, meningiomas and gliomas are the most prevalent BT. Brain metastases present mainly in the sixth and seventh decades of life; as patients survive longer from systemic cancer and therapeutic options are rapidly evolving, the treatment of brain metastases is being recognized increasingly as an emerging area of clinical interest [2]. Meningiomas are tumours of the meninges, mostly benign and often managed by surgical resection, with radiation therapy and chemotherapy reserved for high-risk or refractory disease. High-grade gliomas (HGG), including glioblastoma (GBM), are the most common and malignant BTs in adults, determining significant mortality and morbidity. In both American and European studies, the incidence rate of BT ranges from $17.6/10^5$ to $22.0/10^5$, showing progressively higher incidence with advancing age [3, 4]; the overall incidence is the same in males and females, but GBM is more frequent in men, while meningiomas occur more often in women.

Despite intensive efforts to develop new therapies, the response to standard-of-care treatments is limited and the prognosis is still poor [5, 6].

The clinical manifestations of BT include a variety of signs and symptoms, usually referable to the anatomic area of the brain involved or adjacent structures, and include seizures, headaches, fatigue, motor, sensory and cognitive dysfunction.

M. Bartolo (✉)
Department of Rehabilitation, Neurorehabilitation Unit, HABILITA, Bergamo, Italy
e-mail: michelangelobartolo@habilita.it

I. Springhetti
Functional Recovery and Rehabilitation Unit, Neuromotor/Oncologic Sections, Fondazione Salvatore Maugeri, Pavia, Italy

© Springer Nature Switzerland AG 2019   103
M. Bartolo et al. (eds.), *Neurorehabilitation in Neuro-Oncology*,
https://doi.org/10.1007/978-3-319-95684-8_8

Although surgery, radiation therapy and chemotherapy extend survival, they have a very high likelihood of producing long-term disabling effects with a deep impact on patients' independence in daily living and consequently on patients' quality of life (QoL) [7]. Accordingly, in clinical practice the efforts aim to balance tumour control with treatment-related adverse consequences over the course of the disease process.

As far as public health is concerned, despite the relatively low incidence, BT causes high direct costs (i.e. diagnostic resources, high complexity treatments and rehabilitation) and high-unforeseen costs (i.e. dismissal from work, family and social expenditures). A population-based comparison of cancer survivors with matched controls found a substantially increased burden of illness in cancer survivors, consisting in days lost from work, inability to work, perceived poor general health and the need for help with daily activities. Furthermore, compared with age-matched controls, cancer survivors reported poorer health outcomes, decreased psychological? functioning and higher levels of burden across multiple domains [8].

As the symptoms are complex, multidisciplinary expertise is necessary to evaluate the influence of each variable to plan appropriate support and rehabilitative interventions, so that the persons may reach their optimal physical, sensory, cognitive, psychological and social functional level.

8.2   Symptoms of Brain Tumours

In BT patients symptoms are due to the growth rate and to growth mode of the tumoural lesion [9]. In case of slow-growing lesions such as low-grade gliomas (LGG), the functions of the affected area may remain intact for a long time, as tumour may induce progressive functional compensatory reshaping of brain networks [10, 11]. Conversely, when tumour growth is rapid, symptoms usually occur earlier and may improve after tumour removal if the tumour mass has not completely compromised the surrounding nervous fibres. Patients may present progressive symptoms and signs related to mass effect, displacement of brain tissue and vasogenic oedema. Generalized symptoms, due to expanding mass effect, are manifestation of increased intracranial pressure. In most BT cases the initial presenting symptom is represented by *headache*, with features as non-specific, intermittent, mild intensity, tension-like or mimicking migraine [12]. Epidemiologic data regarding the prevalence of headache are extremely variable, ranging from 33 to 71% of BT patients; moreover patients have at least one neurological symptom in addition to the headache. There is no exact relation between the headache topography and tumour location; when the intracranial pressure is high, headache is referred in widespread areas.

Nausea and *projectile vomiting* may occur as a result of direct or reflex stimulation of the emetic centre of the medulla. Such stimulation often accompanies increased intracranial pressure and occurs most frequently with brainstem dislocation secondary to herniation. Sometimes the lesions of brainstem nuclei may influence the gastrointestinal tract causing altered bowel motility, with slow propagation and incoordination of intestinal motility and prolonged gastric emptying; hiccups and yawning can also occur.

Seizures are a presenting symptom in approximately 20–40% of BT patients, while a further 20–45% of patients will present them during the course of disease. The incidence of seizures is inversely related to malignancy, with the highest incidence for LGG (65–95%) and the lowest incidence (15–25%) occurring in HGG. Furthermore, BT involving the deep white matter and those below the tentorium are less likely to produce seizures than tumours situated in the cortical or subcortical regions of the cerebral hemispheres, thus making seizures' onset a favourable prognosis factor. Generalized seizures may occur with tumours in a variety of locations while focal seizures are more common with tumours in the motor or sensory subcortical regions. The unpredictable responses to seizures after surgical removal of BT suggest that multiple factors are involved [13, 14].

Cognitive and *behavioural changes* accompanying BT are often subtle in onset, usually consisting of progressive disturbances affecting behaviour, emotion and cognitive functioning [15].

A large number of patients with primary or metastatic BT require neurosurgical intervention, being either radical/subtotal resection, palliative debulking or diagnostic biopsy. Maximal possible tumour resection with minimal neurological damage represents the gold standard for BT patients because it reduces symptoms, including epilepsy, due to the mass effects, probably improves survival and efficacy of adjuvant therapies [16–18]. Nevertheless, after surgery, some patients experience more or less significant sensory-motor-cognitive and behavioural deficits as well as general accompanying signs.

Post-craniotomy headache is reported by at least 60% of patients, occurring in the area of surgery; it develops within the first 48 h after surgical intervention and disappears within 7–8 days. This pain is typically somatic, pulsing or pounding, and it has a positive response to common analgesics. On the other hand, headache can be expression of potentially serious complications of neurosurgery including intracerebral abscess, meningitis, haemorrhage and cerebrospinal fluid (CSF)-leakage. Low CSF pressure headache is caused by post-surgery spinal fluid leak: it becomes severe when the patient is upright after getting out of bed, and quickly disappears when the patient is lying flat, and may be accompanied by some neck discomfort and nausea.

In the post-surgery period *electrolyte disorders*, such as hyponatraemia, may present. Hyponatraemia is most commonly due to inappropriate antidiuretic hormone (SIADH) or cerebral salt wasting. Symptoms are highly related with depletion extent and speed of onset. Early symptoms include headache, nausea, vomiting, leading to confusion, seizures, stupor and even coma. It occurs in approximately 50% of patients; exact diagnosis and fast treatment are required.

Vasogenic cerebral oedema strongly contributes to symptoms in BT patents. It could be an additional cause of mass effect, often exceeding the effect induced by the tumour itself. Vasogenic cerebral oedema could be an expression of disease progression, or under-dosing of the steroids therapies, or delayed effects of radiotherapy. Symptoms due to vasogenic cerebral oedema include headache, nausea, vomiting, blurred vision, faintness, and in severe cases, seizures and coma. Corticosteroids and osmotic agents often provide dramatic relief of symptoms caused by cerebral oedema. Surgical treatment, with decompressive craniectomy, is occasionally recommended in case of a rapid deterioration of neurological status.

Sometimes a thalamic tumour or, less commonly, a basal ganglia tumour may produce secondary blockage of cerebrospinal fluid flow and consequently *hydrocephalus*. In these cases, patients typically present with headache, vomiting, sleepiness and visual disturbances, resulting from increased intracranial pressure secondary to trapping of the lateral horn in one of the ventricles. This complication is treated with surgical excision or palliative ventricular–peritoneal liquor derivation.

Fatigue could be considered as a BT symptom and/or as a side effect of surgical, oncologic and medical therapy and/or as expression of depressive state [19]. It may appear at any stage of the disease, representing a disabling condition with negative impact on quality of life in great number of brain? cancer patients; in the case of neurological tumours it is frequently shaded by the presence of sensorimotor and cognitive impairments.

8.2.1 Side Effects of Chemo/Radiotherapy

After surgery some patients are candidates for adjuvant chemotherapy (CT) and/or radiotherapy (RT) which could be a source of additional discomfort [20].

During the course of RT, in a small percentage of cases acute radiation induced encephalopathy may occur, with oedema causing headache, transitory worsening or progressive worsening of preexisting neurologic deficits, and seizures. The steroid therapy must be continued at the minimum effective dose, taking into account that steroids may induce psychiatric symptoms such as anxiety, euphoria, depression, rarely psychosis, in about 6% of patients. Steroids should be gradually discontinued to avoid withdrawal syndrome. In those patients who are too aggressively weaned, recurrence of cerebral oedema and painful mass effect may occur. Furthermore, disturbances of taste and salivation could commonly develop during the course of RT due to damage of afferent receptors. This can worsen a preexisting dysphagia and has to be taken into account and treated during the rehabilitation care.

In long survivors *delayed cerebral radionecrosis*, occurring from 4 months to 4 years after treatment, may present, typically manifesting with headache, personality changes, focal deficits and seizures. *Radiation-related dementia* is a more diffuse late brain injury (after 6 months to several years) in which clinical manifestations are represented by progressive cognitive decline as lack of initiative, short-term memory deficits, fatigue and personality changes. Occasionally gait impairment, incontinence and dysarthria may also occur. In some cases RT may also induce radiation induced endocrine dysfunction and thus affecting brain functioning in an indirect way.

The main goal of CT in BT patients is to control tumour growth while assuring optimal function and quality of life. Chemotherapy agents, such as temozolomide, can induce headache, nausea, vomiting and others non-specific, non-neurologic side effects (decreased appetite, fatigue, etc.) in up to 25% of patients. The selective serotonin receptor antagonists (e.g. ondansetron, granisetron) are used to prevent nausea and vomiting, but these agents are reported to cause headache in 14–39% of patients. The cognitive side effects of CT known as *chemobrain* or *chemofog* have been widely described; this condition encompasses a range of symptoms such as memory loss, inability to concentrate, difficulty in thinking and other subtle, cognitive changes. Although the severity of cognitive difficulty varies among patients, the slightest deterioration in cognitive function can be devastating for the patient's quality of life [21, 22]. Neurotoxicity has been reported with several chemotherapy agents, particularly if multimodal or high-dose regimens are used; however, the late neurotoxic side effects of CT may be difficult to discern from RT, because most patients treated with CT have already been treated with RT or are even treated with radiation concomitantly. In contrast to the late radiation encephalopathy, side effects of CT on the central nervous system tend to arise during, or shortly after, CT.

Finally, one of the most common and often most debilitating effects of cranial RT and/or CT is progressive fatigue. A growing number of cancer control studies have examined the relationships among cancer, CT, RT and fatigue suggesting that symptoms like lack of strength and/or vigour often persist for several weeks beyond the completion of therapy [23, 24].

8.3 The ICF as the Framework for Assessment in Neuro-Oncological Rehabilitation

As for other diseases/impairments, disabilities caused by BT can be described within the conceptual framework of the International Classification of Functioning, Disability and Health (ICF), which was developed by the World Health Organization to describe health and the multidimensional health-related concerns of individuals [25].

The ICF system examines the structural and functional alterations produced by diseases, with regard to the limitations in the individual's activities and to the restriction of participation in social relationships and work. In this perspective, all the environmental variables (structural and relational) acting as a facilitator or a barrier to the person's choices, are integral part of the model. Using a comprehensive approach to humans, the ICF defines three main domains: body function and structures, activity and participation. Body function and structures refer to the anatomical and physiological functions of the body systems, whose alterations are defined "impairments" (e.g. muscle weakness, spasticity, restricted joint motion, pain, visual deficits, seizures, poor cardiorespiratory fitness). All these are then categorized into subdomains. Environment (health professionals, close relatives, as well as workplace) and personal factors (sex, age, social status, life experiences, etc.) interact with health conditions (body functions and structures), determining whether and how impairments result in disability. For example, a cancer treatment, such as chemotherapy, that causes a peripheral neuropathy and consequent ankle weakness (impairments), may limit patient's ability to walk (activity) and to work (participation). Patient may require an orthosis like an ankle brace and/or an external facilitator like an elevator, to maintain both ability and level of participation.

Assuming that each disease has its own pattern, the ICF system built up groups of codes (core set) related to specific and relevant aspects in many ICD diagnosis and conditions. Moreover, some set appeared particularly relevant regardless of the ICD diagnosis, and are considered mandatory: for all diagnosis and for rehabilitation (see: https://www.icf-research-branch.org/download/send/4-icf-core-sets/141-icf-generic-set *accessed on January 2018*).

The development of ICF core sets provides clinicians and researchers with comprehensive but concise measurement categories in each subdomain that help to describe each item from a biopsychosocial point of view. Some ICF core sets have been developed for head and neck and breast cancer.

In neuro-oncology, specific studies in this regard are lacking. The WHO ICF Research Branch has developed a rigorous method of transversal core sets for different conditions, which take into account both patient's and healthcare environment's points of view. Among these, at an early stage of the disease the core set for post-acute neurological conditions (the so-called brief core set for neurological conditions in post-acute care: see https://www.icf-research-branch.org/download/send/8-neurologicalconditions/166-brief-icf-core-set-for-neurological-conditions-in-post-acute-care *accessed on January 2018*) appears suitable for defining the rehabilitation plan immediately after surgery. In this phase priorities are: identifying conditions of patient and its context, impairments and limitations on which to intervene, barriers to be eliminated and facilitators to be created or supported. From this point of view the ICF coding does not differ in neuro-oncology from other neurological conditions (i.e. hemiplegia and aphasia of vascular aetiology). Conversely, relevant items such as quality of life, end-of-life issues are not specifically addressed. So, further studies are necessary to identify appropriate set, able to depict BT patients' condition in which the path from the very beginning to the terminal phase comes frequently to an end in a 12–15 months' timeframe [26].

8.4 Measurements in Neuro-Oncological Rehabilitation

The continuum of care for BT patients is articulated through clinical pathways. The organizational model that we consider evaluates performance both of the health system and of the patient, using validated indicators and assessment tools. In fact, indicators act as a basis for decision-making models oriented to (1) control disease; (2) enhance patients' potential; (3) drive policy planning [27, 28]. Among indicators, some categories seem relevant from a clinical perspective: a brief description will be here outlined.

Performance status indexes are semi-quantitative measures of psycho-physical general performance, obtained through different scoring systems created for the oncological patients. They grossly evaluate personal care, personal activities and work capacity as variables. The *Karnofsky performance status scale* (KPSS) [29] and *Eastern cooperative oncology group performance status* (ECOG) [30] are the most widely adopted in the literature. The maximum attributable value is 100 for KPSS for normal asymptomatic conditions; values decrease proportionally with disability increase, assistance needs in KPSS. ECOG has similar but inverted progression from 0 to 100. In most serious illnesses the lower the Karnofsky score or the higher ECOG score—the lower the likelihood of survival. KPSS and ECOG are the most widespread tools in the world to compare effectiveness of different therapies, to assess the extent of response to therapy, so to assess the prognosis in individual patients.

However, these tools appear extremely approximate (especially in the 40–60 point classes for KPSS and 2/3 for ECOG) in reading the real functional dependence of the patient and therefore scarcely suitable for the rehabilitative use.

Regarding rehabilitation functional outcomes, the most commonly used measures are the Barthel index (BI) [31] and the functional independence measure (FIM) [32], that, even if they do not specifically address the neuroncological patients, are widely used to describe functional and rehabilitation outcomes in this population. The first one is a tool focused on basic mobility function and personal activities of daily living, while the second one represents the evolution of Barthel index adding more quantitative criteria to measure independence in different domains of daily life.

Quality of life can be assessed through different tools. EORTC-QLQ-C30 is a widespread multidimensional questionnaire developed to evaluate cancer-related quality of life, as regards functional outcome and side effects of specific treatments (chemotherapy/radiotherapy) [33]. The EORTC-QLQ-C30 is often used combined with a specific questionnaire, the EORTC QLQ-BN20 validated for BT [34, 35]. This questionnaire consists of 20 items divided into four subsets, concerning future uncertainty, motor dysfunction, communication deficits and visual disorders.

Finally, many tools have been developed to assess pain; most are variation on the unidimensional visual analogical scale (VAS) [36] like a schematic representation of the body for the patient to indicate where their pain is located, or verbal rating scale (VRS) [37], or numerical rating scale (NRS) [38]. Conversely, the McGill pain questionnaire [39] is considered time consuming. The short form consists of 15 qualitative descriptors of the sensory (11 item) and affective (4 item) pain experience. The answers are graded on a scale ranged from 0 to 3 and the score can therefore vary from 0 to 45, due to gravity increase.

Clinical complexity is a common feature of BT patients. Identifying conditions of "greater frailty" enable both the clinician and the administrator to provide adequate therapy and care. Indirect complexity markers can be considered most of the external devices supporting basic life's functions (percutaneously inserted central catheter, port a cath, systems for nutritional support, tracheostomy, oxygen support, non-invasive ventilation, vacuum assisted closure (VAC®)-therapy, among others).

Regarding multi-symptomatic conditions and frailty, in the palliative setting the Edmonton symptom assessment scale (ESAS) [40] is commonly used. This tool was developed in an oncological context, and evaluates the severity of subjective perception in 10 symptoms, of which nine predefined (pain, fatigue, nausea, depression, anxiety, drowsiness, loss of appetite, malaise, dyspnea) and one reported by patient (e.g. itching, hiccup).

Another tool, the brief psychiatric rating scale (BPRS) [41] consists of a semi-quantitative evaluation of psychiatric symptoms. These disturbances may present at any stage of disease, depending on the site of lesion, therapies and previous diseases. This allows for the integration of psychological and clinical evaluation of patients, and it is mostly used in palliative setting.

8.5   The Multidisciplinary Approach

As reported above, BT patients may present complex disabilities, due to the involvement of both sensorimotor and cognitive areas, also affecting personality and behaviour. Overall, functional impairments influence different aspects of the person (activity and participation) and are similar to those seen in patients commonly admitted to rehabilitation programs. Moreover, symptoms and disabilities have a relevant impact on patients' daily life, hindering their ability to function independently and to maintain usual family and social roles, influencing ultimately the QoL of not only patients, but also of their informal caregivers [42].

The role of rehabilitation becomes relevant to favour the highest degree of functional recovery and autonomy for patients and to provide informal caregivers with support, education and coping strategies [43].

In a rehabilitative approach, all these aspects must be included in a global vision of the person, taking in charge all the different aspects of disabilities manifested by the patients, with a multidisciplinary approach recognized in the literature as most appropriate.

Multidisciplinary rehabilitation assumes that besides the anatomical or physiological problems, psychological factors (fear, anxiety, mood disturbance) and social/environmental factors (workplace and social issues) may amplify symptoms and worsen disability and functional independence. These insights have led to the design of interventions that simultaneously address multiple factors, typically involving a combination of physical, psychological, social and/or work-related components, which are delivered by a team of health professionals with different skills [44].

Multidisciplinary rehabilitation can be defined as the coordinated delivery of multidimensional rehabilitation interventions, provided by different disciplines, such as nursing, physiotherapy, psychology, occupational therapy, social work and others, combined with medical professionals which aims to improve patient symptoms, maximize functional independence and social integration (participation) by means of a holistic biopsychosocial model of care, as defined by the ICF.

The multidisciplinary approach prioritizes patient-centred care, focusing on person's functions and disabilities, using a goal-based functionally oriented approach that is time-based. The first hired is that the patient (and his/her caregiver) are the focus. They must be actively involved in the goal setting process. To do this, a number of personal factors (individual's experiences, coping style, self-efficacy, attitudes, values, preferences, knowledge) are to be considered as relevant factors in both the identification of rehabilitation goals and the selection of the rehabilitation programs. Within the context of multidisciplinary rehabilitation, the content, intensity and frequency of rehabilitation therapy can vary, tailoring the programs according to clinical needs and individual personal factors.

As today, the literature reported only low level evidence for the effectiveness of rehabilitation programs specifically for BT patients, but a number of preliminary studies addressed the benefit of multidisciplinary rehabilitation in reducing disability in people with BTs. Performing rehabilitation with a multidisciplinary approach seems to improve functional abilities and cognitive functioning in BT patients more than rehabilitation programs performed with standard care [45].

The model of "simultaneous care", which is deeply multidisciplinary, seems to describe the best approach to neuro-oncological patients because it ensures the continuity of care, but also includes the supportive care (control the side effects of treatments and comorbidities) and palliative care (prevention and the relief from suffering) at the same time as anticancer therapies are administered (simultaneous care) [46].

8.6   Sensory-Motor Rehabilitation

Many studies showed that regular physical exercise aimed to maintain health condition and structured and guided (by professionals) exercise training are useful for primary and secondary disease prevention in different clinical settings. In the light of these considerations, in the last years the clinicians developed greater awareness of the rehabilitation needs of BT patients, although not completely yet.

The main goal of cancer rehabilitation is to maximize patients' functioning, to promote their independence, also by means of adaptation, with the final aim of improving patients' QoL, regardless of the length of residual life. As already mentioned above, since rehabilitation is a holistic and comprehensive approach to the person, the combined expertise of a multidisciplinary team is necessary and goals have to be established through a cooperative effort among health professionals, patients, families and informal caregivers in order to tailor the rehabilitative care on patient's needs (different clinical features, levels of disability).

The early phase of rehabilitation usually aims to restore function [47] while in advanced stages rehabilitation becomes relevant within the context of palliative care to prevent complications, control symptoms, and maintain patients' independence and QoL.

Patient should receive treatment for motor deficits in order to improve mobility and independence and to prevent the negative effects of immobility like pressure ulcers, muscle atrophy and contractures; informal caregiver should be given skills for home assistance and support during a path that is expected to be fast and strenuous (almost in high-grade malignancy as glioblastomas). In case of LGG, and whenever life expectancy is longer (meningiomas, ependymomas, tumours with uncertain behaviour as oligodendrogliomas and others), medium-term and long-term goals can be hazarded, stimulating patient to work toward social and working abilities.

When planning the rehabilitative intervention, specificity of medical treatment, complication of surgery and side effects of RT and CT have to be taken into consideration; also the severity of deficits and the ability to respond to rehabilitation programs may fluctuate during the treatment (e.g. during RT there may be a transitory decline in the patient's neurological functioning). Side effects of drugs such as corticosteroids and anticonvulsants are also relevant, because they can be associated with clinical (myopathy, osteoporosis, etc. and behavioural changes that can influence the rehabilitation process [48]. Furthermore, BT patients are prone to a number of medical complications due to their clinical frailty, such as infectious, thromboembolic complications, nutritional problems that must be managed during the rehabilitation pathway in order to avoid functional worsening.

Methods and specific techniques aimed at increasing function will not be described here; the choice of the appropriate technique is made according to the patients' residual capacities (i.e. quality of deficit and intellectual/cognitive ability).

A number of studies investigated the effects of structured rehabilitation programs, but they were considered with a "low-level" of evidence [45]; however, many authors demonstrated that BT patients may benefit from inpatient rehabilitation, achieving functional improvements comparable to stroke patients or traumatic brain injured patients, irrespective of the tumour type, location and tumour treatments [7, 20, 47, 49]. Recent meta-analyses and systematic reviews reported that exercise training, performed as part of a rehabilitation program is safe, well-tolerated and represents an adjunctive therapeutic strategy associated with significant improvements in a broad range of cancer-related symptoms and QoL. The next step will be to determine whether exercise therapy, in addition to control symptoms, may modulate cancer-specific outcomes (i.e. cancer progression and metastasis), clarifying the potential association between physical exercise, functional capacity and prognosis as well as the cellular and molecular mechanisms underlying these associations [50].

Finally, besides motor impairment, BT patients may experience dysphagia. Common symptoms are pharyngeal pooling or aspiration caused by delayed or pharyngeal swallowing ability or reduced laryngeal elevation. A regular swallowing evaluation should be done together with the execution of a videofluoroscopy to obtain objective information. Rehabilitation techniques may be compensatory or therapeutic; for some patients dietary modification or tube feedings (e.g. percutaneous endoscopic gastrostomy—PEG catheter) may be needed. Devices are often necessary also for neurogenic sphincter disorders and the rehabilitative approach is similar to that adopted for other neurological diseases.

8.7 Cognitive Rehabilitation

Besides motor and functional impairment, a frequent and disabling symptom for BT patients is represented by cognitive decline: in fact, as more effective therapies have prolonged survival cognitive dysfunction has been recognized as one of the most frequent complications among long-term survivors [51, 52]. More extensively discussed in chapter 10.

The aetiology of cognitive deficits following a diagnosis of BT is multifactorial, depending on histology, disease progression and treatment-related neurotoxicity; other potential reported exacerbating factors are represented by related lethargy, endocrine dysfunction, epilepsy and anticonvulsant therapy, as well as mood disorders, that all can contribute to determining the type and severity of cognitive impairment [53, 54]. Moreover, recent literature findings underlined that BT in addition to inducing focal neural disruption and mass effect may cause alterations in brain connectivity, ultimately determining whole brain dysfunction [55–58].

Epidemiological data are extremely variable due to the use of different neuropsychological tests and reference data as well as to the heterogeneity of the studied populations; however, specific cognitive deficits have been described in at least 30% of patients' post-surgical procedure and extending up to 90% at long-term follow-up post-treatment [59, 60]. Among the most common cognitive symptoms psychomotor slowing, attention and memory (working memory) deficits, executive dysfunction or focal deficits such as aphasia or apraxia may occur in most BT patients. In turn cognitive deficits can have a large impact on patients' self-care, social and professional functioning, ability to undertake activities of daily living, as well as on patients' ability to make informed decisions related to their own treatment and care. Therefore cognitive impairment has been demonstrated to be a major factor in health-related quality of life (HRQoL), especially when resulting in loss of functional independence [61–64], despite adequate disease control. Moreover, cognitive status was found to be a stronger prognostic factor for survival than physical state and a reliable index of tumour progression [65].

In consideration of the devastating impact of cognitive impairments and of the lack of pharmacological approaches to prevent or treat cognitive deficits, cognitive rehabilitation (CR) may have an important role to achieve an improvement in cognitive functions and a better quality of life. The term CR includes a variety of interventions, all aimed at relieving patients' cognitive deficits by retraining previously learned skills and/or teaching compensatory strategies, with the ultimate goal of favouring a positive adaptation of the patients to their environment [66]. CR has proven to be effective in other neurological patients [67], but only few studies have analysed the potential benefits of such rehabilitation for BT patients. The studies conducted up to now provide preliminary but encouraging results on the application of CR techniques in BT patients, showing an improvement of cognitive functions, a reduction of mental fatigue, a greater autonomy in everyday life and a lesser burden for family caregivers [68]. However, the extreme heterogeneity of the approaches as well as the differences in study design, in the diagnosis and phase of the disease, in the measures used to assess cognitive functions and to evaluate the outcomes suggests the need for further studies to clarify which are the most effective interventions and the patients who can benefit from the intervention. A better understanding of the mechanisms and of the treatment protocols is now essential to optimize these procedures.

8.8 Occupational Therapy

In the context of a multidisciplinary approach, CR can be combined with occupational therapy (OT) that aims at fostering generalization of re-learned skills to ecological situations to enhance patients' independence in performing activities of daily living (ADL). OT in fact, through the use of a variety of techniques and tools, facilitates patients' engagement in meaningful everyday activities [69]. However, even if OT may reduce cancer-related disability, it still remains severely underused in BT patients, due to the poor awareness of OT by the health professionals, lack of knowledge of whom OT would benefit and the practical accessibility to the service. As soon as the goals of OT become better understood, accessing an occupational therapist will become more standard practice.

8.9 Psychological Support

Feelings of anxiety, depression and future uncertainty represent frequent psychological symptoms in BTs patients, whose origin is not completely understood; either focal brain injury or reactive emotional distress may be responsible [70]. Among patients with HGG shock, sense of helplessness, depression, anxiety and recognition of death are highly prevalent; soon after the diagnosis the experience of a surreal feeling combined with disbelief has also been reported, while powerlessness and suffering often dominate future perspectives [63]. In these phases mechanisms of repression or denial may help patients to keep high motivation. As described, patients in the course of the disease may progressively shift from death anxiety and fear to fatalism and then to a more conscious state of mind characterized by the awareness of the inevitability of death [71].

Soon after receiving the diagnosis, usually patients focus attention and personal resources on the recovery of their own functional autonomy rather than on the disease evolution; coping with restriction in fact seems to be most difficult to deal with and patients generally balance between losing independence and trying to maintain autonomy. Above all, in fact, patients suffer from the lack of independence, the difficulty in accomplishing previous roles, the inability to drive or to work and the reduction of social relationship that may lead to feelings of depression, anxiety and meaningless [71]. Patients often need help to accept their difficulties, stop hiding them and finding a wider way to manage them.

Hope improves patients' QoL, helping them to live better and fight the disease, even if it is very vulnerable especially at diagnosis, at every new scan and when treatment failure with terminal expectations and limited legacy occur [72]. Patients always live in the balance between needing information and keeping hope.

Other than emotional disturbances, the sudden appearance of patients' personality and behavioural alterations become a destabilizing factor for the family context, which initially does not understand and does not know how to react, while having to adapt quickly. That's why compared with caregivers of other BT patients, caregivers of patients with a GBM have a worse quality of life [73] and may have more psychosocial needs because the disease process is faster and they have less time to adapt [74].

Due to the dramatic emotional sequelae of having a BT, it is important that patients are screened routinely for psychological distress, to implement adequate support intervention and to improve their psychological well-being. Health professionals must build a warm, harmonious and yet realistic communication, which must also consider the patients' and family's levels of understanding and capacity for acceptance.

During the last decades, psycho-oncology has been recognized by international literature and guidelines as a relevant topic in the field of oncology, and the psycho-oncologist has often become a full member of the rehabilitation team, though it has not always been implemented as standard care.

The main aim of psycho-oncological care is devoted to retain and improve the persons' perception of the QoL, during the disease evolution, providing existential support to facilitate the acceptation of the diagnosis, the engagement required by the treatments and the end-of-life issues.

Literature evidences reported that BT persons appreciate the opportunity to discuss existential fears and concerns early from the illness diagnosis rather than support only being offered toward the end of life. This is particularly relevant considering that disease progression can greatly compromise people's cognitive and communication skills, often requiring the intermediation of other people (family/caregiver). In this sense, the continuous and constant information by health professionals about the meaning of the patient's behaviour may favour a process of adaptation that is faster, otherwise impossible. The effectiveness of psycho-oncological support (such as psycho-educative interventions or psychotherapeutic interventions) performed both in group and in individual therapies has been shown in various studies.

Professionally or peer-led support groups may provide patients with cancer with a sense of community, unconditional acceptance and information about the disease that they would not experience elsewhere. In particular, therapies based on support groups performed in different settings have shown to increase the well-being of the patients. Moreover, they seem to facilitate the patient's relationship with family and friends by relieving the burden of care and providing a safe place for the emotional expression [75].

8.10 The Family Role

Caring for BT people may be particularly challenging both physically and emotionally for relatives due to the rapid progression of the disease, the coexistence of cognitive impairment and behavioural changes, the rapid physical deterioration and the changes in family life. This is the reason why brain tumour has been defined a family disease [76].

Extensive literature documented the significant burden and distress that caregivers may report as result of providing care without training or psychological support for this role, with significant physical, social and psychological consequences [77].

As for patients, receiving the diagnosis represents a shock for caregivers who feel a loss of safety in everyday life, powerlessness and feeling of being overwhelmed, denial and anger [74, 78]. Caregivers express dramatically the feeling of losing the patient, even before the patient's death [79]; the onset of cognitive and behavioural changes is perceived by caregivers as a bending in their relationship with the patient and they often refer to the patient as someone else than they knew before [80].

From diagnosis on, caregivers report feelings of isolation and solitude as they spend all time to assist the patient, feel reluctant to leave patient alone and therefore take time off at work and neglect friends and social relationship [74]; they feel alone also when are requested to make decisions when patients cannot express their wishes anymore [81].

As disease progresses, the onset of new symptoms, physical, cognitive and neuropsychiatric occur and an ever increasing level of assistance is required in the dimensions of personal daily living tasks. Often caregivers feel inadequately prepared to face these requests, expressing the need for information and guidance to manage patient's symptoms and side effects at home as well as practical support [80]. When patient becomes unable to make conscious choices, caregivers must take on the role of decision-maker in any choice related to therapy and family management, expressing a sense of total responsibility and experiencing a heavy feeling of burden and isolation [74, 81].

Therefore as distress levels are consistently high and cannot be predicted at any time point, caregivers should be monitored over time to promptly identify evolving psychological morbidity. Studies in fact suggest that educational programs and/or cognitive-behavioural therapy may relieve the distress, addressing the caregiver to better identify the main concerns. [RCT by Boele] In turn caregivers' psychological and behavioural responses to caregiving may impact on their own emotional and physical health, also influencing the quality of care delivered to the patient at home as well as the decision to institutionalize patients.

A lot of recommendations from literature suggest that the approach to caregiver should include:

(a) educational programs;
(b) teaching stress reduction techniques and coping strategies;
(c) improvement in communication.

The educational programs for caregiver prepare them for changes in their loved one and to increase understanding of care pathways, including treatment processes. The knowledge of techniques to modulate stress and coping strategies may attenuate the global burden due to continuous caring. Moreover, involving caregivers in communication, such as involving them in family consultations, particularly in the crisis phases may facilitate the caregiver's awareness with respect to the disease progression and care needs. About this, literature reports that the most prevalent caregiver needs, soon after diagnosis, usually regards "getting information about the illness and its evolution" as well as "dealing with fears and worries", while at follow-up visits the needs usually shift on "getting a break from caring", "practical help in the home", "equipment to help care" and "managing patient's symptoms" [77].

Provide a health support, directing the caregiver to conscious choices as well as meeting the emotional needs of caregivers of BT persons, represents a priority commitment in rehabilitation care in order to reduce their burden and maintain the best possible level of well-being for both patients and families.

References

1. McFaline-Figueroa JR, Lee EQ. Brain tumors. Am J Med. 2018;22:pii:S0002-9343(18)30031-7.
2. Tabouret E, Chinot O, Metellus P, Tallet A, Viens P, Gonçalves A. Recent trends in epidemiology of brain metastases: an overview. Anticancer Res. 2012;32(11):4655–62.
3. Crocetti E, Trama A, Stiller C, Caldarella A, Soffietti R, Jaal J, et al. Epidemiology of glial and non-glial brain tumours in Europe. Eur J Cancer. 2012;48:1532–42.
4. Ostrom QT, Gittleman H, Fulop J, Liu M, Blanda R, Kromer C, et al. CBTRUS statistical report: primary brain and central nervous system tumors diagnosed in the United States in 2008–2012. Neuro Oncol. 2015;17(Suppl.4):iv1–62.
5. Sim HW, Morgan ER, Mason WP. Contemporary management of high-grade gliomas. CNS Oncol. 2018;7(1):51–65.
6. Ostrom QT, Gittleman H, Stetson L, Virk S, Barnholtz-Sloan JS. Epidemiology of intracranial gliomas. Prog Neurol Surg. 2018;30:1–11.
7. Vargo M. Brain tumor rehabilitation. Am J Phys Med Rehabil. 2011;90(Suppl):S50–62.
8. Yabroff KR, Lawrence WF, Clauser S, Davis WW, Brown ML. Burden of illness in cancer survivors: findings from a population-based national sample. J Natl Cancer Inst. 2004;96(17):1322–30.
9. Mukand JA, Blackinton DD, Crincoli MG, Lee JJ, Santos BB. Incidence of neurologic deficits and rehabilitation of patients with brain tumors. Am J Phys Med Rehabil. 2001;80: 346–50.
10. Schiffbauer H, Ferrari P, Rowley HA, Berger MS, Roberts TP. Functional activity within brain tumours: a magnetic source imaging study. Neurosurgery. 2001;49:1313–20.
11. Duffau H. Lessons from brain mapping in surgery for low-grade glioma: insights into associations between tumour and brain plasticity. Lancet Neurol. 2005;4(8):476–86.
12. Russo M, Villani V, Taga A, Genovese A, Terrenato I, Manzoni GC, et al. Headache as a presenting symptom of glioma: a cross-sectional study. Cephalalgia. 2017;38(4):730–5.
13. Politsky JM. Brain tumor-related epilepsy: a current review of the etiologic basis and diagnostic and treatment approaches. Curr Neurol Neurosci Rep. 2017;17(9):70.
14. Vecht C, Royer-Perron L, Houillier C, Huberfeld G. Seizures and anticonvulsants in brain tumours: frequency, mechanisms and anti-epileptic management. Curr Pharm Des. 2017;23(42):6464–87.
15. Boele FW, Klein M, Reijneveld JC, Verdonck-de Leeuw IM, Heimans JJ. Symptom management and quality of life in glioma patients. CNS Oncol. 2014;3(1):37–47.
16. Hervey-Jumper SL, Berger MS. Role of surgical resection in low- and high-grade gliomas. Curr Treat Opt Neurol. 2014;16:284.
17. Brown TJ, Brennan MC, Li M, Church EW, Brandmeir N, Rakszawski KL, et al. Association of the extent of resection with survival in glioblastoma: a systematic review and meta-analysis. JAMA Oncol. 2016;2:1460–9.
18. Lara-Velazquez M, Al-Kharboosh R, Jeanneret S, Vazquez-Ramos C, Mahato D, Tavanaiepour D, et al. Advances in brain tumor surgery for glioblastoma in adults. Brain Sci. 2017;7(12):166.
19. Asher A, Fu JB, Bailey C, Hughes JK. Fatigue among patients with brain tumors. CNS Oncol. 2016;5(2):91–100.

20. Kirshblum S, O'Dell MW, Ho C, Barr K. Rehabilitation of persons with central nervous system tumors. Cancer. 2001;92:1029–38.
21. Behrend SW. Patients with primary brain tumors. Oncol Nurs Forum. 2014;41(3):335–6.
22. Argyriou AA, Assimakopoulos K, Iconomou G, Giannakopoulou F, Kalofonos HP. Either called "chemobrain" or "chemofog," the long-term chemotherapy-induced cognitive decline in cancer survivors is real. J Pain Symptom Manage. 2011;41(1):126–39.
23. Bower JE. Treating cancer-related fatigue: the search for interventions that target those most in need. J Clin Oncol. 2012;30(36):4449–50.
24. de Raaf PJ, de Klerk C, van der Rijt CC. Elucidating the behavior of physical fatigue and mental fatigue in cancer patients: a review of the literature. Psychooncology. 2013;22(9):1919–29.
25. World Health Organization. International classification of functioning, disability, and health (ICF). Geneva: WHO; 2001.
26. Bornbaum CC, Doyle PC, Skarakis-Doyle E, Theurer JA. A critical exploration of the international classification of functioning, disability, and health (ICF) framework from the perspective of oncology: recommendations for revision. J Multidiscip Healthc. 2013;6:75–86.
27. Jette DU, Halbert J, Iverson C, Miceli E, Shah P. Use of standardized outcome measures in physical therapist practice: perceptions and applications. Phys Ther. 2009;89(2):125–35.
28. Potter K, Fulk GD, Salem Y, Sullivan J. Outcome measures in neurological physical therapy practice, part I: making sound decisions. J Neurol Phys Ther. 2011;35(2):57–64.
29. Karnofsky DA, Burchenal JH. The clinical evaluation of chemotherapeutic agents in cancer. In: McLeod CM, editor. Evaluation of chemotherapeutic agents. New York: Columbia University Press; 1949. p. 191–205.
30. Oken MM, Creech RH, Tormey DC, Horton J, Davis TE, McFadden ET, et al. Toxicity and response criteria of the Eastern Cooperative Oncology Group. Am J Clin Oncol. 1982;5:649–55.
31. Mahoney FI, Barthel D. Functional evaluation: the Barthel Index. Mar St Med J. 1965;14:61–5.
32. Keith RA, Granger CV, Hamilton BB, Sherwin FS. The functional independence measure: a new tool in rehabilitation. Adv Clin Rehabil. 1987;1:6–18.
33. Aaronson NK, Ahmedzai S, Bergman B, Bullinger M, Cull A, Duez NJ, et al. The European organization for research and treatment of cancer QLQ-C30: a quality of life instrument for use in international clinical trials in oncology. J Natl Cancer Inst. 1993;85:365–76.
34. Osoba D, Aaronson NK, Muller M, Sneeuw K, Hsu MA, Yung WK, et al. The development and psychometric validation of a brain cancer quality-of-life questionnaire for use in combination with general cancer-specific questionnaires. Qual Life Res. 1996;5(1):139–50.
35. Taphoorn MJ, Claassens L, Aaronson NK, Coens C, Mauer M, Osoba D, et al. An international validation study of the EORTC brain cancer module (EORTC QLQ-BN20) for assessing health-related quality of life and symptoms in brain cancer patients. Eur J Cancer. 2010;46(6):1033–40.
36. Scott J, Huskisson EC. Graphic representation of pain. Pain. 1976;2:175–84.
37. Keele KD. The pain chart. Lancet. 1948;2:6–8.
38. Downie WW, Leatham PA, Rhind VM, Wright V, Branco JA, Anderson JA. Studies with pain rating scales. Ann Rheum Dis. 1978;37(4):378–81.
39. Melzack R. The McGill Pain Questionnaire: major properties and scoring methods. Pain. 1975;1(3):277–99.
40. Bruera E, Kuehn N, Miller MJ, Selmser P, Macmillan K. The Edmonton Symptom Assessment System (ESAS): a simple method of the assessment of palliative care patients. J Palliat Care. 1991;7:6–9.
41. Overall JE, Gorham DR. The brief psychiatric rating scale. Psychol Rep. 1962;10:799–812.
42. Ownsworth T, Hawkes A, Steginga S, Walker D, Shum D. A biopsychosocial perspective on adjustment and quality of life following brain tumor: a systematic evaluation of the literature. Disabil Rehabil. 2009;31:1038–55.
43. Khan F, Amatya B. Use of the international classification of functioning, disability and health (ICF) to describe patient-reported disability in primary brain tumour in an Australian community cohort. J Rehabil Med. 2013;45(5):434–45.

44. Langbecker D, Yates P. Primary brain tumor patients' supportive care needs and multidisciplinary rehabilitation, community and psychosocial support services: awareness, referral and utilization. J Neurooncol. 2016;127(1):91–102.
45. Khan F, Amatya B, Ng L, Drummond K, Galea M. Multidisciplinary rehabilitation after primary brain tumour treatment. Cochrane Database Syst Rev. 2015;23(8):CD009509.
46. Meyers FJ, Linder J. Simultaneous care: disease treatment and palliative care throughout illness. J Clin Oncol. 2003;21:1412–5.
47. Bartolo M, Zucchella C, Pace A, Lanzetta G, Vecchione C, Bartolo M, et al. Early rehabilitation after surgery improves functional outcome in inpatients with brain tumours. J Neurooncol. 2012;107(3):537–44.
48. Pace A, Metro G, Fabi A. Supportive care in neurooncology. Curr Opin Oncol. 2010;22:621–6.
49. Giordana MT, Clara E. Functional rehabilitation and brain tumour patients. A review of outcome. Neurol Sci. 2006;27:240–4.
50. Wolff G, Toborek M. Targeting the therapeutic effects of exercise on redox-sensitive mechanisms in the vascular endothelium during tumor progression. IUBMB Life. 2013;65(7):565–71.
51. Correa DD. Neurocognitive function in brain tumors. Curr Neurol Neurosci Rep. 2010;10:232–9.
52. Back M, Back E, Kastelan M, Wheeler H. Cognitive deficits in primary brain tumours: a framework for management and rehabilitation. J Cancer Ther. 2014;5:74–81.
53. Taphoorn MJ, Klein M. Cognitive deficits in adult patients with brain tumors. Lancet Neurol. 2004;66:159–68.
54. Giovagnoli AR. Investigation of cognitive impairments in people with brain tumors. J Neurooncol. 2012;108(2):277–83.
55. Martino J, Honma SM, Findlay AM, Guggisberg AG, Owen JP, Kirsch HE, et al. Resting functional connectivity in patients with brain tumors in eloquent areas. Ann Neurol. 2011;69(3):521–32.
56. Harris RJ, Bookheimer SY, Cloughesy TF, Kim HJ, Pope WB, Lai A, et al. Altered functional connectivity of the default mode network in diffuse gliomas measured with pseudo-resting state fMRI. J Neurooncol. 2014;116(2):373–9.
57. Ghumman S, Fortin D, Noel-Lamy M, Cunnane SC, Whittingstall K. Exploratory study of the effect of brain tumors on the default mode network. J Neurooncol. 2016;128(3):437–44.
58. Bahrami N, Seibert TM, Karunamuni R, Bartsch H, Krishnan A, Farid N, et al. Altered network topology in patients with primary brain tumors after fractionated radiotherapy. Brain Connect. 2017;7(5):299–308.
59. Gehrke AK, Baisley MC, Sonck ALB, Wronski SL, Feuerstein M. Neurocognitive deficits following primary brain tumour treatment: systematic review of a decade of comparative studies. J Neurooncol. 2013;115(29):135–42.
60. Day J, Gillespie DC, Rooney AG, Bulbeck HJ, Zienius K, Boele F, et al. Neurocognitive deficits and neurocognitive rehabilitation in adult brain tumours. Curr Treat Options Neurol. 2016;18(5):22.
61. Klein M, Duffau H, Hamer PD. Cognition and resective surgery for diffuse infiltrative glioma: an overview. J Neurooncol. 2012;108:309–18.
62. Piil K, Jarden M, Jakobsen J, Christensen KB, Juhler M. A longitudinal, qualitative and quantitative exploration of daily life and need for rehabilitation among patients with high- grade gliomas and their caregivers. BMJ Open. 2013;3(7):e003183.
63. Sterckx W, Coolbrandt A, Dierckx de Casterlé B, Van den Heede K, Decruyenaere M, Borgenon S, et al. The impact of a high-grade glioma on everyday life: a systematic review from the patient's and caregiver's perspective. Eur J Oncol Nurs. 2013;17(1):107–17.
64. Flechl B, Sax C, Ackerl M, Crevenna R, Woehrer A, Hainfellner J, et al. The course of quality of life and neurocognition in newly diagnosed patients with glioblastoma. Radiother Oncol. 2017;125(2):228–33.
65. Meyers CA, Hess KR. Multifaceted end points in brain tumour clinical trials: cognitive deterioration precedes MRI progression. Neuro Oncol. 2003;5:89–95.

66. Wilson BA. Neuropsychological rehabilitation. Ann Rev Clin Psychol. 2008;4:141–62.
67. Cicerone KD, Langenbahn DM, Braden C, Malec JF, Kalmar K, Fraas M, et al. Evidence-based cognitive rehabilitation: updated review of the literature from 2003 through 2008. Arch Phys Med Rehabil. 2011;92(4):519–30.
68. Bergo E, Lombardi G, Pambuku A, Della Puppa A, Bellu L, D'Avella D, et al. Cognitive rehabilitation in patients with gliomas and other brain tumors: state of the art. Biomed Res Int. 2016;2016:3041824.
69. Chan V, Xiong C, Colantonio A. Patients with brain tumors: who receives postacute occupational therapy services? Am J Occup Ther. 2015;69(2):1–6.
70. Richter A, Woernle CM, Krayenbühl N, Kollias S, Bellut D. Affective symptoms and white matter changes in brain tumor patients. World Neurosurg. 2015;84(4):927–32.
71. Molassiotis A, Wilson B, Brunton L, Chaudhary H, Gattamaneni R, McBain C. Symptom experience in patients with primary brain tumours: a longitudinal exploratory study. Eur J Oncol Nurs. 2010;14:410–6.
72. Rosenblum ML, Kalkanis L, Goldberg W, Rock J, Mikkelsen T, Remer S, et al. Odyssey of hope: a physician's guide to communicating with brain tumor patient across the continuum of care. J Neurooncol. 2009;92:241–51.
73. Janda M, Steginga S, Langbecker D, Dunn J, Walker D, Eakin E. Quality of life among patients with a brain tumor and their carers. J Psychosom Res. 2007;63:617–23.
74. Schubart JR, Kinzie MB, Farace E. Caring for the brain tumor patient: family caregiver burden and unmet needs. Neuro Oncol. 2008;10(1):61–72.
75. Ford E, Catt S, Chalmers A, Fallowfield L. Systematic review of supportive care needs in patients with primary malignant brain tumors. Neuro Oncol. 2012;14:392–404.
76. Fox S, Lantz C. The brain tumor experience and quality of life: a qualitative study. J Neurosci Nurs. 1998;30(4):245–52.
77. Sherwood PR, Cwiklik M, Donovan HS. Neurooncology family caregiving: review and directions for future research. CNS Oncol. 2016;5(1):41–8.
78. Wideheim AK, Edvardsson T, Pählson A, Ahlström G. A family's perspective on living with a highly malignant brain tumor. Cancer Nurs. 2002;25(3):236–44.
79. Schmer C, Ward-Smith P, Latham S, Salacz M. When a family member has a malignant brain tumor: the caregiver perspective. J Neurosci Nurs. 2008;40(2):78–84.
80. Sherwood PR, Given BA, Doorenbos AZ, Given CW. Forgotten voices: lessons from bereaved caregivers of persons with a brain tumour. Int J Palliat Nurs. 2004;10(2):67–75.
81. McConigley R, Halkett G, Lobb E, Novak A. Caring for someone with high grade glioma: a time of rapid change for caregivers. Palliat Med. 2010;24(5):473–9.

Assessment of Neurocognitive Functioning in Clinical Practice and for Trial Purposes

Martin Klein

9.1 Introduction

Patient-oriented outcome measures, such as symptoms, physical functioning, and health-related quality of life, are pertinent outcome measures for patients who cannot be cured of their disease. This is the case for virtually all patients with primary or metastatic brain tumors for whom palliation of symptoms and the maintenance or improvement of health-related quality of life are important goals of treatment earlier or later in the disease trajectory. Brain tumors greatly impact on an individual, as well as their family members and friends. The tumor or its treatment (i.e., chemotherapy, radiation, pharmacological treatment) may directly or indirectly cause neurological impairments that affect the physical, social, vocational, and emotional capabilities of the individual. The available treatment options for both primary and metastatic brain tumors have improved and brought with them modest improved patient survival. Evaluation of treatment in brain tumor patients should therefore not only focus on survival improvement, but should also aim at determining neurological functioning and adverse treatment effects on the normal brain. In this respect, neurocognitive functioning (NCF) is a highly critical outcome measure for brain tumor patients [1]. Apart from a prognostic significance of baseline NCF [2, 3], deterioration in NCF in brain tumor patients may herald tumor progression, even before signs of disease recurrence are evident on CT or MRI [4–6].

Compared to traditional outcome measures like progression-free and overall survival, evaluation of NCF as treatment outcome measure may be time-consuming and burdensome for both the patient and the healthcare professionals involved in the care of these patients. Moreover, given the relatively low incidence of brain tumors

M. Klein (✉)

Department of Medical Psychology, Amsterdam UMC, Vrije Universiteit Amsterdam,
Brain Tumor Center Amsterdam, Amsterdam, The Netherlands
e-mail: m.klein@vumc.nl

© Springer Nature Switzerland AG 2019
M. Bartolo et al. (eds.), *Neurorehabilitation in Neuro-Oncology*,
https://doi.org/10.1007/978-3-319-95684-8_9

and the ultimately fatal outcome of the disease, the interest in NCF emerged relatively late in these patients.

Indices of neurocognitive functioning may be helpful in clinical decision-making for the individual patient in daily practice. In clinical trials for patients with brain tumors, NCF is a useful outcome measure of efficacy and neurotoxicity across experimental treatment arms. Therefore, this chapter will discuss important aspects of assessment of NCF both in clinical practice and for clinical trial purposes.

9.2 Impact of Neurocognitive Deficits on Daily Life

According to Hippocrates (460 BC – 370 BC) "It's far more important to know what person the disease has than what disease the person has." To a large extend this very much applies to patients with primary or metastatic brain tumors. Estimating the impact of neurocognitive deficits on an individual patient's functioning, however, is more complex than measuring survival or tumor response to treatment on imaging, which are considered to be "hard" measures.

One approach to characterize the impact of neurocognitive deficits on daily life is by using the framework of the International Classification of Functioning, Disability, and Health (ICF) developed by the World Health Organization [7]. Unlike traditional medical approaches to health, the ICF framework (see Fig. 9.1) recognizes that a person's level of functioning is the outcome of a dynamic interaction between his or her health condition and the *context* in which an individual functions. Figure 9.1 identifies the three levels of human functioning classified by ICF:

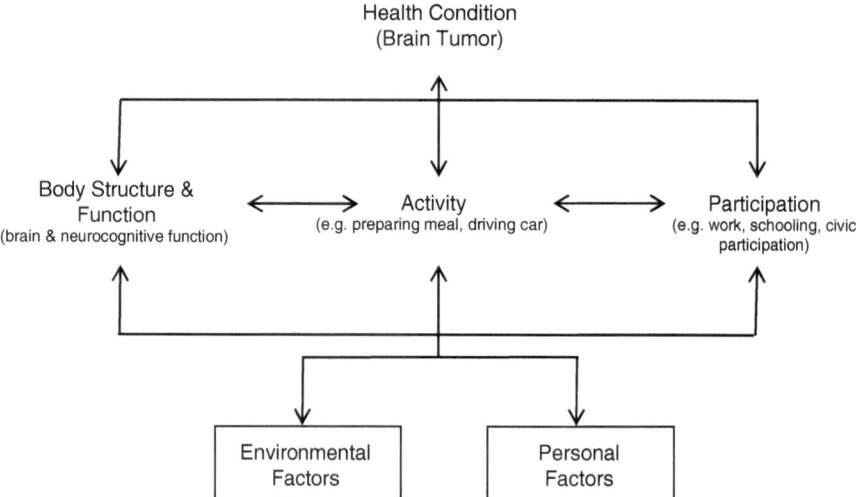

Fig. 9.1 The WHO International Classification of Functioning, Disability, and Health model of functioning

functioning at the level of body or body part, the whole person, and the whole person in his or her context.

Regarding NCF, patient's functioning on the first level, body structure and function (e.g., a memory deficit or generalized neurocognitive decline), can be measured by a comprehensive neuropsychological battery or coarsely by screening instruments like the MMSE [8] or Montreal cognitive assessment (MoCA) [9]. On the second and higher level, patient's *activity* reflects the consequences of the NCF impairment in daily life activities. Agnosia (i.e., failure to recognize a sensory stimulus that is not attributable to dysfunction of peripheral sensory mechanisms or to other cognitive impairments associated with brain damage), for instance, may prevent recognition of kitchen utensils and identification of their use, or impact safety awareness, resulting in significant difficulty carrying out instrumental activities of daily living (IADL). IADLs are tasks that require both motor and neurocognitive skills for successful completion and include more complex everyday tasks such as using the phone, shopping, driving, and managing finances. Since IADL comprises higher order activities, it may identify areas of greater disability and dependency than ADL tasks (e.g., bathing, toileting, dressing, walking, eating). Brain tumor patients who are ADL independent may still be dependent on others for the performance of IADL tasks, suggesting that IADL may represent an early indicator of loss of function in patients with primary brain tumors. Among contextual factors that affect the individual activity level of patients are *environmental factors* (e.g., social support, marital status, living conditions, legal and social structures) and internal *personal factors*, like gender, age, coping styles, social background, education, profession, past and current experiences, character, and other factors that determine how disability is experienced by the individual. Finally, how the activity level affects the patient's well-being and his social interactions may be reflected in the third level—the patient's *participation* level (e.g., the patient who forgets his appointments is forced to stop working and becomes socially isolated). Disability involves dysfunctioning at one or more of these same levels: impairments, activity limitations, and participation restrictions.

While IADL instruments are available for subgroups of neurological patients (e.g., dementia [10], Parkinson's disease [11], and multiple sclerosis [12]), such an instrument specifically addressing issues in patients with primary brain tumors is still under development [13].

Although there are many scales and questionnaires that address the three ICF levels of functioning, ICF is operationalized optimally through the WHO disability assessment schedule (WHODAS 2.0) covering levels of functioning in 6 different major life domains—cognition, mobility, self-care, getting along, life activities (household and work), and participation [14]. These domains directly correspond with ICF's activity and participation dimensions.

It should be noted that the impact of brain tumors on functioning is multifaceted [15]. Brain tumor patients, for example, not only experience the impact of a greatly reduced life expectancy, but at the same time also experience the direct neurological effects of the tumor and treatment on physical, neurocognitive, and behavioral function, not to mention the psychosocial adjustment associated with change in life circumstances [16]. In fact, the psychosocial challenges associated with brain tumors and their treatment range from general behavioral problems to depressive symptoms and poor understanding to more severe symptoms such as personality change and even psychosis [15]. Additionally, cancer and its treatment can alter social roles and limit social activities of patients [17]. As studies of long-term surviving brain tumor patients accumulate, like the international study among 5-year glioblastoma survivors [18], it will become apparent how enduring restrictions in social functioning and participation associated with reduced NCF may be following treatment completion.

9.3   Assessment of Neurocognitive Functioning in Clinical Practice

Neurocognitive deficits in patients with brain tumors, more extensively discussed elsewhere in this volume, can be caused by the tumor, by tumor-related epilepsy and its treatment (surgery, radiotherapy, antiepileptics, chemotherapy, or corticosteroids), and by psychological distress. More likely, a combination of these factors will contribute to neurocognitive dysfunction [1]. Also, local or diffuse tumor regrowth, leptomeningeal metastasis, or metabolic disturbances can negatively affect NCF. While neurological symptoms tend to be specific to the brain structure impacted by disease, individuals with primary or metastatic brain tumors can also present with more generalized symptoms that are not tied to neuropathology in specific brain structures. Such symptoms are common and include headache, seizures, attention deficits, poor memory, impaired reasoning, difficulties with speech and language, visual-perceptual deficits, mood disorders, and fatigue [19]. In a more recent study [20], fatigue, drowsiness, difficulty remembering, disturbed sleep, and distress were the most severe symptoms reported by patients with primary brain tumors, regardless tumor grade. The presence of mood disorders in particular, such as anxiety and depression, can lead to additional complications of their own. That is, mood symptoms have been associated with neurocognitive impairments and fatigue in multiple populations and the effective alleviation of such symptoms is essential to improve overall quality of life.

Comprehensive neurocognitive evaluations in brain tumor patients are usually carried out to address a number of clinical issues. Neurocognitive evaluations might, for instance, be performed to determine the consequences of neurosurgery or the impact of a neurocognitive rehabilitation training program. Neurocognitive evaluations might also be performed to delineate the nature of neurocognitive impairment and its impact on the individual as a means of devising, for instance, a rehabilitation program or offering advice as to an individual's suitability to drive a vehicle or return to the previous employment. Depending on the aim of the referral, specific questions might be addressed to substantiate known risk factors for NCF compromise from the scientific literature: (1) Is there evidence of cognitive decline secondary to radiation therapy? [21] (2) Is there evidence of cognitive decline secondary to chemotherapy or can cancer-related neurocognitive impairment [22] be substantiated?

(3) Is there evidence of neurocognitive decline secondary to tumor recurrence? [23] (4) Does rehabilitation improve (or affect) neurocognitive outcome? [24–26] (5) Can survival be predicted using estimates of baseline neurocognitive functioning? [2, 3] An important consequence of these different goals of assessment is that the crucial features of the assessment process and selection of tests will vary with the goal. It is fairly obvious that the sensitivity to detect small changes in the level of NCF is a much more important characteristic of an instrument used to monitor change as a result of a rehabilitation program, than is the case for a test used purely for diagnostic purposes.

Neuropsychological assessments need to be a cooperative effort between the neuropsychologist and the referring physician, usually the neurologist or neurosurgeon. The referring physician needs to be as specific as possible when formulating the referral questions. Depending on the purpose of testing, pertinent patient information should also be available. This information helps guide the neuropsychologist in the selection of testing materials and approach to the patient:

- The patient's demographic variables (e.g., age, handedness, education/qualifications, current/previous profession, cultural background), in order to set the context for the interpretation of current test performance.
- The patient's previous medical history as well as the current treatment of the tumor (including antiepileptic medication), as this may also be relevant to the development of neurocognitive impairment.
- The results of previous investigations (e.g., neurological examination, EEG, CT/MRI, or functional imaging), and previous (as well as current) psychiatric diagnoses, all of which can assist in the formation of hypotheses about the patient's likely deficits, and so guide the assessment and its interpretation. Since varying degrees of depression in mood and psychiatric symptoms are a frequent accompaniment, or result, of brain tumors, it is important to have this information available. Depression in mood in patients treated for primary intracranial tumors is associated with high levels of physical disability and neurocognitive dysfunction.
- The results of previous neuropsychological assessments—these can guide the choice of current tests and permit evaluation of change.

In the clinical setting there is no standard battery of tests specific for brain tumors. Although test selection ultimately depends on the referral questions, common neuropsychological domains to be assessed include (1) attention/concentration, (2) language (receptive and expressive), (3) memory/learning, (4) visual-perceptual/spatial skills, (5) executive functions, and (6) mood/personality variables.

If testing is to be conducted in the clinical setting, the patient's schedule needs to include blocks of time when no other clinical tests are scheduled (e.g., radiology, discharge planning) so that the patient may be tested without interruptions and when maximally alert and attentive. After the assessment is completed, but before submitting the written report, the neuropsychologist generally contacts the referring physician to provide preliminary feedback. The written report, delivered shortly thereafter, should be brief but complete, including a listing of the tests administered, some form of score report, usually a percentile or standard score for each test, a summary of the findings, and an interpretation of these findings. The brevity of the report depends on the nature of the referral and the questions the referring physician has posed.

Because neurocognitive assessments are not always feasible, several alternatives to the use of formal neurocognitive testing have been tried. These include self-reports of NCF asking about memory, attention, etc. or on how NCF affects daily life—IADL, which can be reliable in patients with low-grade gliomas without or with only mild NCF deficits [27], but tends to be invalid in brain tumor patients with serious neurocognitive deficits and thus often cannot accurately evaluate their own performance. Furthermore, self-perceived NCF seems to be more related to depression than to the results of objective neurocognitive tests [28]. Therefore, subjective data on NCF (e.g., obtained from self-report questionnaires like the six-item medical outcome studies NCF scale) [29] should be interpreted with caution and alongside objective assessments.

When self-reported NCF of outpatients may be difficult to interpret because of disease, or treatment-related decrements in self-awareness, reports of neurocognitive changes made by the partner or a proxy may offer an alternative to neurocognitive testing. Informants can provide important information about the areas to be explored in the neuropsychological assessment, although it should be noted that patient-proxy agreement tends to be lower in patients with neurocognitive deficits than in cognitively intact patients [30]. Nevertheless, this is one of the most common methods for measuring IADLs, and a large number of potentially useful informant-based questionnaires exist, such as the Lawton-Brody IADL scale [31], the Bristol ADL scale [32], and the more recently developed Amsterdam IADL questionnaire [10].

The choice of which particular method of assessment to be used will depend, in addition to practical considerations such as time, on the purpose of the assessment. Real-word observations and performance-based measures provide information about what the person is capable of doing. Questionnaires and other self-reports, on the other hand, measure what the individual is actually doing in his or her day-to-day life.

9.4 Assessment of Neurocognitive Functioning in Clinical Trials

Hippocrates, an early proponent of personalized medicine, wrote about the "individuality" of disease and the importance of prescription of "different" medicines to "different" patients. To help his decision-making when prescribing treatment, Hippocrates assessed several factors, such as a patient's constitution, age, and build, and the time of year to help his decision-making when prescribing treatment.

Failure of conventional therapy to control brain tumors and the recognition of molecular heterogeneity of brain tumors at the genetic, proteomic, and epigenetic levels raised stresses the need for a more personalized approach to treatment development. Interestingly, isocitrate dehydrogenase 1 (IDH1), a key metabolic enzyme that converts isocitrate to α-ketoglutarate, is both a prognostic factor of treatment efficacy in patients with low-grade gliomas and secondary glioblastomas and a factor affecting NCF functioning. In a recent study [33], it was hypothesized that patients with malignant gliomas and the IDH1-wild-type (IDH1-WT) would have poorer NCF compared with those with IDH1-mutant (IDH1-M) tumors. IDH1-WT tumors are more proliferative and aggressive and thus their lesion momentum will be higher than IDH1-M tumors, potentially limiting the potential for plastic reorganization and resulting in more frequent and severe impairment of NCF. Indeed, this is what they found: significantly more pronounced NCF deficits in patients with IDH1-WT tumors than in patients with IDH-M tumors. Interestingly, while tumor size did not differ between IDH1-WT and IDH-M tumor patient groups, there was a lack of correlation between tumor size and NCF deficits in the IDH1-mutated group, confirming that the most important issue is the different pattern of tumor growth. Given these findings, stratifying patients based on their tumor subtype in clinical trials incorporating NCF as primary or secondary outcome measure needs to be considered [34].

If NCF is an important outcome measure in brain tumor clinical trials, the use of comprehensive series of tests has advantages in that it allows for the collection of vast amounts of information on neurocognitive status in a highly standardized manner. These series cover neurocognitive domains representing functions of both the dominant and the non-dominant hemisphere (see Table 9.1 for commonly used tests) [6, 35, 36]. However, the time required for a complete assessment is time-consuming and may fatigue patients with brain tumors, thereby influencing results. Moreover, compliance of both patients and investigators may decrease significantly because of time-consuming procedures, which makes the test results unrepresentative of the trial population. Exclusion of patients at the lower end of the neurocognitive spectrum from analyses obviously introduces undesirable bias in the evaluation of patients' NCF during experimental treatments. Alternatives like IQ measurement or a screening tool like the mini-mental state examination [8] are less adequate for neurologically intact adults with brain tumors. Although the MMSE is the most commonly used mental status test and might have prognostic value for progression-free and overall survival of patients with low-grade gliomas [37], it has a number of limitations [38, 39]. First, one must accept the basic limitation of any screening battery. Since the test has a limited number of questions, adequate testing of cognitive function is not possible. Practically, however, the MMSE score is used as an indicator of intact or impaired performance. The cutoff score of 24 is associated with relatively high false-negative rates (test indicates the absence of impairment when impairment is present) and relatively high false-positive rates (test indicates impairment when no impairment is present). Given its limited sensitivity, declines on the MMSE may be underestimates of the proportion of patients with true decline; subtle changes in cognition related to tumor and/or treatment effects on cognition may thus be missed. Additionally, MMSE scores are affected by educational level, race, and gender. Despite these limitations, the MMSE provides a "quick-and-dirty"

Table 9.1 Neuropsychological tests commonly used in brain tumor patients

Perception/information processing

Line Bisection Test. A device for measuring unilateral neglect, which is usually a sequel of massive right hemisphere lesions.

Benton Facial Recognition Test. This task was designed to detect impairment in the discrimination of faces, a disorder associated with right hemisphere lesions. Since both the target and matching face are seen together, memory requirements are minimized.

Judgment of Line Orientation Test. A test of spatial judgment, also designed to detect right hemisphere dysfunction.

Digit Symbol. This test provides a measure of psychomotor performance that is relatively unaffected by intellectual prowess. This test may not be appropriate for patients with marked motor impairment. A variant of this test is available that requires a verbal response only, thus decreasing motoric demands.

Grooved Pegboard Test. It assesses motor speed and dexterity (dominant and non-dominant hand)

Memory

Rey Auditory Verbal Learning Test. This test provides information on immediate verbal memory, rate of learning, occurrence of retroactive and proactive interference, delayed recall, and recognition.

Hopkins Verbal Learning Test, which is a list of 12 words in 3 semantic categories that measures immediate recall across 3 trials, recognition of the words from distractors, and delayed recall.

Working Memory Task. This task is designed to measure the speed of memory processes and involves working on short-term memory.

Attention and executive function

Stroop Color–Word Test. This test is a selective attention task aiming at measuring interference susceptibility.

Categoric Word Fluency Task. A simple task requiring the generation of words from specific semantic categories within a limited time.

Controlled Oral Word Association, which requires the production of words beginning over a specific letter for three 1-min trials.

Trail Making Test. This test predominantly measures functions associated with executive function. The Trail Making Test is highly dependent upon motor speed, and may not be appropriate for brain tumor patients with marked motor impairment.

Digit Span, which requires the repetition of numbers forward and backward.

Brief Test of Attention. Designed to assess the severity of attentional impairment among nonaphasic hearing adult patients.

Premorbid estimates of intellectual functioning

National Adult Reading Test. This test relies on current performance of reading ability or vocabulary knowledge to estimate premorbid abilities. Both reading ability and vocabulary knowledge tend to be less affected by brain damage than other cognitive abilities. By using these abilities to estimate premorbid IQ, the examiner is able to get an estimate of a lower-bound to previous IQ.

Barona Index. Weighted composite score on the basis of age, gender, race, residence, education, and occupation.

Depending on availability of specific tests, normative data, and ease of administration many local modifications of these tests are in use. The suggested definition of cognitive impairment to be used in clinical trials is a test score ±1.5 SDs worse than the mean of a given test's normative age-adjusted distribution, and when available gender and education-adjusted distribution assessment of overall cognitive function, and in most contexts a score of 22 or lower is considered an accurate mark of clinically significant cognitive impairment as is usually the case in patients with tumor progression [5].

Since a combination of cortical and subcortical lesions, epilepsy, surgery, radiotherapy, AEDs, corticosteroids, and psychological distress is likely to contribute to neurocognitive dysfunctioning in an individually unpredictable way, it would be most pragmatic to choose a core clinical trial testing battery that gauges a broad range of neurocognitive functions. Additionally, the neuropsychological measures have to meet the following criteria: (1) assess several domains found to be most sensitive to tumor and treatment effects; (2) have standardized materials and administration procedures; (3) have published normative data; (4) have moderate to high test–retest reliability; (5) have alternate forms or are relatively insensitive to practice effects, and are therefore suitable to monitor changes in neurocognitive function over time; (6) include tests that have been translated into several languages (i.e., Catalan, Dutch, English (UK and US), French (France and Canada), German, Hebrew, Italian, Spanish (Spain and the USA), Turkish) or require translation primarily of test directions; and (7) total administration time is 30–40 min. The neurocognitive domains deemed essential to be evaluated include attention, executive functions, verbal memory, and motor speed. The test battery that meets most of the afore-mentioned criteria has successfully been used and is still being used in a number of EORTC, NCCTG, NCI-C, RTOG, MRC, and HUB multisite clinical trials. This battery assesses: memory, Hopkins verbal learning test [40], which is a list of 12 words in 3 semantic categories that measure immediate recall across 3 trials, recognition of the words from distractors, and delayed recall; verbal fluency, controlled oral word association [41], which requires the production of words beginning over a specific letter for three 1-min trials; visual-motor scanning speed, trail making test part A [42], which requires the subject to connect dots in numerical order as rapidly as possible; executive function, trail making test part B [42], which requires the subject to connect dots with alternating numbers and letters as rapidly as possible. Evidently, local modifications of this battery can be made by adding tests depending on the goal of the neuropsychological assessment. Data that can thus be gathered systematically both for clinical and research purposes, additionally facilitate comparisons over patient groups and/or treatment regimens.

9.5   Conclusion

With the development in treatment options for brain tumor patients, neurocognitive functioning is an increasingly important outcome measure, next to traditional measures as progression-free and overall survival, because neurocognitive impairments can have a large impact on self-care, social, and professional functioning, and consequently on health-related quality of life. New treatment options and combinations of standard treatments for brain tumor patients warrant the further use of NCF as outcome measure to guide the physician in clinical decision-making and in determining the treatment-related neurotoxicity in clinical trials. In long-term surviving patients with brain tumors assessment of NCF has also become crucial because the prevention of side effects of brain tumor treatment is becoming another challenge now that subgroups of these patients live longer. Likewise, concerted action into studying the costs and benefits of neurocognitive assessments related to outcome of these patients is warranted.

References

1. Taphoorn MJB, Klein M. Cognitive deficits in adult patients with brain tumours. Lancet Neurol. 2004;3:159–68.
2. Klein M, Postma TJ, Taphoorn MJB, et al. The prognostic value of cognitive functioning in the survival of patients with high-grade glioma. Neurology. 2003;61:1796–9.
3. Johnson DR, Sawyer AM, Meyers CA, O'Neill BP, Wefel JS. Early measures of cognitive function predict survival in patients with newly diagnosed glioblastoma. Neuro-oncology. 2012;14:808–16.
4. Armstrong CL, Goldstein B, Shera D, Ledakis GE, Tallent EM. The predictive value of longitudinal neuropsychologic assessment in the early detection of brain tumor recurrence. Cancer. 2003;97:649–56.
5. Brown PD, Jensen AW, Felten SJ, et al. Detrimental effects of tumor progression on cognitive function of patients with high-grade glioma. J Clin Oncol. 2006;24:5427–33.
6. Meyers CA, Hess KR. Multifaceted end points in brain tumor clinical trials: cognitive deterioration precedes MRI progression. Neuro-oncology. 2003;5:89–95.
7. World Health Organization. International classification of functioning, disability and health: ICF. Geneva, Switzerland: WHO; 2001.
8. Folstein MF, Folstein SE, McHugh PR. Mini-mental state: a practical method for grading the cognitive state for the clinician. J Psychiatric Res. 1975;12:189–98.
9. Nasreddine ZS, Phillips NA, Bedirian V, et al. The Montreal cognitive assessment, MoCA: a brief screening tool for mild cognitive impairment. J Am Geriatrics Soc. 2005;53:695–9.
10. Sikkes SA, de Lange-de Klerk ES, Pijnenburg YA, et al. A new informant-based questionnaire for instrumental activities of daily living in dementia. Alzheimers Dement. 2012;8:536–43.
11. Brennan L, Siderowf A, Rubright JD, et al. The Penn Parkinson's daily activities questionnaire-15: psychometric properties of a brief assessment of cognitive instrumental activities of daily living in Parkinson's disease. Parkinsonism Relat Disord. 2016;25:21–6.
12. Hohol MJ, Orav EJ, Weiner HL. Disease steps in multiple sclerosis: a simple approach to evaluate disease progression. Neurology. 1995;45:251–5.
13. Oort Q, Dirven L, Meijer W, et al. Development of a questionnaire measuring instrumental activities of daily living (IADL) in patients with brain tumors: a pilot study. J Neuro-Oncol. 2017;132:145–53.
14. Ustun TB, Chatterji S, Kostanjsek N, et al. Developing the World Health Organization disability assessment schedule 2.0. Bull World Health Organ. 2010;88:815–23.
15. Ownsworth T, Hawkes A, Steginga S, Walker D, Shum D. A biopsychosocial perspective on adjustment and quality of life following brain tumor: a systematic evaluation of the literature. Disabil Rehabil. 2009;31:1038–55.
16. Lidstone V, Butters E, Seed PT, et al. Symptoms and concerns amongst cancer outpatients: identifying the need for specialist palliative care. Palliat Med. 2003;17:588–95.
17. Syrjala KL, Stover AC, Yi JC, Artherholt SB, Abrams JR. Measuring social activities and social function in long-term cancer survivors who received hematopoietic stem cell transplantation. Psycho-Oncology. 2010;19:462–71.
18. Happold C, Felsberg J, Clarke J, et al. Molecular genetic, host-derived and clinical determinants of long-term survival in glioblastoma: first results from the Brain Tumor Funders'

Collaborative Consortium. In: 22nd annual scientific meeting and education day of the society for neuro-oncology. November 16–19 2017, San Francisco, CA.

19. Gilbert M, Armstrong T, Meyers C. Issues in assessing and interpreting quality of life in patients with malignant glioma. Semin Oncol. 2000;27:20–6.

20. Armstrong TS, Vera-Bolanos E, Acquaye AA, et al. The symptom burden of primary brain tumors: evidence for a core set of tumor- and treatment-related symptoms. Neuro Oncology. 2016;18:252–60.

21. Makale MT, McDonald CR, Hattangadi-Gluth JA, Kesari S. Mechanisms of radiotherapy-associated cognitive disability in patients with brain tumours. Nat Rev Neurol. 2017;13:52–64.

22. Vannorsdall TD. Cognitive changes related to cancer therapy. Med Clin N Am. 2017;101:1115–34.

23. Bosma I, Vos MJ, Heimans JJ, et al. The course of neurocognitive functioning in high-grade glioma patients. Neuro-oncology. 2007;9:53–62.

24. Hassler MR, Elandt K, Preusser M, et al. Neurocognitive training in patients with high-grade glioma: a pilot study. J Neuro-Oncol. 2010;97:109–15.

25. Gehring K, Sitskoorn MM, Gundy CM, et al. Cognitive rehabilitation in patients with gliomas: a randomized, controlled trial. J Clin Oncol. 2009;27:3712–22.

26. Gehring K, Aaronson NK, Taphoorn MJ, Sitskoorn MM. Interventions for cognitive deficits in patients with a brain tumor: an update. Expert Rev Anticancer Ther. 2010;10:1779–95.

27. Boele FW, Zant M, Heine ECE, et al. The association between cognitive functioning and health-related quality of life in low-grade glioma patients. Neuro-Oncol Pract. 2014;1:40–6.

28. Cull A, Hay C, Love SB, et al. What do cancer patients mean when they complain of concentration and memory problems? Br J Cancer. 1996;74:1674–9.

29. Stewart AL, Ware JE, editors. Measuring functioning and well-being: the medical outcomes study approach. Durham, NC: Duke University Press; 1992.

30. Ediebah DE, Reijneveld JC, Taphoorn MJ, et al. Impact of neurocognitive deficits on patient-proxy agreement regarding health-related quality of life in low-grade glioma patients. Qual Life Res. 2017;26:869–80.

31. Lawton MP, Brody EM. Assessment of older people: self-maintaining and instrumental activities of daily living. Gerontologist. 1969;9:179–86.

32. Bucks RS, Haworth J. Bristol activities of daily living scale: a critical evaluation. Expert Rev Neurother. 2002;2:669–76.

33. Wefel JS, Noll KR, Rao G, Cahill DP. Neurocognitive function varies by IDH1 genetic mutation status in patients with malignant glioma prior to surgical resection. Neuro Oncology. 2016;18:1656–63.

34. Klein M. Lesion momentum as explanation for preoperative neurocognitive function in patients with malignant glioma. Neuro-oncology. 2016;18:1595–6.

35. Correa DD, Maron L, Harder H, et al. Cognitive functions in primary central nervous system lymphoma: literature review and assessment guidelines. Ann Oncol. 2007;18:1145–51.

36. Klein M, Taphoorn MJ, Heimans JJ, et al. Neurobehavioral status and health-related quality of life in newly diagnosed high-grade glioma patients. J Clin Oncol. 2001;19:4037–47.

37. Brown PD, Buckner JC, O'Fallon JR, et al. Importance of baseline mini-mental state examination as a prognostic factor for patients with low-grade glioma. Int J Radiat Oncol Biol Phys. 2004;59:117–25.

38. Meyers CA, Wefel JS. The use of the mini-mental state examination to assess cognitive functioning in cancer trials: no ifs, ands, buts, or sensitivity. J Clin Oncol. 2003;21:3557–8.

39. Klein M, Heimans JJ. The measurement of cognitive functioning in low-grade glioma patients after radiotherapy. J Clin Oncol. 2004;22:966–7.

40. Benedict RHB, Schretlen D, Groninger L, Brandt J. Hopkins verbal learning test–revised: normative data and analysis of inter-form and test-retest reliability. Clin Neuropsychol. 1998;12:43–55.

41. Benton AL, Hamsher K. Multilingual aphasia examination. Iowa City: AJA Associates; 1989.

42. Lezak MD, Howieson DB, Loring DW. Neuropsychological assessment. New York: Oxford University Press; 2004.

Cognitive Rehabilitation

10

Chiara Zucchella

10.1 Epidemiology of Cognitive Disorders in Brain Tumours

In the last decades in western countries, the advances in diagnostic and therapeutic options have extended average life expectancies of neuro-oncological population [1]; specifically for patients affected by low to intermediate grade tumours the expected survival may reach 10–15 years, while for patients diagnosed with glioblastoma multiforme the median survival has increased to 18–24 months from 9 to 12 months in the years before the introduction of temozolomide in 2006 [2–4].

As survival has improved, long-term treatment and disease-related morbidity has gained more attention and cognitive dysfunction has been recognized as the most frequent complication among long-term survivors [5–7]. A growing literature in fact shows that impairment of cognitive functions, such as psychomotor slowing, attention and memory (working memory) deficits, executive dysfunction (cognitive control and flexibility, planning, and foresight) or focal deficits such as aphasia or apraxia may occur in most patients with brain tumours (BT) [8–11].

Rates of patients suffering from cognitive disorders evaluated through neuropsychological test assessments range from 29% in patients with non-irradiated low-grade glioma (LGG) to 50–90% in patients with diverse BT [12–16]. The lack of homogeneity in study populations and treatments as well as methodological issues such as the insensitivity of the assessment methods used, the duration of follow-up, the variability of normative data used to detect patients with cognitive impairments explain the variability of literature data.

Although the pathophysiology of cognitive impairment is not completely understood, several causes have been recognized, suggesting a multifactorial aetiology of neuropsychological deficits [5, 17–18].

First of all, the tumour itself, tumour progression, tumour-related neurological complications such as epilepsy can cause cognitive deficits. Although tumour type or

C. Zucchella (✉)
Neurology A – Verona University Hospital, Verona, Italy

© Springer Nature Switzerland AG 2019
M. Bartolo et al. (eds.), *Neurorehabilitation in Neuro-Oncology*,
https://doi.org/10.1007/978-3-319-95684-8_10

volume has not always been found to predict cognitive performance [19], cognitive impairments have been detected more frequently at diagnosis in rapid-growing tumours such as glioblastomas than in slow-growing ones such as LGG [20]. Nevertheless, recent literature underlined that also LGG can't be considered "tumour mass" as reported in the classic literature; instead, they represent an infiltrating chronic disease that invades the central nervous system, especially the subcortical connectivity known to be critical for brain and cognitive functions [21, 22]. Moreover, deficits in cognitive functions may indicate tumour recurrence, even before structural changes are evident on computerized tomography or magnetic resonance imaging [23, 24].

Apart from the tumour itself, also medical treatments contribute largely to the cognitive side effects: a wide literature in fact has documented that surgery, radiotherapy, chemotherapy, and antiepileptic drugs can all have adverse effects on cognitive functioning [5]. Cognitive impairments due to the damage to tumour surrounding tissue after surgical resection have been reported to be mild and transient in most cases [25]; however, the paucity of studies including pre- and post-surgical cognitive evaluations prevents from drawing definitive conclusions about the effect of surgery on cognitive functioning. Conversely, treatment-related neurotoxicity has been more widely explored. Radiation encephalopathy has been classified into three phases depending on the between the administration of radiotherapy and symptoms onset [26]. Actually, in a few days after the beginning of radiotherapy, acute radiation encephalopathy may occur, producing headache, somnolence, and worsening of pre-existing neurological deficits; similarly, within the first 6 months after completion of radiotherapy, early delayed radiation encephalopathy may develop. In both cases however, a return to normal baseline has been described. Conversely, late-delayed encephalopathy is an irreversible and serious disorder, occurring several months to many years after radiotherapy, that can manifest as local radionecrosis or diffuse leucoencephalopathy and cerebral atrophy. Cognitive disturbances are the hallmark of the diffuse encephalopathy [27–30]. Chemotherapy-related cognitive impairment, referred to as "chemobrain" (or chemofog), is the most widely reported source of cognitive deficits in neuro-oncological population. Animal models suggest vulnerability of neural stem cells to specific chemotherapy agents (carmustine, cisplatin, cytarabine, and methotrexate) with resultant cognitive deterioration [31, 32]; moreover, demyelination, inflammation, and microvascular injury have all been postulated as mechanisms underlying neurotoxicity of therapy [33, 34]. Combined injury may occur with concomitant or sequential administration of brain radiotherapy and chemotherapy because of alterations in blood brain barrier permeability and drug distributions.

Finally, the impact of emotional disturbances can't be neglected as emotional distress may affect attention, vigilance, and motivation, subsequently impairing cognitive performance [35].

10.2   Cognitive Impairments: Function, Participation, and Quality of Life

Although the severity of cognitive difficulty varies among patients, even the slightest deterioration in cognitive function can be devastating for the patient's quality of life (QOL), interfering with the patient's ability to function at premorbid levels professionally and socially and therefore resulting in loss of functional independence [18]. The limited ability to undertake activities of daily living, reduced autonomy and inability to return to work may create an even greater restriction than a physical disability [36]. According to the International Classification of Functioning, Disability and Health proposed by the World Health Organization [37], functioning should be considered at three perspectives: body, person, and societal. At the most basic level, a problem in body function or structure is noted as *impairment* (i.e., cognitive impairment such as memory deficits, dysexecutive syndrome…) as a result of disease or injury. At the personal level, the patient's *activity limitations* reflect the consequences of the impairment in daily life (i.e., the patient with cognitive deficits is unable to remember things, to plan activities, to produce or to understand verbal messages…), whereas patient's *participation restrictions* reflects how the disability affects the patient's social interactions (i.e., the patient who suffers from cognitive impairments will be forced to leave work, school…).

Therefore the comprehensive concept of health-related QOL (HRQOL) that covers physical, psychological, and social domains, as well as symptoms induced by the disease and its treatment has been proposed to fully describe patients' functioning and well-being [38, 39]. In fact it is increasingly recognized that the benefits of treatments have to be carefully weighed against the side effects they produce [40] and that measures of HRQOL are important (secondary) outcome measure in clinical trials for BT patients, complementing traditional measures of survival or disease stability [41–43].

Considering the limited survival of neuro-oncological patients, this is an even more urgent issue.

10.3   Cognitive Rehabilitation

10.3.1 Main Features

In broad terms, rehabilitation principally focuses on the improvement of functioning and quality of life. While other branches of health care aim at the prevention and treatment of the disease, rehabilitation assumes that disability may be reduced even in presence of a permanent injury or chronic disease. Therefore, according to McLellan [44] rehabilitation may be defined as "an interactive process whereby people who are disabled by injury or disease work together with professional staff, relatives, and members of the wider community to achieve their optimum physical, psychological, social, and vocational well-being".

Despite most of rehabilitative studies and techniques addressed motor disability, rehabilitation is not only limited to improving physical deficits: Cognitive rehabilitation (CR) aims at enhancing cognitive functioning and independence through interventions that reduce the impairments or lessen the disabling impact of those impairments [45–48].

Differences among definitions of CR depend on theoretical differences regarding the underlying cognitive mechanisms that result in functional and behavioural deficits as well as on the contents of treatments. However, some basic distinctions, despite not mutually exclusive, are common among the different approaches, including modular versus comprehensive, restorative (or remedial) versus compensative (or adaptive), and contextualized versus decontextualized approaches.

In *modular* approach usually the intervention focuses on the treatment of specific cognitive disturbances, while the term *comprehensive* approach refers to the treatments of patients suffering with multiple impairments (both cognitive and emotional or behavioural) by means of a combination of modular cognitive treatments as well as interventions addressing self-awareness of the impact of cognitive deficits and cognitive-behavioural intervention for emotional disturbances. This latter holistic approach is defined "neuropsychological rehabilitation" that, according to the definition proposed by Wilson [49], is broader than cognitive rehabilitation, as it is concerned with the amelioration of cognitive, emotional, psychosocial, and behavioural deficits caused by an insult to the brain.

Restorative interventions focus on the cause rather than the effect of a deficit and are aimed at reducing the severity of the deficit, enhancing (or normalizing if possible) specific impaired cognitive functions. These kind of interventions usually are based on the direct training of the impaired function through the repetitive and intensive use of exercises with growing levels of complexity and cognitive demands. Conversely, *adaptive or compensatory* therapies don't aim to correct the underlying deficit but to minimize its impact on everyday activities through the development of compensatory strategies or through the use of tools and aids to overcome the impairment [50, 51]. Ideally, the possibility to restore functions represents an appealing option affecting a broad range of activities damaged by the same impairment; on the contrary, compensatory strategies tend to be linked to specific activities, representing therefore more local solutions (although sometimes the only ones realistically achievable).

Finally, the distinction between contextualized versus decontextualized approaches refers to the degree in which they take place in the real world and use materials, activities, and tasks related to patient's everyday life. While *decontextualized* interventions are simpler to standardize but are more "artificial", *contextualized* approaches are more likely to enhance motivation and improve patient's self-awareness because they deal with personally relevant tasks within a familiar environment. Establishing meaningful and functionally relevant goals for rehabilitation linked to day-to-day activities represents a key point to restore patient's social participation.

Obviously, these attributes of CR are not mutually exclusive but can be combined in different ways: modular treatments, for example, may be aimed to either restoration or compensation as well as they can also be either contextualized or decontextualized; in any case, each patient should be carefully evaluated before starting the intervention in order to plan realistic rehabilitation goals, identify priorities for intervention, evaluate progress, break rehabilitation down into achievable steps, resulting in better outcomes [52]. Additionally as described by Sohlberg and Mateer [53] "there should be an emphasis to provide functional endpoints to a rehabilitation programme, so that impact on activities of daily living can be optimized. The ultimate measure of success of any cognitive rehabilitation program is

Table 10.1 Main components of cognitive rehabilitation

Component	Contents and aims
Education	Improvement of patient's understanding of the problem and its consequences as well as enhancement of awareness of cognitive weaknesses and strengths.
Process training	Improvement of skills through direct retraining of the impaired cognitive abilities to restore functions.
Strategy training	Use of environmental, internal, and external strategies to compensate the existing deficits, favouring an effective adaptation.
Functional activities training	Application of the other three components in everyday life to favour generalization of the improvements to activity of daily living.

Modified from Society of Cognitive Rehabilitation

improvement in an individual's ability to manage work, daily living or leisure activities, not simply on practiced therapy tasks".

Table 10.1 summarizes the main components of CR according to the Society for Cognitive Rehabilitation [54].

10.3.2 Literature Evidence

Despite CR programmes have been proven to be effective in the treatment of cognitive deficits in various populations of patients with neurological disorders, including those with traumatic brain injury, stroke, neurodegenerative disease, mainly Alzheimer's disease [48], few studies have investigated strategies to prevent or treat cognitive deficits in patients with BT [1, 55], likely because they are not seen as potential candidates due to their poor prognosis.

A single case study of a patient who suffered from cognitive deficits after right temporal lobectomy for an astrocytoma was the first report of a cognitive rehabilitation intervention in neuro-oncological patients [56]. After a 4-month intervention combining cognitive retraining with psychoeducational and compensation techniques, improvements were observed on follow-up neuropsychological data, behavioural observations made by the patient's wife, and efficiency on work-related tasks.

Subsequently, preliminary support for the effectiveness of postacute brain injury rehabilitation in the management of neuro-oncological patients was offered by a retrospective study published in 1997. Sherer and colleagues [57] showed that after an average of 2.6 ± 1.9 months of vocational rehabilitation performed both in individual and group sessions, primary BT outpatients enjoyed favourable community independence and employment outcomes. Moreover, gains made during treatment were generally maintained at follow-up evaluations performed an average of 8 months after discharge.

In the randomized controlled 2-week trial by Locke et al. [58] 13 pairs of BT patients and their caregivers underwent a combined cognitive-rehabilitation and problem-solving therapy intervention. After receiving the intervention, 88% of patients were able to learn the study specific strategies and to continue using the strategies to some degree at the follow-up after 3 months. Also, 88% of those who received the intervention described it as helpful and indicated that they would recommend the intervention to other patients. Caregivers were similarly enthusiastic about the intervention strategies.

In a Dutch trial 140 patients with LGG and anaplastic gliomas, clinically stable (i.e., without any evidence of disease progression) for a minimum of 6 months before study entry, were recruited from 11 hospitals in the Netherlands and randomly assigned to an intervention group or to a waiting-list control group [59]. The intervention consisted of six weekly, individual sessions of 2 h each and included both computer-based attention retraining and compensatory skills training of attention, memory, and executive functioning. The weekly therapy sessions were combined with homework tasks including computer-based attention retraining exercises and of logs kept about experiences with applying compensatory strategies in daily life. The waiting-list control group received usual care and contact with the research staff was at similar intervals as the intervention group. At the immediate post-treatment evaluation, statistically significant intervention effects were observed for measures of subjective cognitive functioning and perceived burden, while at the 6-month follow-up, the intervention group performed significantly better on tests of attention and verbal memory and reported less mental fatigue.

In 2010 Hassler and colleagues [60] performed a small pilot study involving 11 patients with high-grade gliomas (HGG) to evaluate the effectiveness of 10 weekly group training sessions of 90 minutes, according to an holistic mnemonic training in which all aspects of mental activity were separately addressed, using exercises to train perception, concentration, attention, memory, retentiveness, verbal memory, and creativity. In the intervention group, comparison of mean group differences between baseline and at post-training evaluation after 12 weeks revealed improvement across all neurocognitive variables, especially attention and memory skills.

These positive results were further confirmed by an Italian randomized trial published in 2013 [61] that included 58 patients with primary BT who were randomly assigned to a rehabilitation group or to a control group, early after surgery. The intervention consisted of 16 one-hour individual sessions of therapist-guided cognitive training, spread over 4 weeks, combining computer exercises (remedial approach) and metacognitive training (compensatory approach). Patients in the control group received usual care without cognitive training. At the end of the intervention patients in the rehabilitation group showed a significant improvement of cognitive functions, especially in attentive and mnesic domains, while the control group exhibited only a slight, not statistically relevant, enhancement of cognitive performances.

To investigate whether virtual reality (VR) training will help the recovery of cognitive function in BT patients, a Korean group of researchers enrolled 38 patients with cognitive impairment who were randomly assigned to either VR group ($n = 19$) or control group ($n = 19$) [62]. Both VR training (30 min a day for 3 times a week) and computer-based cognitive rehabilitation program (30 min a day for 2 times) for 4 weeks were given to the VR group. The control group was given only the computer-based cognitive rehabilitation program (30 min a day for 5 days a week) for 4 weeks.

The VR group showed significantly ($p < 0.05$) better improvements than the control group in attentive measures, memory tests, and concentration, suggesting that VR training can have beneficial effects on cognitive improvement.

In the observational pilot study carried out by Maschio et al. [63] 16 patients affected by primary BT or cerebral metastases and tumour-related epilepsy performed a computerized remedial training consisting in one weekly individual session of 1 h, for a total of 10 weeks. Patients were evaluated with the same battery of tests used at baseline, directly after cognitive rehabilitation (T1), and at 6-month follow-up (T2). Statistical analysis showed that short-term verbal memory, episodic memory, fluency and long-term visuospatial memory improved immediately after the T1 and remained stable at T2.

Finally, Lo Buono et al. [64] described the effectiveness of a rehabilitative training based on cognitive retraining and motivational techniques performed by a young man after the removal and the treatment of a fibrillary grade II astrocytoma. After 3 months of training (2 times/week for a total of 24 sessions) the authors documented an improvement in memory, attention, shifting, and visual activities, in writing and reading, and in the ability to access the linguistic register.

The considered studies highlight the extreme heterogeneity of the available approaches that are included under the broad term of CR as well as the differences regarding the study design, the number of patients included in the trials, the diagnosis and the phase of the disease, and the measures used to assess cognitive functions and to evaluate the outcome. Despite such dissimilarity, all studies found evidence that CR was more effective than no rehabilitation or control to improve cognitive functions of BT patients, suggesting the need for further well-conceptualized, executed, and reported randomized controlled trials to clarify which are the most effective approach and the patients who can benefit from the intervention. Last but not least, also the impact of CR on daily function and quality of life is an urgent issue to deal with: in fact even highly efficacious treatments may induce enhancement only on specific measures of the targeted impairment but may fail to show improvement in real-world activities, participation or quality of life, resulting therefore scarcely useful. Actually some cognitive interventions appear to be more concerned with improving test scores than with reducing everyday problems [65], likely assuming that reducing impairments will reduce everyday problems. To date, however, there is little evidence that this actually happens [66].

The main results and limitations of the above-mentioned studies are listed in Table 10.2.

Based on evidence about CR and expert opinion, the Society for Cognitive Rehabilitation [54] provided a comprehensive list of recommendations for best practice whose main points are summarized below:

- The cognitive treatment plan must be defined on the basis of the results of a comprehensive neuropsychological assessment, that underlines patient's cognitive weaknesses and strengths.
- Whenever possible, assessment results and treatment plans should be explained and agreed with the patient and the caregiver; all rehabilitative

Table 10.2 Main studies on cognitive rehabilitation for brain tumour patients

Authors	Study design	Sample size and population	Type of training	Timing of training	Main Results	Limitations
Lo Buono et al. [64]	Case study	1 (grade II Astrocytoma)	Cognitive and motivational techniques	3 months (2 times/week for a total of 24 sessions)	Improvement in memory, attention, shifting, and visual activities, in writing and reading, and in the ability to access the linguistic register.	Non-generalizable data
Maschio et al. [63]	Observational study	16 (4HGG, 2 GBM, 5 LGG, 2 MEN, 3 MET) + related epilepsy	Computerized remedial training (Training NeuroPsicologico—TNP®) software	Once a week for 10 weeks	Improvement in short-term verbal memory, episodic memory, fluency and long-term visuospatial memory after the training and at 6 month follow-up	No control group Small sample size
Yang et al. [62]	RCT	38 (5 GBM, 2 AST, 10 MEN, 6 MET, 15 other	SG: Virtual reality training + computer-based cognitive rehabilitation CG: computer-based cognitive rehabilitation	SG: VR training (30 min a day for 3 times a week) and computer-based cognitive rehabilitation program (30 min a day for 2 times) for 4 weeks CG: computer-based cognitive rehabilitation program (30 min a day for 5 days a week) for 4 weeks.	SG showed significant better improvements than the CG in attentive and memory tests and concentration	Small sample size No follow-up

Authors	Study design	Sample size and population	Type of training	Timing of training	Main Results	Limitations
Zucchella et al. [61]	RCT	58 (25 HGG, 7 LGG, 16 MEN, 5 other)	*SG*: combining computer exercises (remedial approach) and metacognitive training (compensatory approach) *CG*: usual care without cognitive training	16 one-hour individual sessions spread over 4 weeks	SG: significant improvement in attentive and mnesic domains CG: mild enhancement of cognitive performances, not statistically relevant	No follow-up
Hassler et al. [60]	Clinical trial	11 (6 GBM, 5 HGG)	*SG*: holistic mnemonic training	10 weekly group training sessions of 90 min	At post-training evaluation improvement across all neurocognitive variables, especially attention and memory skills.	No control group Small sample size
Gehring et al. [59]	RCT	140 (117 LGG, 23 HGG)	*SG*: both computer-based attention retraining and compensatory skills training of attention, memory, and executive functioning + weekly homework assignments *CG*: The waiting-list control group received usual care without cognitive intervention	6 weekly, individual sessions of 2 h each.	At the post-treatment evaluation, measures of subjective cognitive functioning and perceived burden significantly improved. At the 6-month follow-up, the SG performed significantly better on tests of attention and verbal memory and reported less mental fatigue	Patients with mild cognitive deficits

(continued)

Table 10.2 (continued)

Authors	Study design	Sample size and population	Type of training	Timing of training	Main Results	Limitations
Locke et al. [58]	RCT	19 pairs patient (13 HGG, 6 LGG)/ caregiver	SG: cognitive rehabilitation and problem-solving. CG: no cognitive training	6 sessions over the course of 2 weeks	88% of patients were able to learn to study specific strategies and to continue using the strategies to some degree after 3 months	Small sample size
Sherer et al. [57]	Retrospective study	13 (1 GBM, 9 LGG, 1 embryonal choriocarcinoma, 1 pineoblastoma, 1 anaplastic ependymoma)	Individualized vocational rehabilitation designed to decrease the impact of the patient's impairments on his/her functioning	Therapy was conducted in both individual and group settings The typical therapy day lasted 5 h. Patients received an average of 2.6 ± 1.9 months of rehabilitation	Patients enjoyed favourable community independence and employment outcomes. Gains were maintained at the follow-up after 8 months	Small sample size No control group No standardization of the training
Rao et al. [56]	Case study	1 (grade II–III Astrocytoma)	Retraining of simple cognitive capacities at home + psychoeducational and compensation techniques	4 months	Improvements in neuropsychological data, behavioural observations, and efficiency on work-related task	Non-generalizable data

HGG high-grade glioma, *GBM* glioblastoma, *LGG* low-grade glioma, *MEN* meningioma, *MET* metastasis, *RCT* randomized controlled trial, *SG* study group, *CG* control group goals should be specific, measurable, and realistic as well as valuable and meaningful for the patient.

- CR treatments should encompass both attempts at restoration of impaired functions and teaching compensatory strategies to minimize cognitive deficits;
- The therapy has to be systematic, structured, and repetitive according to the patient's needs and it must be part of a multidisciplinary approach.
- Treatment goals should be directed towards enhancing the individual's ability to function as independently as possible; the goals of the intervention must focus on functional competence in real life.
- Opportunities to practice in real-life settings should be provided as part of the intervention to favour generalization and transfer of learning.
- Patient's awareness regarding the presence or severity of cognitive deficits represents the key to successful rehabilitation and should be directly worked on.
- Although cognitive deficits are the major focus of CR, emotional and psychosocial consequences of brain injury need to be addressed in rehabilitation programs. There is an interaction between these different functions, and it is not always easy to separate them from one another.

10.4   Theoretical Framework and Neural Plasticity

The heterogeneous array of interventions that are included within the term CR reflects the lack of a unified theoretical framework able to explain normal cognitive processes, how these are affected by brain injury and how recovery of cognitive processes may occur. In fact most of the neuropsychological models proposed by cognitive neuropsychologists try to explain the working of a normal brain and can detect if something is wrong, but are quite silent with respect to what to do about it [67]; conversely, a useful theory of cognitive rehabilitation should inform clinicians as when, how, and how much to treat to maximize recovery of functions.

As cognitive recovery requires re-learning of skills, theories of learning and memory are crucial for rehabilitation according to Baddeley [68] who claimed that "a theory of rehabilitation without a model of learning is a vehicle without an engine" (p. 235). In the last decades, behavioural experiments as well as careful and repeatable observations have clarified a lot of important principles about how people can learn and retain new information (operant and classical conditioning, shaping behaviours, intermittent reinforcement...); recently, the principle of errorless learning (i.e. preventing people, as far as possible, from making mistakes while they are learning a new skill or acquiring new information) has been highly influential in memory rehabilitation, proving to be particularly effective [69]. Models and theories from behavioural psychology have provided some of the most useful and influential theoretical contributions to rehabilitation, not only for the understanding, management, and remediation of disruptive behaviours, but also for the remediation of cognitive deficits [67]. Moreover, behavioural theories are especially valuable in cognitive rehabilitation because they inform assessment, treatment, and the measurement of rehabilitation efficacy.

Another approach that have revealed quite useful to simulate the mechanisms of learning of new information and specific cognitive tasks is represented by the connectionist models of learning that describe mental and behavioural phenomena as the emergent processes of interconnected networks of simple units. Among many forms of connectionism, the most common forms use neural network models, where units in the network represent neurons and the connections represent synapses. At any time, a network can change through the activation of a neural unit (or group of neural units) in the networks and the spread of the activation to all the other units connected to it. Memory, for instance, is created by modifying the strength of the connections between neural units, based on the principles of Hebb [70] who links learning to the synchronous firing of pre-and post-synaptic cells that leads to inter-neuron linkages through changes in synaptic strengths (*cells that fire together, wire together*), building a bridge between the behavioural/cognitive and the neurophysiological level of analysis.

However, considering the complexity of the field and the range of issues to be dealt with, CR needs a broad theoretical base incorporating frameworks, theories, and models from different areas in order to consider all the important aspects (cognitive, psychological, physical, social, and vocational) of patients' lives [67].

Starting from the concept of Hebbian learning, the following assumptions have been proposed by Robertson and Murre [71] to explain recovery after brain damage:

– The brain is capable of a large degree of self-repair through synaptic turnover (change in the dendritic branches of neurons and in the pattern of synaptic connectivity) and may be engaged in this, even in the absence of overt damage.
– This synaptic turnover is to some extent experience-dependent and is a key mechanism underlying both learning and recovery of function following brain damage.
– Recovery processes following brain damage share common mechanisms with normal learning and experience-dependent plasticity processes.
– Experience and inputs available to damaged neural circuits will shape synaptic interconnections and hence influence recovery.

Therefore, two neurons or groups of neurons that have been disconnected by an injury may become reconnected if they are activated together. Simultaneous activation will take place if both neurons are separately connected to a circuit whose neurons themselves are functionally interconnected. With several repetitions of this process, partially damaged neural circuits thus may become reconnected and cortical functions may be restored.

The capacity of the central nervous system to reorganize itself and adapt in response to changes in the environment or lesions is called *neural plasticity* [72]: results from neurophysiological and neuroanatomical experiments in animals and noninvasive neuroimaging and electrophysiological studies in humans in fact showed considerable plasticity of cortical representations with use or non-use, skill learning, or injury to the nervous system [73, 74].

Although plasticity has been mainly investigated in humans with acute strokes, a growing literature demonstrated that when a tumour invades part of the brain affecting the underlying functions, the brain attempts to compensate for the functional deficit through cortical reorganization, or plasticity [75, 76]. Neural plasticity is therefore a continuous process allowing short-, middle-, and long-term remodelling with the aim to optimize the functioning of brain networks. To explain the pathophysiological mechanisms underlying cerebral plasticity, several hypotheses have been proposed involving both the microscopic (modulations of synaptic efficiency, unmasking of latent connections, phenotypic modifications, neurogenesis) and the macroscopic level (diaschisis, functional redundancies, compensatory recruitment of areas not initially dedicated to the impaired function) as well as morphological changes [25].

Functional imaging studies have shown that slow-growing lesions may induce major neural reorganization and are compensated for much more efficiently than acute lesions [77, 78]. Rearrangements observed in pre-operative studies in fact explain why most LGG patients appear either normal or only slightly impaired under standard neurological assessments [79, 80]. To compensate for LGG invasions different plastic processes have been described that seem to follow a hierarchic model, involving local compensation first with intrinsic reorganizations occurring within the injured and perilesional structures, and only at a later time the remote recruitment in the ipsi- and contra-lesional hemispheres [77, 81]. The postoperative literature reinforces the pre-surgical observations by suggesting that functional recovery involves a large array of complementary mechanisms.

Cerebral plasticity therefore represents the neural basis underlying any rehabilitative intervention and in the past few years it has become more and more evident that the understanding of these neuroplastic principles will address the development of more rational, hypothesis-driven strategies to promote and guide recovery of functions, likely resulting in improvements in patients' care.

10.5 Conclusions

Cognitive impairment is increasingly recognized as a relevant issue to consider in regard to the assessment of the impact and morbidity of a primary brain tumour. In the light of the deep impact of cognitive disturbances on patients' participation and quality of life, continued efforts are needed to assess the efficacy of interventions to improve cognitive functions. Although still preliminary, evidence suggests that multidisciplinary approaches to rehabilitation that encompasses adaptive, remedial, functional, and metacognitive interventions can optimize cognitive outcome.

References

1. Back M, Back E, Kastelan M, Wheeler H. Cognitive deficits in primary brain tumours: a framework for management and rehabilitation. J Cancer Ther. 2014;5:74–81.
2. Stupp R, Hegi ME, Mason WP, van den Bent MJ, Taphoorn MJ, Janzer RC, et al. Effects of radiotherapy with concomitant and adjuvant temozolomide versus radiotherapy alone on survival in glioblastoma in a randomised Phase III study: 5-year analysis of the EORTC-NCIC Trial. Lancet Oncol. 2009;10(5):459–66.

3. Cairncross G, Wang M, Shaw E, Jenkins R, Brachman D, Buckner J, et al. Phase III trial of chemoradiotherapy for anaplasticoligodendroglioma: long-term results of RTOG 9402. J Clin Oncol. 2013;31(3):337–43.
4. van den Bent MJ, Brandes AA, Taphoorn MJ, Kros JM, Kouwenhoven MC, Delattre JY, et al. Adjuvant procarbazine, lomustine, and vincristine chemo- therapy in newly diagnosed anaplastic oligodendroglioma: long-term follow-up of EORTC brain tumour group study 26951. J Clin Oncol. 2013;31(3):344–50.
5. Taphoorn MJ, Klein M. Cognitive deficits in adult patients with brain tumours. Lancet Neurol. 2004;3:159–68.
6. Fliessbach K, Rogowski S, Hoppe C, Sabel M, Goeppert M, Helmstaedter C, et al. Computer-based assessment of cognitive functions in brain tumor patients. J Neurooncol. 2010;100:427–37.
7. Bergo E, Lombardi G, Pambuku A, Della Puppa A, Bellu L, D'Avella D, et al. Cognitive rehabilitation in patients with gliomas and other brain tumors: state of the art. Biomed Res Int. 2016;2016:3041824. https://doi.org/10.1155/2016/3041824.
8. Giovagnoli AR. Investigation of cognitive impairments in people with brain tumors. J Neurooncol. 2012;108(2):277–83.
9. Monje M, Dietrich J. Cognitive side effects of cancer therapy demonstrate a functional role for adult neurogenesis. Behav Brain Res. 2012;227(2):376–9.
10. Gehrke AK, Baisley MC, Sonck ALB, Wronski SL, Feuerstein M. Neurocognitive deficits following primary brain tumour treatment: systematic review of a decade of comparative studies. J Neurooncol. 2013;115(29):135–42.
11. Day J, Gillespie DC, Rooney AG, Bulbeck HJ, Zienius K, Boele F, et al. Neurocognitive deficits and neurocognitive rehabilitation in adult brain tumours. Curr Treat Options Neurol. 2016;18(5):22.
12. Tucha O, Smely C, Preier M, Lange KW. Cognitive deficits before treatment among patients with brain tumours. Neurosurgery. 2000;47:324–33.
13. Klein M, Taphoorn MJ, Heimans JJ, van der Ploeg HM, Vandertop WP, Smit EF, et al. Neurobehavioural status and health-related quality of life in newly diagnosed high-grade glioma patients. J Clin Oncol. 2001;19:4037–47.
14. Meyers CA, Smith JA, Bezjak A, Mehta MP, Liebmann J, Illidge T, et al. Neurocognitive function and progression in patients with brain metastases treated with wholebrain radiation and motexafin gadolinium: results of a randomized phase III trial. J Clin Oncol. 2004;22:157–65.
15. van Nieuwenhuizen D, Klein M, Stalpers LJ, Leenstra S, Heimans JJ, Reijneveld JC. Differential effect of surgery and radiotherapy on neurocognitive functioning and health-related quality of life in WHO grade I meningioma patients. J Neurooncol. 2007;84:271–8.
16. Zucchella C, Bartolo M, Di Lorenzo C, Villani V, Pace A. Cognitive impairment in primary brain tumors outpatients: a prospective cross-sectional survey. J Neuro-Oncol. 2013;112(3):455–60.
17. Bosma I, Vos MJ, Heimans JJ, Taphoorn MJ, Aaronson NK, Postma TJ, et al. The course of neurocognitive functioning in high-grade glioma patients. Neuro-Oncology. 2007;9(1):53–62.
18. Correa DD. Neurocognitive function in brain tumours. Curr Neurol Neurosci Rep. 2010;10:232–9.
19. Kayl AE, Meyers CA. Does brain tumour histology influence cognitive function? Neuro Oncology. 2003;5:255–60.
20. Hahn CA, Dunn RH, Logue PE, King JH, Edwards CL, Halperin EC. Prospective study of neuropsychologic testing and quality-of-life assessment of adults with primary malignant brain tumours. Int J Radiat Oncol Biol Phys. 2003;55:992–9.
21. Correa DD, Shi W, Thaler HT, Cheung AM, DeAngelis LM, Abrey LE. Longitudinal cognitive follow-up in low grade gliomas. J Neurooncol. 2008;86:321–7.
22. Ius T, Angelini E, Thiebaut de Schotten M, Mandonnet E, Duffau H. Evidence for potentials and limitations of brain plasticity using an atlas of functional resectability of WHO grade II gliomas: towards a "minimal common brain". NeuroImage. 2011;56:992–1000.
23. Meyers CA, Hess KR. Multifaceted end points in brain tumour clinical trials: cognitive deterioration precedes MRI progression. Neuro-oncology. 2003;5:89–95.

24. Armstrong CL, Goldstein B, Shera D, Ledakis GE, Tallent EM. The predictive value of longitudinal neuropsychologic assessment in the early detection of brain tumour recurrence. Cancer. 2003;97:649–56.
25. Duffau H. Lessons from brain mapping in surgery for low-grade glioma: insights into associations between tumour and brain plasticity. Lancet Neurol. 2005;4:476–86.
26. Sheline G, Wara WM, Smith V. Therapeutic irradiation and brain injury. Int J Rad Oncol Biol Phys. 1980;6:1215–28.
27. Surma-aho O, Niemela M, Vilkki J, Kouri M, Brander A, Salonen O, et al. Adverse long-term effects of brain radiotherapy in adult lowgrade glioma patients. Neurology. 2001;56:1285–90.
28. Postma TJ, Klein M, Verstappen CC, Bromberg JE, Swennen M, Langendijk JA, et al. Radiotherapy-induced cerebral abnormalities in patients with low-grade glioma. Neurology. 2002;59:121–3.
29. Brown PD, Pugh S, Laack NN, Wefel JS, Khuntia D, Meyers C, et al. Memantine for the prevention of cognitive dysfunction in patients receiving whole-brain radiotherapy: a randomized, double-blind, placebo-controlled trial. Neuro-Oncology. 2013;15(10):1429–37.
30. Makale MT, McDonald CR, Hattangadi-Gluth JA, Kesari S. Mechanisms of radiotherapy-associated cognitive disability in patients with brain tumours. Nat Rev Neurol. 2017;13(1):52–64.
31. Dietrich J, Han R, Yang Y, Mayer-Pröschel M, Noble M. CNS progenitor cells and oligodendrocytes are targets of chemotherapeutic agents in vitro and vivo. J Biol. 2006;5(7):22.
32. Dietrich J, Monje M, Wefel J, Meyers C. Clinical patterns and biological correlates of cognitive dysfunction associated with cancer therapy. Oncologist. 2008;13:1285–95.
33. Saykin AJ, Ahles TA, McDonald BC. Mechanisms of chemotherapy-induced cognitive disorders: neuropsychological, pathophysiological, and neuroimaging perspectives. Semin Clin Neuropsychiatry. 2003;8:201–16.
34. Abrey LE. The impact of chemotherapy on cognitive outcomes in adults with primary brain tumours. J Neurooncol. 2012;108:285–90.
35. Anderson SI, Taylor R, Whittle IR. Mood disorders in patients after treatment for primary intracranial tumours. Br J Neurosurg. 1999;13:480–5.
36. Piil K, Jarden M, Jakobsen J, Christensen KB, Juhler M. A longitudinal, qualitative and quantitative exploration of daily life and need for rehabilitation among patients with high-grade gliomas and their caregivers. BMJ Open. 2013;3(7):e003183.
37. World Health Organization. International classification of functioning, disability, and health (ICF). Geneva: WHO; 2001.
38. Aaronson NK. Quality of life: what is it? How should it be measured? Oncology (Williston Park). 1988;2(5):69–76.
39. Dirven L, Reijneveld JC, Aaronson NK, Bottomley A, Uitdehaag BMJ, Taphoorn MJ. Health-related quality of life in patients with brain tumours: limitations and additional outcome measures. Curr Neurol Neurosci Rep. 2013;13(7):359.
40. Cheng J, Zhang X, Liu BL. Health-related quality of life in patients with high-grade glioma. Neuro-Oncology. 2009;11(1):41–50.
41. Bosma I, Reijneveld JC, Douw L, Vos MJ, Postma TJ, Aaronson NK, et al. Health-related quality of life of long-term high-grade glioma survivors. Neuro-Oncology. 2009;11(1):51–8.
42. Veilleux N, Goffaux P, Boudrias M, Mathieu D, Daigle K, Fortin D. Quality of life in neurooncology—age matters. J Neurosurg. 2010;113:325–32.
43. Giovagnoli AR, Meneses RF, Silvani A, Milanesi I, Fariselli L, Salmaggi A, et al. Quality of life and brain tumours: what beyond the clinical burden? J Neurol. 2014;261:894–904.
44. McLellan DL. Functional recovery and the principles of disability medicine. In: Swash M, Oxbury J, editors. Clinical neurology. Edinburgh, UK: Churchill Livingstone; 1991. p. 768–90.
45. Harley JP, Allen C, Braciszewski TL, Cicerone KD, Dahlberg C, Evans S, et al. Guidelines for cognitive rehabilitation. Neurorehabilitation. 1992;2(3):62–7.
46. Wilson BA. Cognitive rehabilitation: how it is and how it might be. J Int Neuropsychol Soc. 1997;3(5):487–96.

47. Katz DI, Ashley M, O'Shanick GJ, Connors SH. Cognitive rehabilitation: the evidence, the funding and case for advocacy in brian injury. Mc Lean, VA: Brain Injury Association of America; 2006.
48. Cicerone KD, Langenbahn DM, Braden C, Malec JF, Kalmar K, Fraas M, et al. Evidence-based cognitive rehabilitation: updated review of the literature from 2003 through 2008. Arch Phys Med Rehabil. 2011;92(4):519–30.
49. Wilson BA. Neuropsychological Rehabilitation. Annu. Rev. Clin. Psychol. 2008;4:141–62.
50. Sohlberg M, Mateer C. Introduction to cognitive rehabilitation theory and practice. New York: The Guilford Press; 1989.
51. Vargo M. Brain tumour rehabilitation. Am J Phys Med Rehabil. 2011;90(5):S50–62.
52. Nair KT, Wade DT. Satisfaction of members of interdisciplinary rehabilitation teams with goal planning meetings. Arch Phys Med Rehabil. 2003;84(11):1710–3.
53. Sohlberg M, Mateer C. Cognitive rehabilitation: an integrative neuropsychological approach. New York: The Guildford Press; 2001.
54. Society for Cognitive Rehabilitation, "What Is Cognitive Rehabilitation?" 2013. www.society-forcognitiverehab.org.
55. Gehring K, Sitskoorn MM, Aaronson NK, Taphoorn MJB. Interventions for cognitive deficits in adults with brain tumours. Lancet Neurol. 2008;7:548–60.
56. Rao SM, Bieliauskas LA. Cognitive rehabilitation two and one-half years post right temporal lobectomy. J Clin Neuropsychol. 1983;5:313–20.
57. Sherer M, Meyers CA, Bergloff P. Efficacy of postacute brain injury rehabilitation for patients with primary malignant brain tumours. Cancer. 1997;80:250–7.
58. Locke DEC, Cerhan JH, Wu W, Malec JF, Clark MM, Rummans TA, et al. Cognitive rehabilitation and problem-solving to improve quality of life of patients with primary brain tumours: a pilot study. J Support Oncol. 2008;6:383–91.
59. Gehring K, Sitskoorn MM, Gundy CM, Sikkes SA, Klein M, Postma TJ, et al. Cognitive rehabilitation in patients with gliomas: a randomized, controlled trial. J Clin Oncol. 2009;27(22):3712–22.
60. Hassler MR, Elandt K, Preusser M, Lehrner J, Binder P, Dieckmann K, et al. Neurocognitive training in patients with high-grade glioma: a pilot study. J Neurooncol. 2010;97(1):109–15.
61. Zucchella C, Capone A, Codella V, De Nunzio AM, Vecchione C, Sandrini G, et al. Cognitive rehabilitation for early post-surgery inpatients affected by primary brain tumour: a random-ized, controlled trial. J Neurooncol. 2013;114(1):93–100.
62. Yang S, Chun MH, Son YR. Effect of virtual reality on cognitive dysfunction in patients with brain tumour. Ann Rehabil Med. 2014;38(6):726–33.
63. Maschio M, Dinapoli L, Fabi A, Giannarelli D, Cantelmi T. Cognitive rehabilitation training in patients with brain tumour-related epilepsy and cognitive deficits: a pilot study. J Neurooncol. 2015;125:419–26.
64. Lo Buono V, Corallo F, De Cola MC, Chillemi A, Grugno R, Bramanti P, et al. Effect of cognitive rehabilitation in a case of thalamic astrocytoma. Appl Neuropsychol Adult. 2016;23(4):309–12.
65. Carney N, Chesnut RM, Maynard H, Mann NC, Patterson P, Helfand M. Effects of cognitive rehabilitation on outcomes for persons with traumatic brain injury: a systematic review. J Head Trauma Rehabil. 1999;14:277–307.
66. Wilson BA, Herbert CM, Shiel A. Behavioural approaches in neuropsychological rehabilita-tion: optimising rehabilitation procedures. Hove, UK: Psychology Press; 2003.
67. Wilson BA. Neuropsychological rehabilitation: theory and practice. Lisse, The Netherlands: Swets & Zeitlinger BV; 2003.
68. Baddeley AD. A theory of rehabilitation without a model of learning is a vehicle without an engine: a comment on Caramazza and Hillis. Neuropsychol Rehabil. 1993;3:235–44.
69. Kessels RP, de Haan EH. Implicit learning in memory rehabilitation: a meta-analysis on error-less learning and vanishing cues methods. J Clin Exp Neuropsychol. 2003;25(6):805–14.
70. Hebb DO. The organization of behavior; a neuropsychological theory. New York: Wiley and Sons; 1949.

71. Robertson IH, Murre JMJ. Rehabilitation of brain damage: brain plasticity and principles of guided recovery. Psychol Bull. 1999;125(5):544–75.
72. Sharma N, Classen J, Cohen LG. Neural plasticity and its contribution to functional recovery. Handb Clin Neurol. 2013;110:3–12.
73. Bütefisch CM. Plasticity in the human cerebral cortex: lessons from the normal brain and from stroke. Neuroscientist. 2004;10(2):163–73.
74. Nudo RJ, McNeal D. Plasticity of cerebral functions. Handb Clin Neurol. 2013;110:13–21.
75. Matthews PM, Honey GD, Bullmore ET. Applications of fMRI in translational medicine and clinical practice. Nat Rev Neurosci. 2006;7:732–44.
76. Fisicaro RA, Jost E, Shaw K, Brennan NP, Peck KK, Holodny AI. Cortical plasticity in the setting of brain tumours. Top Magn Reson Imaging. 2016;25(1):25–30.
77. Desmurget M, Bonnetblanc F, Duffau H. Contrasting acute and slow-growing lesions: a new door to brain plasticity. Brain. 2007;130:898–914.
78. Ghinda CD, Duffau H. Network plasticity and intraoperative mapping for personalized multi-modal management of diffuse low-grade gliomas. Front Surg. 2017;4:3.
79. Duffau H, Capelle L. Functional recuperation following lesions of the primary somatosensory fields. Study of compensatory mechanisms. Neurochirurgie. 2001;47:557–63.
80. Duffau H, Capelle L, Denvil D, Sichez N, Gatignol P, Lopes M, et al. Functional recovery after surgical resection of low grade gliomas in eloquent brain: hypothesis of brain compensation. J Neurol Neurosurg Psychiatry. 2003;74:901–7.
81. Heiss WD, Thiel A, Kessler J, Herholz K. Disturbance and recovery of language function: correlates in PET activation studies. Neuroimage. 2003;20(Suppl 1):S42–9.

Managing Challenging Behaviour in Brain Tumour (BT) Patients

11

Wolfgang Grisold, Simon Grisold, Alla Guekht, and Roberta Ruda

11.1 Introduction

Despite many new developments and efforts, the management of malignant brain tumour (BT), in particular glioblastoma (GBM), remains a challenge in many ways. This chapter will consider the behavioural challenges in BT patients and different possibilities of management and may contribute to an often neglected area of management in these patients. Changes in behaviour and personality are the most frequent changes.

Mental changes can be subtle, and may be recognizable only for the patients, or the caregivers might become aware of the changes and note that something is "different". Subtle changes can affect language and communication, resulting in reduced verbal fluency, attention and concentration and reduced memory and learning and, in particular, personality and emotional changes.

Behavioural changes in BT patients cover a wide range and are poorly defined. Mental and psychopathological changes can occur in patients with BTs. As BTs encompass variable numbers of different tumours, with a broad range of clinical courses and therapeutic options, this chapter will focus on the most frequent tumour occurring in adults, GBM.

Authors cooperate on international level, and add their local and international experience.

W. Grisold (✉)
Ludwig Boltzmann Institute for Experimental und Clinical Traumatology, Vienna, Austria

S. Grisold
Sozialpsychiatrisches Ambulatorium Landstraße, Vienna, Austria

A. Guekht
Moscow Research and Clinical Center for Neuropsychiatry and Russian National Research Medical University, Moscow, Russia

R. Ruda
Department of Neuro-Oncology, University and City of Health and Science Hospital of Turin, Turin, Italy

© Springer Nature Switzerland AG 2019
M. Bartolo et al. (eds.), *Neurorehabilitation in Neuro-Oncology*,
https://doi.org/10.1007/978-3-319-95684-8_11

GBM and anaplastic glioma (World Health Organization; WHO III [1]) have a similar time course. Low-grade gliomas have a much longer life expectancy and affect a younger age group than GBM, and will therefore only be mentioned in regard to possible radiotherapy damage and seizures.

The larger group of generally "benign tumours", such as as meningiomas and others, as well as cancer-associated intracranial and intracerebral tumours (metastases) will not be discussed.

Despite the attempt to classify the behavioural changes in BT patients in regard to the cause and their temporal occurrence, patients need a thorough individual assessment. There is also the possibility that, in an individual patient, different causes may overlap. For example, a personality trait may be accentuated in a situation of crisis. The patient may be aged, and a concomitant infection may occur, which, in addition to the strategic localization of the tumour (e.g., frontal), may complicate the search for the etiology of the behavioral changes.

11.1.1 Time Course of the Disease

The typical presentation of a BT can be with neurological signs (e.g., hemiparesis, hemisensory symptoms) and also with speech or neuropsychological symptoms, seizures, or cognitive and personality changes. Rarely, the presentation is confined to anxiety and psychosis.

In general, the acute or subacute onset of a personality change, mood swings or psychotic behaviour in a middle-aged or mature or elderly person should point to the possibility of a BT [1]. From the practical point of view the temporal aspects of the course of GBM are classified into four phases.

P1 At diagnosis
P2 During active treatment
P3 Progression and cessation of active tumour treatment
P4 End of life.

P1, the first phase, is the time of diagnosis, where patients can have behavioural abnormalities. These abnormalities can be the initial presentation of the tumour, or they may be behavioural patterns related to the tumour and the diagnosis. This initial phase can often be compared with the previously described pattern of the stages described by Kübler-Ross [2] where there is denial, not acknowledgement, and often procrastination in regard to the awareness of the disease. As the diagnosis of a fatal disease has immediate and unexpected changes in the life of the person, major psychological and even psychiatric reactions may occur.

P2, the second phase, is the time of active tumour treatment, which is usually standardized. Both the patients and the medical team aim to improve and preserve the patient's status quo. In this timely context, focal organic and drug symptoms, as well as seizures, can appear.

Brain organic symptoms, and seizure-related and psychiatric symptoms can overlap and at times cannot be distinguished from one another. The time of active anti-tumour therapy is a busy time for patients and their health care professionals (HCPs), and the patients often suffer not only treatment effects, but also gradual worsening of their symptoms and competencies. Denial often changes, with the recognition of reality, and patients and their carers may feel the increasing burden of the disease.

However, the continuation of denial and often unreal expectations may have a strong influence on the relations with the HCPs. Suggestions from friends, relatives, or internet searches seem to open new possibilities, and the usual course of evidence-based behaviour of BTs and the value of common treatment procedures are denied.

In addition, there may be a tendency to request a second and even "multi" opinions, and this can often be a burden in the relations between the HCPs and the patient and carers.

An analytic, open approach from the patient/carer and the HCPs is necessary to face these situations, as patients and carers will often return for help in advanced stages, after the failure of what seemed to be promising alternative therapies. A door of understanding must be kept wide open, even after severe difficulties.

However, the slope can be slippery, and patients and carers may demand, from the HCPs, support to convince insurance providers and medical institutions to finance and pay for their often irrational therapeutic wishes. This can create difficult relations.

P3 The third phase usually marks a time point when the tumour has progressed and often cognitive changes dominate. Cognitive changes are often diffuse and have multifactorial causes. The common presentation is a global reduction of mentation and cognition; reduced tenacity; and impairment of speech, often accompanied by loss of activity, lack of initiative and sometimes apathy, which can also be a potential frontal lobe sign. Conversely, but more rarely, patients can present with mood swings, mania, dysphoria, anxiety and irritability. Often patients who suffer from speech disorders are very irritable. At this stage the HCPs often make the decisive step to reduce treatment, which can be quite excessive, to supportive measures that are aimed to improve or maintain the patient's quality of life.

The expectations now shift from cure and healing towards prolonged life expectancy and survival. In this stage severe cognitive and mental changes develop, which make life at home and maintenance and care of the patient difficult. There is often a need for counselling and advice for the carers, to support them in their difficult task. Depending on the site of the tumour, motor, sensory and neuropsychological handicaps may also complicate the management of the patient.

There can be several behavioural changes, often rather resembling depression and apathy, more rarely more exogenic behaviours such as anxiety, restlessness and even manic behaviour.

P4 Phase 4 is the "end of life" where most patients veer towards an apathetic state, while some have a more agitated behaviour, which can make the last phases quite difficult. Often also somatic symptoms such as the "death rattle" and diffuse "all body pain" create a difficult environment and not only have an uncertain impact on the patients, but are also difficult to bear for the carers.

The interactions between the HCPs, the carers and the patients now have several variations. Ideally, when the patients and carers are well prepared and accepting, the transition into the final stage can be smooth. There are many aspects of this transition, which will be discussed subsequently. Important interactions also occur in the context of cultural differences.

11.2 Causes of behavioral

11.2.1 Focal and Diffuse Brain Damage

These considerations refer to diffuse and focal brain lesions. Due to their diffuse effect, or the strategic location, they can be the cause for behavioural changes. Local tumors, recurrence, cysts, hydrocphalus and leptomeningeal tumor spread need to be evaluated and if feasible treated.

Among all cancer patients, BT patients are considered at higher risk of developing neuropsychiatric symptoms during the course of their disease. Although this occurs rarely, some BTs may present with neurobehavioural or psychiatric symptoms only.

Symptoms of anger, loss of emotional control, indifference and changes in behaviour are commonly reported by BT patients [3–7]. Personality changes can result directly from the presence of the tumour or from its treatment, including cranial irradiation, chemotherapy, corticosteroids, and antiepileptic drugs.

The precise extent to which tumour location impacts on psychopathology is not well understood. Neuropsychiatric symptoms are, per se, nonspecific in terms of tumour localization, and also do not strictly correlate with the degree of tumor malignancy.

Brain tumours in the frontal and temporal lobes may produce varying degrees of neurobehavioural changes, including mood alterations, impaired judgement, inattentiveness, irritability, memory deficits, and frank dementia 1. Quantitative studies indicate that behavioural problems are more evident in patients with frontal tumours than in controls without neurological compromise. Patients with frontal tumours report more executive dysfunction, apathy and disinhibition than patients with nonfrontal tumours.

Classically, three "frontal lobe syndromes" have been proposed to arise in patients with BTs located in specific prefrontal areas. Damage to dorsolateral prefrontal areas is associated with impaired executive functioning, orbitofrontal damage may cause disinhibition and impulsiveness, and lesions in the medial frontal areas may result in apathy or abulia [8, 9]. Disinhibition and aggression may be due to structural damage or may represent physiological alterations of critical neurotransmitter pathways.

However, clinically significant levels of apathy and executive dysfunction are reported by many patients with BTs located outside the frontal lobes. When the paralimbic structures are involved, mood problems are important.

Patients with tumours affecting the corpus callosum, cingulate gyrus and deep and midline brain areas frequently demonstrate neurobehavioural symptoms, personality changes and affective disorders, and these changes are reported in up to 90% of the patients [10] Neurocognitive and mood disorders have also been described in patients with cerebellar tumours and brainstem lesions, supporting the notion that the cerebellum has important functions in the neural network system relevant to higher cognitive function [11]. Patients with pituitary lesions and associated neuroendocrine dyscrasias are subject to mood and vegetative symptoms that mimic a primary depression.

The impacts of BT location on emotion and personality [12] have to be considered. Right hemispheric BT lesions, in addition to focal symptoms such as neglect, also seem to have a higher association with psychiatric symptoms. There is a wide range of focal pathology in regard to speech, coordination and apraxia, and there are also subtle changes in detecting intonation in prosody or loss of the ability to recognize the prosodic speech of others. Depending on the tumour site, cortical blindness, prosopagnosia and rare individual neuropsychological symptoms can also appear. Organic brain changes result in neuropsychological disorders. Also, a Wernicke-like state can be produced by the involvement of parts of the limbic system [13].

In addition, tumour growth and brain oedema may have a significant influence on behaviour.

Whereas motor and sensory functions can often be easily tracked, correlated personality and behavioural changes are more difficult to localize and deviate significantly from the "classical" localizing topography. This can be explained by the often diffuse growth and oedema, and also by the effect of a focal lesion on the network of the brain [14].

Differential diagnosis of behavioural changes may be difficult. A patient who is apathetic, withdrawn, and lacks motivation may be depressed or may have an organic brain syndrome. Patients with BT and delirium may be misdiagnosed as depressed. Levine et al. [15] reported that 64% of general cancer patients with delirium were misdiagnosed as depressed. This number may be even greater for patients with primary BTs. The distinction is important, as misdiagnosis and subsequent treatment of depression in a patient with an organic brain syndrome might worsen the condition.

Problems with memory or the inability to initiate activity can negatively impact adherence to treatment regimens. Patients may be offered experimental treatments, and the decision to participate and give informed consent requires intact reasoning, the ability to weigh risks and benefits, and the appreciation of long-term consequences.

11.2.2 Different Psychiatric conditions in BT Patients: Depression, Mania, Denial, Delusional Ideation, Perception of Reality, Psychosis

Although BTs can have several psychiatric manifestations, comparatively few recent publications discuss these common topics. There are two comprehensive papers on psychiatric symptoms in BT [1, 16]. Most efforts to describe psychiatric changes in BT patients focus on the role of tumour location in patients with psychiatric symptoms and BT [17–19]. Another approach is the masking of a BT by psychiatric symptoms [20, 21], the orientation of the BT in regard to symptoms [22] and neurobehavioural presentations [23].

For practical use, a comprehensive summary of likely psychiatric manifestations is of value. It is useful to aim to make a distinction between a "psychiatric reaction (towards the disease)", and an organic psychosis (if this terminology can be maintained).

Psychological/psychiatric/personality/coping reactions and traits can be equally caused by focal and diffuse organic brain damage and electrophysiological phenomena; these traits may also be drug- and treatment-related and in the progressive disease stages may be due to often multifactorial changes. Apart from psychosis, denial, irritability, depression and apathy also occur.

The classification of psychiatric conditions will be discussed according to the current ICD 10 classification.

Descriptions of frequently occurring psychiatric phenomena discussed in the scientific papers "Psychiatric aspects of brain tumour: a review" [ref1] and "Psychiatric symptoms in Glioma patients" [ref16] will be discussed.

11.2.2.1   International Classification of Diseases 10 (ICD 10)

The International Classification of Diseases 10 (ICD 10), noted in Chap. 4 "Mental and behavioural disorders", lists psychiatric diseases in ten categories (F00–F99) and defines the criteria for valid diagnosis. Concerning this topic, the items F0 "Organic, including symptomatic, mental disorders", F2 "Schizophrenia, schizotypal and delusional disorders", F3 "Mood [affective] disorders", F4 "Neurotic, stress-related and somatoform disorders" and F5 "Behavioural syndromes associated with physiological disturbances and physical factors" will be of further interest. A distinction is made between psychiatric diseases with an organic correlate (F0) and others with the focus on the psychopathology and the psychiatric manifestations (F2–F5). Treatment options in part overlap and in part differ.

11.2.2.2   F0 Cluster (Organic Diseases)

The psychiatric diseases listed in this cluster share the same essential definition: They are defined through cerebral dysfunction and the resulting psychiatric symptoms. The cerebral impairment may be permanent, e.g., some definite loss of function due to severe brain injury, or may be transient, e.g., systemic disease or endocrine disorders affecting the brain secondarily. Concerning the latter, the psychiatric symptoms diminish when the primary cause of disease is successfully treated.

An example of the first group (i.e., 11.2.2.1) would be an organic personality disorder resulting in a significant alteration of the habitual patterns of behaviour displayed by the subject.

The second group is more unspecific and includes such entities as delirium not induced by alcohol, or the postencephalitic syndrome [24]. Treatment of psychiatric afflictions due to permanent damage may be symptomatic, and treatment of the underlying disease is essential for recovery.

Psychiatric disorders without evident organic connection: F2–F5.

This section describes psychiatric diseases using symptoms and time criteria, excluding external and differential diagnosis. However, organic damage of brain function or structures is, by definition, excluded from this section.

The diseases in F2–F5 include some diseases from the F2 cluster, e.g., acute psychotic disorders; the F3 cluster, e.g., depressive or bipolar disease; the F4 cluster, e.g., panic disorder or general anxiety disease, and the F5 cluster.

Particularly interesting are three entities in the F4 cluster: acute stress reaction (F43.0), adjustment disorders (F43.2) and finally posttraumatic stress disorder (F43.1).

Anxiety is a recognized prodromal and post-event symptom associated with seizures. Other physical causes of anxiety symptoms are similar to those considered in the etiology of delirium: hypoxia of any cause (including anemia or evolving pulmonary embolus), electrolyte and endocrine abnormalities, sepsis, and unrelieved pain. Many drugs (e.g., corticosteroids) used in primary or supportive treatment of cancer in the nervous system often cause anxiety symptoms. Various phenothiazine antiemetics and other neuroleptics (e.g., haloperidol) can cause akathisia, which is described by patients as "anxiety." In addition, drugs of any class with significant anticholinergic effects can cause anxiety and agitation, as can benzodiazepine anxiolytics and opioid analgesics.

This summary demonstrates not only the wide spectrum of psychiatric manifestations, according to the "F" classification of the ICD 10, but also illustrates the often nonspecific manifestations, which do not allow us to determine the underlying "organic" or mental background.

11.2.3 Influence of Seizures/Epilepsy on Behaviour

Brain tumours are one of the main causes of acquired epilepsies (around 12% of all cases) and are associated with 3–6% of all new cases of epilepsy [25]. Rapidly growing tumours, such as GBMs, are associated with seizures in 37% of cases, while low-grade gliomas and dysembryoplastic neuroepithelial tumours are even more frequently (up to 70–100% of cases) the cause of seizures and epilepsy.

The clinical and neuroimaging features of these tumours that are associated with the early onset of spontaneous seizures have been reviewed recently by Kasper and Kasper [26] Clinically, these tumours present with seizures usually in adolescence (mean age of 16.5 years). The lateralization and location of the tumours (in the majority temporal or frontal regions) determine the ictal presentation, as well the interictal abnormalities, including behavioural features.

In patients with epilepsy caused by low-grade gliomas, cognitive impairment and emotional dysfunctions are prevalent. These manifestations may be due to the effects of the tumour itself, seizures, psychological stress, chemotherapy, radiotherapy, and the effect of antiepileptic drugs (AEDs) on brain function. Depression occurs frequently in patients with epilepsy and BTs, probably being a sequela of both conditions, as well as being a sequela of therapeutic interventions and psychiatric aspects. According to the recent study by Rahman et al. [27], in a cohort of patients with primary BTs, with epilepsy in 68% of them, cognitive impairment was documented in 50.6%, and abnormal scores were documented on the anxiety scale in 33%, and on the depression scale in 34%. Importantly, there were no statistically significant differences between patients with and without epilepsy and seizures, so the presence of BTs itself could be attributed to cognitive impairment/depression/anxiety irrespective of the presence of epilepsy. However, a high seizure burden was an independent risk factor for poor health-related quality of life in patients with primary BTs.

Rarely, in patients with epilepsy, violent acts occur [28], which may be considered as ictal or postictal behavioural abnormalities. Postictal violence is characterized by resistive behaviour towards attempts of restraint, or—in rare cases—the behavior is due to postictal psychosis. Aggressive acts, rage and confusion have been described in children with epilepsy secondary to ganglioglioma or meningioma in the temporal lobe. The involvement of the amygdala was considered to play the key role [29]. Abnormal behaviour has been associated with left as well as right hemispheric lesions. Left temporal focuses seem to be more frequently involved [29] in behavioural changes. Surgical interventions are curative for the seizures as well as the behavioural abnormalities in the majority of cases, [29]; however, there might be no behavioural improvement, and in some patients the behaviour may even worsen [30, 31].

Brinkman et al. [32] evaluated the prevalence and predictors of suicidal ideation in youth and adult survivors of paediatric brain tumours. Suicidal ideation was significantly associated with mental health variables, treatment modality and history of seizures; these findings are concordant with numerous studies on the complex and multidirectional association between depression, epilepsy and suicidality [33].

Brain tumours sometimes are the cause of status epilepticus, including nonconvulsive status epilepticus (NCSE). In adults with NCSE, 4–12% have a tumoural origin [34, 35]. In addition, patients with BTs and altered mental status were demonstrated to have NCSE in 6% of all the cases [36].

Another significant diagnostic challenge in patients with BT-related seizures is peri-ictal pseudoprogression, which might result in transient clinical, including behavioural, and magnetic resonance imaging abnormalities that can incorrectly suggest tumour progression [37].

Although carefully controlled studies are lacking, newer AEDs such as levetiracetam, lamotrigine, pregabalin, and lacosamide have more favourable adverse effect profiles in patients with tumour-related epilepsies; minimal/or no interactions with chemotherapeutic agents are mandatory [38]. The psychiatric adverse effects of AEDs are well described [39–41].

Topiramate, vigabatrin, levetiracetam and zonisamide have been more frequently associated with adverse psychotropic effects than gabapentin, pregabalin, lacosamide and lamotrigine. The following adverse effects might be especially relevant for the treatment of patients with tumour-related epilepsies: depression (topiramate, zonisamide, perampanel); agitation, aggression, irritability (levetiracetam, perampanel); and somnolence (topiramate, gabapentin, pregabalin).

11.2.4 Oncological (Tumour) Treatment

In addition to focal brain damage, seizures and treatment-induced effects need to be considered at any stage of the disease. Radiation can induce acute or delayed effects, but usually induces late effects, which are as important in LGG as in ?, and are less frequent in GBM; however, late important in LGG due to the long survival, and are less frequent in GBM, however may be important in longterm survivors.

Very frequently steroids can have psychotropic effects, which range from a nonspecific excitatory state, anxiety, irritability, and sleeplessness to overt psychosis, and also depressive states, as observed by Stiefel et al. (1989). Patients may become anxious, with psychomotor agitation and racing thoughts consistent with mania. They may also become dysphoric, with negative or nihilistic ruminative thoughts, sometimes escalating to the point of psychosis. Because these reactions are idiosyncratic, it is difficult to predict which patients will have adverse reactions to steroids.

High-dose and prolonged steroid treatment always needs to be carefully monitored and, as a rule, should be tapered. Generally there is a tendency to have patients on steroids for too long [42, 43]. Conversely, sudden discontinuation of prolonged steroid therapy may also result in mood swings and depression.

Interferons are associated with depressive reactions, usually at high doses or over long treatment periods. On rare occasions, acute depressive reactions occur shortly after treatment begins. Interferon-β is most likely to cause neuropsychiatric side effects. Interferon-alpha, which is used more often in neuro-oncology, is generally less problematic [44].

The issue of chemobrain has been attracting attention [45], in particular in low-grade gliomas [46]. The clinical correlation of slowing of mentation and cognition is also termed "chemofog" and is not well defined. In elderly patients in particular the influence of chemotherapy on cognition can be substantial [47].

Most drugs used in the treatment of GBM, such as temozolamide, do not seem to have psychotropic effects, although psychotropic effects due to several causes have been suspected in association with chemotherapy [38].

However, patients treated with older drugs, such as procarbazine (a monoamine oxidase inhibitor) can present with psychiatric symptoms. Also, during treatment with vascular endothelial growth factor inhibitors, acute mental changes can be caused by the development of posterior reversible encephalopathy syndrome [48].

Perioperative situations, such as the influence of sedation and anesthesia, can induce transient confusion and states of delirium in patients, in particular with increasing age.

At any time, as an effect of therapy, or concomitant infections causing, pneumonia and rarely sepsis may occur. Oral mucusatoxic effects, may have an influence on reduced fluid intake and subsequently dehydration. Rarely antibiotics as the chinolones can have psychotropic effects. [49].

Anemia can be caused by several circumstances, such as a drug side effect, or as a result of bone marrow damage or other causes. Anaemia usually occurs in the later stages of therapy, after several cycles of chemotherapy and bone marrow toxicity.

Also, increasing age needs to be considered as a cause of confusion [38].

However, the cumulation of benzodiazepines, antidepressants and, rarely, anti-dementia drugs, also needs to be considered, as well as the buildup of opioids [50, 51] causing delirium. These presentations usually resolve or decrease in intensity with dose reduction or discontinuation of the relevant medication.

Anti-dementia drugs such as memantine and donezepil have been proposed to improve cognitive function in BT patients. As delirium can be a rare side effect of such drugs [52], the indication has to be carefully considered.

11.3 Management and treatment of behavioural disorders

Depending on the time of occurrence and the cause of the ? manifestation, several management suggestions can be made:

11.3.1 Communication with Patients and Caregivers

Communication with patients and caregivers is one of the most important tasks in the management of ?. This means that not only does the patient need attention and communication, but often co-management for the needs and behaviour of relatives is necessary. This can be made more complicated by cultural issues and will need adjustment of care.

Communication can be a concern for any of the health care professionals (HCPs) or member of the HCP group. Often the barriers to communication are lower with healthcare groups such as nurses and other members of the HCP, in particular with "lower ranks" of the medical hierarchy, than the barriers with physicians [53]. The members of the HCP group will either be exposed to communication difficulties, or they will pick up problems in their patient contacts and counselling.

11.3.2 Drugs and Psychotherapy

For the ICD 10 F0 cluster; cerebral dysfunction has to be treated if possible either symptomatically (e.g., impulsive behaviour following a permanent brain lesion) or by treatment of the underlying reversible cause (e.g., delirium arising from different causes or endocrine malfunction).

Psychiatric symptoms might also be treated with psychopharmacological medication, e.g., antidepressants or antipsychotics.

Additionally, some modification or adaptation of behavioural disorders by means of different treatment settings, some specialized institutions, or special care through professionals at home or in nursing homes is suggested.

11.3.2.1 Regarding the F2–F5 Cluster

Psychiatric treatment should combine medical treatment and psychotherapy. Whereas there are guidelines and state-of-the-art consensus statements for the medical treatment, e.g., selective serotonin reuptake inhibitors for depression, first-generation tricyclic antidepressants are hardly used, although amitriptyline (which has a strong anticholinergic effect) still has a role in the treatment of neuropathic pain.

For psychosis preferably second-generation neuroleptic medication is used. Psychotherapy is a wide field and there are several methods to be chosen from.

Behavioural therapies show a rapid improvemenst of the altered psychic state and behavioural problems; however, the long-term effect seems to be inferior to other psychotherapies (e.g., psychoanalytical methods).

Mood stabilizers are rarely an issue in patients with glioma; however, if the patient also needs anticonvulsant therapy, valproate, carbamazepine, and oxcarbazepine can also act as mood stabilizers. Mood swings can be disconcerting, and can be treatment-dependent; for example, the effects of steroids may appear as unrest, agitation and anxiety.

The choice of drugs follows the same principles as those applying in patients with other psychiatric symptoms [16, 54].

11.3.3 The Final Stages

The management of "end of life" situations requires the full attention of all health care participants. Usually, if patients are treated by a continuous-care team, the experienced team will have a good feeling when the final part of the disease is reached. This is often managed in hospital or hospice care, and models of terminal home care [55] have also been developed. Not infrequently patients are sent to hospital care in the last phase of their life, which is often due to difficult or unmanageable situations, or the irrational thought that some intervention may still help.

Usually patients become lethargic and apathetic; rarely, a final delirium develops [56]. Somatic issues such as breathing abnormalities, hypersalivation, "all body pain", and an increase in or the first appearance of seizures create difficulties for the carers and the HCP. The recent paper by Pace et al. and the European Association of Neuro-Oncology Palliative Care Task Force on palliative care and end-of-life care, tackles several aspects of these issues [57].

The HCP often has to make difficult decisions in the selection of symptomatic treatment of fever and infections. Also, there are issues of hydration and nutrition and the avoidance of therapeutic actions, which can appear to hasten death.

In these situations, an additional focus of attention is directed towards the carers, who can have a wide range of behavioural patterns, also depending on their cultural background.

11.3.4 Further Considerations

11.3.4.1 Patients

On the patients' side, multiple factors concerning treatment, social implications and support and long-term quality of life should be considered. Patients have to be assured of support, and the demoralization syndrome needs to be avoided [58].

Not infrequently a social decline precedes or follows the patient's physical decline. Family resources are very important. It is important to give patients many opportunities to plan their future care. Also, caregivers need to be involved in the circumstances of the patient's life care. It is important to communicate the patient's plans and wishes.

11.3.4.2 Resilience

Somasundaram and Devamani [59], in a comparative study, focus on the factors of resilience, perceived social support and hopelessness among cancer patients. They concluded that patients with stronger social support and higher rates of resilience in curative care experienced less hopelessness and showed fewer psychiatric symptoms, e.g., depression. Resilience is defined as the ability to recover from psychic stress due to traumatic life events to the former level of psychic functioning. Following this study it might be important to support factors that increase resilience and coping and provide or encourage social support. Thus, relatives or other persons important for the patient should be integrated in the patient's treatment, given care and encouragement and be strongly supported by professionals.

11.3.4.3 On Death and Dying

Kübler-Ross [2] primarily described the stages in the process of imminent death as denial, anger, bargaining, depression and acceptance. Subsequently, Kübler-Ross expanded the theory beyond dying and included other life events such as (the onset of) diseases [60]. Also phases of extreme fear of death can occur [61].

It is important to support or accompany the patient through these different phases, whether after diagnosis, through critical times until recovery or in the process of dying.

Psychiatric diseases may occur or may exacerbate the different phases. or in some aspects or phases are identical (e.g., a depressive episode). Support can be psychological or medical, and can involve relatives and social contacts, or it can even occur on a religious or spiritual level.

11.3.5 Organizational Aspects

11.3.5.1 Consultation: Liaison Psychiatry

If psychiatric symptoms occur, a medical examination by a professional psychiatrist is essential. The symptoms and underlying diseases should be treated by a multiprofessional team [62, 63]. Regular examinations by a psychiatrist should be obligatory, whether before and after diagnoses or throughout the treatment and perhaps the eventual recovery or stabilization with some quality of life. Furthermore, psychiatrists or psychologists should have an important role concerning the instruction, teaching and training of staff (doctors and nurses and other members of the HCP group) to deal with the psychiatric symptoms and reactions of the ill.

11.4 Debriefing Carers/Bereavement

The end of life of the patient is not the end of the process for the carers.

Also, the HCP group may be emotionally affected after the patient's death. However, the professionalism of the HCP group and their need to be available for other persons usually mean that these emotional effects are usually manageable. For the HCP group, interventions such as supervision post-case, or PM (post portem) [64] (Fearey) discussion and PM analysis may be helpful and will give incentives for the management of patients. It is important to look at possible complications and interactions. Also, the issue of "compassion fatigue" [65] has to be considered.

The situation is more complex for the carers, whose engagement often increases towards the final stages of the disease and then comes to an end. Positive emotional engagement, but also anxieties, fears and often guilt come to a sudden halt. These feelings can be aggravated in difficult final medical situations, and the final acceptance of the patient's death may be difficult.

Relatives and carers need debriefing [66] from their responsible position, and therapies and coaching can be useful to help with the bereavement [67] process.

11.5 Summary and Conclusion

Behavioural changes can occur in BT patients; these changes have a wide range, from subtle ones to major personality changes, anxiety, mood swings, psychosis and apathy.

The changes are dependent on tumour stage, tumour localization and size, treatment effects, seizures, and a variety of neuropsychological and psychiatric manifestations; often the causes overlap but they may need distinct therapeutic strategies, which are not confined to drug therapy, but must involve the HCP team and the carers in addition to the patient.

In addition to the more technical aspects, such as care, treatment issues and drugs, interactive communication between the patients, the HCP team and the carers, and also between the carers and patients, are major issues. The patient's behavioural changes can be temporary, permanent, and decreasing or increasing and escalating. They can be caused by "organic brain" issues, seizures, neuropsychological issues, and psychiatric interactions.

In addition to drug therapy, a communication strategy, counselling, and psychiatric interventions such as liaison services are helpful in the treatment of BT patients.

Conflict of Interest The authors report no conflict of interest and have contributed equally to the chapter.

References

1. Madhusoodanan S, Ting MB, Farah T, Ugur U. Psychiatric aspects of brain tumors: a review. World J Psychiatry. 2015;5:273–85.
2. Kübler-Ross E. On death and dying. London: Routledge; 1969. ISBN 0-415-04015-9.
3. Andrewes DG, Kaye A, Murphy M, Harris B, Aitken S, Parr C, Bates L. Emotional and social dysfunction in patients following surgical treatment for brain tumour. J Clin Neurosci. 2003;10:428–33.
4. Cavers D, Hacking B, Erridge SE, Kendall M, Morris PG, Murray SA. Social, psychological and existential well-being in patients with glioma and their caregivers: a qualitative study. CMAJ. 2012;184:E373–82.
5. Cummings JL. Frontal-subcortical circuits and human behavior. Arch Neurol. 1993;50:873–80.
6. Lucas MR. Psychosocial implications for the patient with a high-grade glioma. J Neurosci Nurs. 2010;42:104–8.
7. Sterckx W, Coolbrandt A, Dierckx de Casterle B, Van den Heede K, Decruyenaere M, Borgenon S, Mees A, Clement P. The impact of a high-grade glioma on everyday life: a systematic review from the patient's and caregiver's perspective. Eur J Oncol Nurs. 2013;17:107–17.
8. Fuster JM. The prefrontal cortex – an update: time is of the essence. Neuron. 2001;30:319–33.
9. Gregg N, Arber A, Ashkan K, Brazil L, Bhangoo R, Beaney R, Gullan R, Hurwitz V, Costello A, Yaguez L. Neurobehavioural changes in patients following brain tumour: patients and relatives perspective. Support Care Cancer. 2014;22:2965–72.
10. Nasrallah HA, Mcchesney CM. Psychopathology of corpus callosum tumors. Biol Psychiatry. 1981;16:663–9.
11. Schmahmann JD. Disorders of the cerebellum: ataxia, dysmetria of thought, and the cerebellar cognitive affective syndrome. J Neuropsychiatry Clin Neurosci. 2004;16:367–78.
12. Campanella F, Shallice T, Ius T, Fabbro F, Skrap M. Impact of brain tumour location on emotion and personality: a voxel-based lesion-symptom mapping study on mentalization processes. Brain. 2014;137:2532–45.
13. Oberndorfer S, Urbanits S, Lahrmann H, Kirschner H, Kumpan W, Grisold W. Akinetic mutism caused by bilateral infiltration of the fornix in a patient with astrocytoma. Eur J Neurol. 2002;9:311–3.
14. Bourdillon P, Apra C, Lévêque M, Vinckier F. Neuroplasticity and the brain connectome: what can Jean Talairach's reflections bring to modern psychosurgery? Neurosurg Focus. 2017;43(3):E11. https://doi.org/10.3171/2017.6.FOCUS17251.
15. Levine PM, Silberfarb PM, Lipowski ZJ. Mental disorders in cancer patients: a study of 100 psychiatric referrals. Cancer. 1978;42:1385–91.
16. Boele FW, Rooney AG, Grant R, Klein M. Psychiatric symptoms in glioma patients: from diagnosis to management. Neuropsychiatr Dis Treat. 2015;11:1413–20.
17. Betul O, Ipek M. Brain tumor presenting with psychiatric symptoms. J Neuropsychiatry Clin Neurosci. 2011;23:E43–4.
18. Madhusoodanan S, Opler MG, Moise D, Gordon J, Danan DM, Sinha A, Babu RP. Brain tumor location and psychiatric symptoms: is there any association? A meta-analysis of published case studies. Expert Rev Neurother. 2010;10:1529–36.
19. Uribe VM. Psychiatric symptoms and brain tumor. Am Fam Physician. 1986;34:95–8.
20. Munjal S, Pahlajani S, Baxi A, Ferrando S. Delayed diagnosis of glioblastoma multiforme presenting with atypical psychiatric symptoms. Prim Care Companion CNS Disord. 2016;18:6.
21. Pool JL, Correll JW. Psychiatric symptoms masking brain tumor. J Med Soc N J. 1958;55:4–9.
22. Mardaga S, Al Bassir M, Bracke J, Dutilleux A, Born JD. Which psychiatric symptoms must raise suspicion about a possible brain tumor? Rev Med Liege. 2017;72:399–405.
23. Filley CM, Kleinschmidt-Demasters BK. Neurobehavioral presentations of brain neoplasms. West J Med. 1995;163:19–25.
24. Confusion: delirium and dementia. http://www.victoriahospice.org/sites/default/files/imce/Delirium-Section-MedCareOfDying.pdf. p. 455–83.

25. Annegers JF, Rocca WA, Hauser WA. Causes of epilepsy: contributions of the Rochester epidemiology project. Mayo Clin Proc. 1996;71:570–5.
26. Kasper BS, Kasper EM. New classification of epilepsy-related neoplasms: the clinical perspective. Epilepsy Behav. 2017;67:91–7.
27. Rahman Z, Wong CH, Dexter M, Olsson G, Wong M, Gebsky V, Nahar N, Wood A, Byth K, King M, Bleasel AB. Epilepsy in patients with primary brain tumors: the impact on mood, cognition, and HRQOL. Epilepsy Behav. 2015;48:88–95.
28. Delgado-Escueta AV, Mattson RH, King L, Goldensohn ES, Spiegel H, Madsen J, Crandall P, Dreifuss F, Porter RJ. Special report. The nature of aggression during epileptic seizures. N Engl J Med. 1981;305:711–6.
29. Van Elst LT, Woermann FG, Lemieux L, Thompson PJ, Trimble MR. Affective aggression in patients with temporal lobe epilepsy: a quantitative MRI study of the amygdala. Brain. 2000;123(Pt 2):234–43.
30. Andermann LF, Savard G, Meencke HJ, Mclachlan R, Moshe S, Andermann F. Psychosis after resection of ganglioglioma or DNET: evidence for an association. Epilepsia. 1999;40:83–7.
31. Guimaraes CA, Franzon RC, Souza EA, Schmutzler KM, Montenegro MA, Queiroz Lde S, Cendes F, Guerreiro MM. Abnormal behavior in children with temporal lobe epilepsy and ganglioglioma. Epilepsy Behav. 2004;5:788–91.
32. Brinkman TM, Liptak CC, Delaney BL, Chordas CA, Muriel AC, Manley PE. Suicide ideation in pediatric and adult survivors of childhood brain tumors. J Neuro-Oncol. 2013;113:425–32.
33. Hecimovic H, Salpekar J, Kanner AM, Barry JJ. Suicidality and epilepsy: a neuropsychobiological perspective. Epilepsy Behav. 2011;22:77–84.
34. Casazza M, Gilioli I. Non-convulsive status epilepticus in brain tumors. Neurol Sci. 2011;32(Suppl 2):S237–9.
35. Cavaliere R, Farace E, Schiff D. Clinical implications of status epilepticus in patients with neoplasms. Arch Neurol. 2006;63:1746–9.
36. Hormigo A, Liberato B, Lis E, DeAngelis LM. Non-convulsive status epilepticus in patients with cancer: imaging abnormalities. Arch Neurol. 2004;61:362–5.
37. Rheims S, Ricard D, Van den Bent M, Taillandier L, Bourg V, Desestret V, Cartalat-Carel S, Hermier M, Monjour A, Delattre JY, Sanson M, Honnorat J, Ducray F. Peri-ictal pseudoprogression in patients with brain tumor. Neuro-Oncology. 2011;13:775–82.
38. Schiff D, Lee EQ, Nayak L, Norden AD, Reardon DA, Wen PY. Medical management of brain tumors and the sequelae of treatment. Neuro-Oncology. 2015;17:488–504.
39. Chen B, Choi H, Hirsch LJ, Katz A, Legge A, Buchsbaum R, Detyniecki K. Psychiatric and behavioral side effects of antiepileptic drugs in adults with epilepsy. Epilepsy Behav. 2017;76:24–31.
40. Piedad J, Rickards H, Besag FM, Cavanna AE. Beneficial and adverse psychotropic effects of antiepileptic drugs in patients with epilepsy: a summary of prevalence, underlying mechanisms and data limitations. CNS Drugs. 2012;26:319–35.
41. Weintraub D, Buchsbaum R, Resor SR Jr, Hirsch LJ. Psychiatric and behavioral side effects of the newer antiepileptic drugs in adults with epilepsy. Epilepsy Behav. 2007;10:105–10.
42. Roth P, Happold C, Weller M. Corticosteroid use in neuro-oncology: an update. Neuro-Oncol Pract. 2015;22(1):6–12.
43. Lee EQ, Wen PY. Corticosteroids for peritumoral edema: time to overcome our addiction? Neuro-Oncology. 2016;18:1191–2.
44. Valentine AD, Meyers CA, Kling MA, Richelson E, Hauser P. Mood and cognitive side effects of interferon-alpha therapy. Semin Oncol. 1998;25:39–47.
45. Simoa M, Rifa-Rosa X, Rodriguez-Fornellsa A, Bruna J. Chemobrain: a systematic review of structural and functional neuroimaging studies. Neurosci Biobehav Rev. 2013;37(8):1311–21.
46. Behrend SW. Patients with primary brain tumors. Oncol Nurs Forum. 2014;41:335–6.
47. Gaman AM, Uzoni A, Popa-Wagner A, Andrei A, Petcu EB. The role of oxidative stress in etiopathogenesis of chemotherapy induced cognitive impairment (CICI)-"Chemobrain". Aging Dis. 2016;7:307–17.

48. Kamiya-Matsuoka C, Cachia D, Olar A, Armstrong TS, Gilbert MR. Primary brain tumors and posterior reversible encephalopathy syndrome. Neurooncol Pract. 2014;1:184–90.
49. Golomb BA, Koslik HJ, Redd AJ. Fluoroquinolone-induced serious, persistent, multisymptom adverse effects. BMJ Case Rep. 2015;2015:bcr2015209821. https://doi.org/10.1136/bcr-2015-209821.
50. Estfan B, Yavuzsen T, Davis M. Development of opioid-induced delirium while on olanzapine: a two-case report. J Pain Symptom Manag. 2005;29:330–2.
51. Swart LM, Van der Zanden V, Spies PE, de Rooij SE, Van Munster BC. The comparative risk of delirium with different opioids: a systematic review. Drugs Aging. 2017;34:437–43.
52. Mollazadeh-Moghaddam K, Jamali A, Adili-Aghdam F, Akhondzadeh S. Delirium associated with donepezil in a patient with Alzheimer's disease: a case report. Iran J Psychiatry. 2013;8:59–60.
53. Jors K, Tietgen S, Xander C, Momm F, Becker G. Tidying rooms and tending hearts: an explorative, mixed-methods study of hospital cleaning staff's experiences with seriously ill and dying patients. Palliat Med. 2017;31(1):63–71.
54. Moore DP. Textbook of clinical neuropsychiatry. London: Hodder Arnold; 2008.
55. Pompili A, Telera S, Villani V, Pace A. Home palliative care and end of life issues in glioblastoma multiforme: results and comments from a homogeneous cohort of patients. Neurosurg Focus. 2014;37(6):E5. https://doi.org/10.3171/2014.9.FOCUS14493.
56. Bush SH, Kanji S, Pereira JL, Davis DHJ, Currow DC, Meagher D, Rabheru K, Wright D, Bruera E, Hartwick M, Gagnon PR, Gagnon B, Breitbart W, Regnier L, Lawlor PG. Treating an established episode of delirium in palliative care: expert opinion and review of the current evidence base with recommendations for future development. J Pain Symptom Manag. 2014;48:231–48.
57. Pace A, Dirven L, Koekkoek JAF, Golla H, Fleming J, Ruda R, Marosi C, Le Rhun E, Grant R, Oliver K, Oberg I, Bulbeck HJ, Rooney AG, Henriksson R, Pasman HRW, Oberndorfer S, Weller M, Taphoorn MJB, European Association of Neuro-Oncology Palliative Care Task Force. European Association for Neuro-Oncology (EANO) guidelines for palliative care in adults with glioma. Lancet Oncol. 2017;18:e330–40.
58. Kissane DW, Clarke DM, Street AF. Demoralization syndrome – a relevant psychiatric diagnosis for palliative care. J Palliat Care. 2001;17:12–21.
59. Somasundaram RO, Devamani KA. A comparative study on resilience, perceived social support and hopelessness among cancer patients treated with curative and palliative care. Indian J Palliat Care. 2016;22:135–40.
60. Kübler-Ross E. On grief and grieving: finding the meaning of grief through the five stages of loss. London: Simon & Schuster; 2005.
61. Adelbratt S, Strang P. Death anxiety in brain tumour patients and their spouses. Palliat Med. 2000;14:499–507.
62. Ramirez AJ. Liaison psychiatry in a breast cancer unit. J R Soc Med. 1989;82:15–7.
63. De Giorgio G, Quartesan R, Sciarma T, Giulietti M, Piazzoli A, Scarponi L, Ferrari S, Ferranti L, Moretti P, Piselli M. Consultation-Liaison Psychiatry-from theory to clinical practice: an observational study in a general hospital. BMC Res Notes. 2015;8:475.
64. Fearey P, Collier B, DeMarco T. A defined process for project post mortem review. Browse J Mag IEEE Softw. 1996;13(4):65–72. https://doi.org/10.1109/52.526833.
65. Cetrano G, Tedeschi F, Rabbi L, Gosetti G, Lora A, Lamonaca D, Manthorpe J, Amaddeo F. How are compassion fatigue, burnout, and compassion satisfaction affected by quality of working life? Findings from a survey of mental health staff in Italy. BMC Health Serv Res. 2017;17:755. https://doi.org/10.1186/s12913-017-2726-x.
66. Ma C. The importance of debriefing in clinical simulations. Clin Simul Nurs. 2008;4(2):e19–23. https://doi.org/10.1016/j.ecns.2008.06.006.
67. Keene EA, Hutton N, Hall B, Rushton C. Bereavement debriefing sessions: an intervention to support health care professionals in managing their grief after the death of a patient. Pediatr Nurs. 2010;36:185–9. quiz 190.

Neuropathic Pain in Nervous System Tumours

12

Augusto Tommaso Caraceni and Fabio Formaglio

12.1 Cancer Pain

Pain is one of most frequent symptoms in cancer. About 30% of cancer patients complain of pain directly due to the tumour from the beginning of the disease. Pain prevalence rises to almost 50% in the active treatment phase and reaches 70% in advanced cancer patients. In spite of significant therapy improvements occurred in the last 20 years, still about 66% of advanced cancer patients suffer from pain which is not optimally controlled [1].

Pain in advanced cancer is associated with symptoms as fatigue, dyspnoea, anorexia, and psychosocial and spiritual elements of suffering, such as anxiety, depression and loss of autonomy. Pain is directly associated with the degree of deterioration of functionality and of quality of life in patients affected by tumours. The complexity of the needs of cancer pain patients are better met switching the goal of the therapeutic interventions from a just pain intensity reduction to a global palliative care strategy. This comprehensive management requires both a general palliative care approach and specialized multidisciplinary palliative care teams [2].

The mainstay of cancer pain treatment is the use of pharmacological therapies, integrated with physical interventions and psychological and social supports when appropriate. Pharmacological treatment of cancer pain is mainly based on the World Organization of Health analgesic ladder method: drugs should be given "by the clock", rather than "on demand"; preferred way to assume drugs is by the mouth, rather than invasive routes; clinicians should avoid fixed doses of analgesics and adapt drugs doses to the individual patient response; careful management of analgesic unwanted side effects is warranted. This guideline recommends to choose the analgesic according to pain intensity: non-opioids (Paracetamol, Aspirin

A. T. Caraceni (✉) · F. Formaglio
Palliative Care, Pain Therapy and Rehabilitation Center, Fondazione IRCCS Istituto Nazionale dei Tumori, Milan, Italy
e-mail: augusto.caraceni@istitutotumori.mi.it; fabio.formaglio@istitutotumori.mi.it

© Springer Nature Switzerland AG 2019
M. Bartolo et al. (eds.), *Neurorehabilitation in Neuro-Oncology*,
https://doi.org/10.1007/978-3-319-95684-8_12

Table 12.1 Analgesics used in cancer pain management with initial typical doses

Drug	Suggested dosages
Paracetamol	500–1000 mg, as needed or every 4–6 h Maximal dose: 4000 mg/day
Ibuprofen	600 mg as needed or every 6 h Maximal dose 2400 mg/day
Ketorolac	10–30 mg as needed or every 6–8 h Maximal dose 120 mg/day. Only for short-periods treatment
Codeine (in association with Paracetamol 500 mg)	30–60 mg as needed or every 4–6 h Maximal Paracetamol daily dose: 4000 mg day
Tramadol	50 mg as needed or every 6 h or 100 mg every 12 or 24 h (extended release tablets) Use lower dosage when other serotoninergic drugs are administered Consider halved dose in parenteral administration Maximal daily dose 400 mg
Tapentadol	50–100 twice a day up to 500 mg/day Titrate every 2–3 days from lower dosage Consider Tramadol or other opioids analgesics as rescue
Morphine	5–10 mg every 4 h (immediate release formulation) or 10 every 12 h (slow release tablets) Titrate to effect every 24 h, increasing of 30–50% of daily dose
Oxycodone	5 mg (associated to Paracetamol 325 mg) every 4 h or 5–10 mg (alone or associated to Naloxone), extended release tablets every 12 h Maximum dose in Naloxone—associated tablets, 160 mg/day
Fentanyl	12–100 mcg/h, 3 days patch

and non-steroidal anti-inflammatory drugs) for mild pain management; non-opioids and second step opioids (Codeine, Tramadol, and low doses of Oxycodone or Morphine) for moderate pain; non-opioids and step III opioids (such as Morphine, Oxycodone, Fentanyl) for severe pain treatment (Table 12.1). Additional—"adjuvants"—drugs should be added at any steps for specific pain syndromes, such as neuropathic pain and pain arising from cancer bone invasion. A rapid onset analgesic should be available for the management of pain exacerbations, also known as breakthrough pains, such as in the case of incident pain due to movement or weight bearing.

12.2 Neuropathic Pain and Central Pain

Neuropathic pain is defined as the pain arising as a direct consequence of a lesion or disease affecting the somatosensory system [3]. According to this statement, pain experts developed a consensus definition of the characteristics required for neuropathic pain diagnosis (Table 12.2) [4, 5].

Table 12.2 Criteria for neuropathic pain diagnosis

Neuropathic pain criteria	Pain has a plausible neuroanatomical distribution
	There is a clinical history of neurological disease or injury in a localization that can explain pain distribution
	During examination are detected positive or negative sensory signs confined on the boundary of pain distribution and concordant with neurological lesions
	Diagnostic neuroimaging and/or neurophysiological tests confirm neurological lesion or disease consistent with pain and sensory disorder distribution
Central neuropathic pain	Pain due to a lesion of the central nervous system
Peripheral neuropathic pain	Pain due to a lesion of the peripheral nervous system

Central pain syndromes are specific neuropathic pain conditions, arising from injuries or diseases of the brain and spinal cord [6, 7]. Central pain is an ominous complication of neurological diseases, as stroke and multiple sclerosis [8]. About one third of the patients with spinal cord injuries is affected by central pain [6]. Difficulties to investigate brain and spinal cord with neurophysiologic and neuroanatomical techniques in vivo have prevented an appropriate knowledge of the central pain mechanisms. A combination of neuronal excitability and loss of inhibitory inputs, both caused by the neurosensorial net damage, is postulated to cause central pain [6]. Some recent observations attribute to the glia a primary role to sustain and augment neuropathic pain afferents [9].

The management of neuropathic pain generally is focused to reduce pain severity and to sustain patients about the disabling aspects of their diseases, since a direct intervention on the pain mechanisms only rarely can be implemented. Furthermore, the management of aetiological conditions typically does not lead to the pain remission. In recent years, several clinical studies on large neuropathic pain patients' populations, mainly based on peripheral neuropathy induced pain syndromes, have permitted to define consistent guidelines on neuropathic pain therapy. Standard neuropathic pain treatment is mainly pharmacological, based on a few antidepressants (Duloxetine and tryciclic antidepressants) and anticonvulsants (gabapentinoids) [10–13]. Data supporting combination drugs therapies are inconsistent [13]. Patients with neuropathic pain generally do not respond to Paracetamol and NSAID. In peripheral neuropathic pain opioids are considered a fourth line treatment, reserved to selected poor-responding patients, for short period of therapy only [13]. In fact, at least one well conducted randomized controlled clinical trial shows benefits in combining Morphine with Gabapentin for peripheral neuropathic pain [14]. In the last years, a surge in United States hospital admissions, and even deaths, provoked by opioids over-dosage consequences, mainly in patients with chronic nonmalignant pain conditions, has kicked off a heated debate about long term opioid treatments for many chronic pain patients [15]. Sedative adverse effects of the opioids may impact with the functionality and hamper cognitive and physical neurorehabilitation programmes in patients suffering from neurological diseases. However, pain

Table 12.3 Pharmacological therapies for central neuropathic pain (modified from [13])

Drug	Suggested dosages
Gabapentin	Start: 100–300 mg nocte Standard doses: 300–600 mg TID Maximal dose: 1.200 mg TID
Pregabalin	Start: 25–75 mg nocte Standard doses: 150 mg BID or TID Maximal dose: 300 mg BID
Amytriptiline	Start: 10 mg nocte Standard doses: 25–50 mg nocte or BID Maximal dose: 50 mg morning—100 mg nocte
Duloxetine	Start: 30 mg day Standard doses: 60 mg day Maximal dose: 120 mg day

itself is one of the major factors of poor efficiency of rehabilitation. Thus, when appropriate, an opioid based treatment, managed by experienced clinicians, is warranted also into a non-palliative context [16]. Non-pharmacological treatments could be considered in selected non-responders cases, added or in substitution to the standard drug therapies. Approaches based on psychology may enforce pain tollerance. Overall, there is a significant effect for placebo to reduce central pain [17]. Several physical therapies may result in a pain decrease [18]. Mirror movements after limb amputation may decrease phantom limb pain. Thus, descendant motor neural efferents inhibit nociceptive afferent signals. Motor cortex brain stimulation techniques (direct electric cortex stimulation or transcranial magnetic stimulation, particularly into a repetitive fashion) reduce controlateral central pains, and support a weak recommendation for the use of motor cortex electrical stimulation in central post-stroke pain [19] and for repetitive transcranial magnetic stimulation in central pain from spinal cord lesions [20]. Data are inconclusive to recommend spinal cord stimulation, deep brain stimulation and dorsal roots neurolesions in spinal cord injury pain [12].

There are no conclusive central pain management guidelines. Duloxetine and tryciclic antidepressants, Pregabalin and Gabapentin, are considered first-line treatments on the basis of favourable results into studies on specific central pain syndromes, such as post stroke pain, pain in multiple sclerosis and post spinal cord injury (Table 12.3) [21–25]. Non steroidal anti inflammatory drugs and opioids lack of efficacy in these pain syndromes [26]. However, even with the best available treatments, central pain may often be reduced only of some degree and several patients fail any analgesic strategies [6, 27].

12.3 Neuropathic Cancer Pain

Neuropathic pain is a rather common complication of cancer. One out five cancer patient suffers from neuropathic pain. This prevalence rises to about 40% when are included patients with mixed neuropathic and nociceptive pain, both stemming from pain mechanism peculiar to cancers, and also considering patients affected by more than one pain [28]. Neuropathic pain in cancer patients is difficult to manage, and often requires a specific expertise. Neuropathic pain is a major responsible of cancer pain therapy failure and significantly impact on quality of life [29–31].

Neuropathic cancer pain is the painful syndrome directly caused by the impact of growing cancers on nervous structures [28] (Fig. 12.1). Several characteristics of neuropathic cancer pain, such as the distribution, qualities and the generating mechanisms of the pain, distinguish this syndrome from non-oncological neuropathic pain. Common neuropathic cancer pain treatment also differs from that of neuropathic pain not caused by cancer. When directly caused by cancer it is common clinical practice to manage pain mainly with opioid medications, while antidepressants and anticonvulsants are used as adjuvants analgesics. A few clinical trials show a small but significant evidence of superiority of the treatments based on

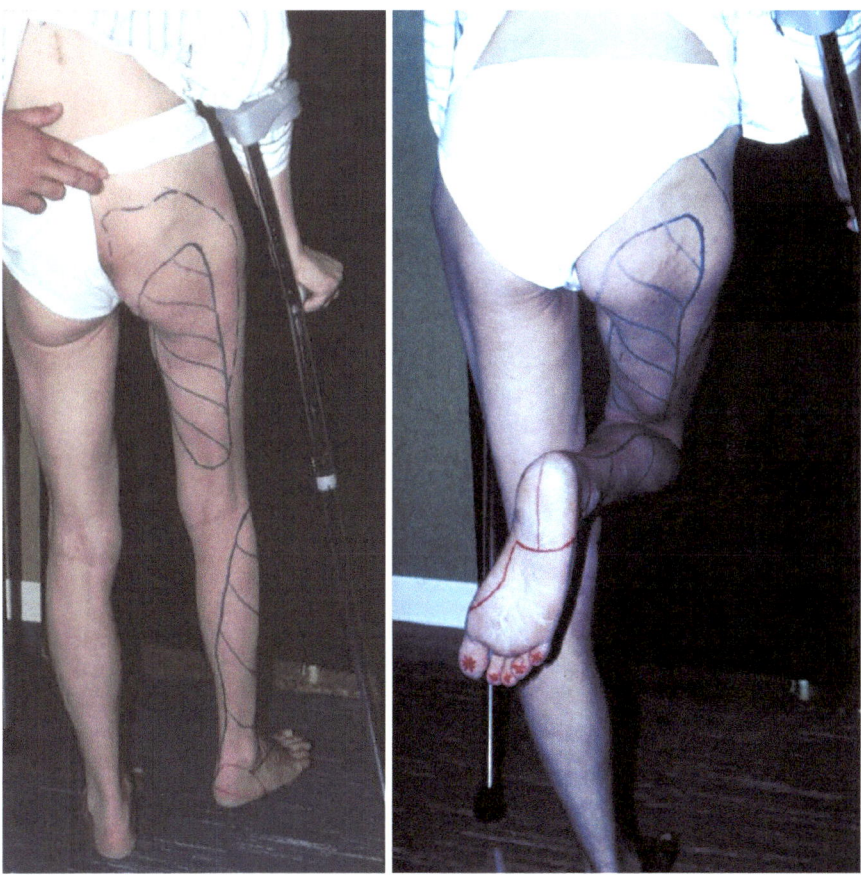

Fig. 12.1 Patient with carcinoma of the cervix infiltrating the lumbar plexus which generates: lancinating pain episodes; continuous burning pain; dysesthesia to touch. Regions of the skin with sensory loss (blue line) and allodynia to the touch (red line) are outlined

Gabapentin or Pregabalin in addition to an opioids therapy taken at regular time over an opioid treatment alone [32–34]. Duloxetine analgesic effect into neuropathic cancer pain is postulated and currently investigated [35]. However robust clinical studies on this syndrome are still lacking and strong clinical recommendations cannot be given [34].

12.4 Pain in Brain and Brainstem Tumours

Brain and other intracranial tumours involving the brain and the brain stem can generate complex pain syndromes. Within a large survey on pain caused by cancers of different types, complains of non-neuropathic pain of the head, due to intracranial hypertension and meningeal disease, are rare conditions, and neuropathic pains, due to cerebral and brain stem tumours, are even less frequent [36].

However, in selected populations of brain tumours patients, bodily pain and headache are between the main disturbing symptoms, showing a surge in frequency and severity during the last phases of the disease [37–39].

In these patients headache is largely the most prevalent type of pain, occurring in 30–90%, showing higher occurrence during the last weeks of life [37, 39–45]. Headache is mainly caused by raised intracranial liquoral pressure, due to growing tumours and surrounding edema, and to obstruction of liquoral reabsorption pathways. This pain is dull, diffused to the head, it has daily recurrence, worst in the early morning and lying down, and is typically aggravated by Valsalva manoeuvres [46]. The main treatment for raised liquoral pressure headache are steroids, for their anti edema effect [47]. Dexamethasone is largely the most used steroid [37, 42, 45]. Dexamethasone, at the usual dosage of 4–8 mg/day, provides pain relief in the majority of the patients. Higher dosage of 16 mg/day can be given in treatment failure cases, sometimes together or substituted by Mannitol in urgent situations, waiting for radiotherapy or surgical treatment and chemotherapy of the tumour [43, 48–50]. However, robust confirmatory investigation studies on the appropriate steroid dosages and duration of the therapies are not available [49]. In two small studies Dexamethasone dosages of 4, 8 and 16 mg/day showed overlapping effects [51, 52]. Long-period Dexamethasone therapy is associated with side effects, which include oral thrush, dysphoria, Cushing dysmorphism, steroid myopathy, more accentuated to proximal limbs, osteoporosis, gastric lesions and diabetes mellitus [43, 53]. When necessary, a slow steroid tapering, done into 2 weeks or more time, is recommended, due to the high frequency of symptoms recurrence [49].

Leptomeningeal spread of brain tumours [54], but also sometimes invasion of other skull tissues, as dura mater [55], can cause pain [56, 57]. Pain is typically referred to neck and to retro orbital regions [56, 58]. Steroids, along with standard analgesic therapy and radiotherapy are usually indicated.

Intracranial tumours localized into the cerebellopontine angle may be the cause of trigeminal neuralgia-like syndromes. The larger prevalence come from neurinomas of the Acoustic nerve [59]. Surgical resection is the standard of care. In selected cases stereotactic radiosurgery could be a valid alternative [60]. Trigeminal pain therapy is based on anticonvulsants, specifically Carbamazepine, or in some refractory patients Oxcarbazepine, Lamotrigine or Baclofen, while there is no role for opioids and anti-inflammatory drugs [11, 61].

Central neuropathic pain is a peculiar, but infrequent, feature of brain and brain stem tumours. Central pain existence is documented from a few case reports and by a small survey. Cheek and Taveras reported the features of some patients affected by tumours involving the thalamus [62]. Gan and Choksey described the case of a patients with facial pain, which they hypothesized was due to an irritative state of the brain cortex produced by a parafalcine meningioma [63]. Patel et al. reported the case of a patient suffering from central pain due to a thalamic metastasis [64]. In a wide survey on cancer pain, excluding cases provoked by raised intracranial pressure, no patients suffered from pain due to intracerebral metastatic lesions [36].

A few surveys on the last period of life in patients with cerebral gliomas report a prevalence of non-cephalic pain between 10% and 30% [37, 44]. These pain syndromes are no further described, but they could account for central neuropathic mechanisms, with pain projected to the body. Gonzales et al., from the New York Memorial Sloan-Kettering Cancer Center, investigated the prevalence of central pain in hospitalized patients with cancer, seen as consults by the Pain Service or by the Neurological Service. Sixteen patients (4%), from a total of 388 cancer pain patients visited from a neurologist pain consultant, and 11 (2%), from 557 patients with cancer pain admitted to the neurological ward, had a diagnosis of central pain. Six patients only, from the 27 central pain patients, had an history of brain tumours, 3 with thalamic injuries, 2 with a left parietal and 1 with a right parietal brain injuries. No patient with brainstem lesion and central pain has been reported [65].

The hypothesis that only afferent nociceptive neural pathway lesions may generate neuropathic pain is respected by these scarce clinical reports [5, 6]. Thalamus is the main hub of the somatosensory system in the brain, and it projects pain perceptions to the insula and to the parietal cortex. Thus, it does not surprise that these structures injuries only are associated with central pain. Central pain in cancer patients is idiosyncratic: only a few of patients with apparently identical lesions will develop neuropathic pain. Pain generating mechanisms are still greatly unknown. In the survey previously described, neoplasms injuring parietal cortex (3 cases) were metastatic: two of breast type and one of laryngeal origin. Thalamic lesions (3 cases) were the consequences of a an oligodendroglioma invasion of the right basal brain in one case, of the bilateral thalamic region spread of an anaplastic astrocytoma in the second case and of a cerebral lymphoma mass in the left thalamic region in the third case. This latter patient experienced an exacerbation of a burning sensation to the deep regions of the controlateral hemibody immediately after every intravenous Methotrexate injection [65]. Thus, the hypothesis that central pain is maintained by glial activation in association with a specific neoplasm cytology is clinically unproven [6]. Central pain in cancer patients may also rarely arise from surgical lesions of the brain and brainstem.

Neuropathic pain due to brain neoplasms onset may be delayed, from days to several years, after the cerebral injuries; it may last even for years, or have a duration of a few days only [65]. Usually there is not a clear-cut relation between pain and tumor progression. Sometimes neoplasm treatments, as surgery, radiotherapy or chemotherapy, alleviates neuropathic pains, but in some other cases these interventions can exacerbate, or even generate, central pains. However, all the patients in the Memorial Sloan Kettering Cancer Center survey received these treatments, and also steroids, with the intention to alleviate pain [65].

Central pain in brain neoplasms patients respect the plausible neuroanatomical distribution rule [6]. Pain is projected to the contralateral to the brain injury side: limbs and trunk, in variable pattern, plus sometimes to the controlateral side of the face, but also to the homolateral side in dissociated sensory syndromes caused by brainstem neoplasms. The prevalent clinical literature reports pain syndromes characterized by a dull and aching qualities, continuous and non-paroxysmal duration, diffuse to deep tissues and poorly localizable. Central pain diagnostic criteria include the detection of sensory abnormalities confined in the painful regions [5]. Often central pain patients show an exacerbation of pain provoked by cold stimuli— cold allodynia [8]. All central pain cancer patients examined by Gonzales and co-authors presented abnormal temperature sensations, including cold allodynia and impaired sensitivity to cold and heat stimuli [65].

12.5 Pain in Spinal Tumours

Central neuropathic pain from spinal cord lesions could be severe and refractory to standard pharmacological therapies. Moreover it is usually associated with highly disabling neurological conditions, such as paraparesis/tetraparesis and loss of bladder and bowel control, which contribute to aggravate global quality of life [66].

Tumours of the spine and spinal cord more often provokes mixed neuropathic and nociceptive pain syndromes, the latter from bone and meningeal structures involvement. Neuropathic pain itself often share central and peripheral characteristics, from the involvement of both spinal cord and nervous roots [67]. In a survey on central pain from cancer, spinal cord lesions were by far more often associated with pain than brain or brain stem lesions, occurring in a total of 21 of 27 patients [65].

Pain is the predominant presenting symptom in neoplastic epidural space invasion [68, 69]. Leptomeningeal seeding of neuroaxial tumours very often presents with radicular pain or pain projected to the neck or to the back [56, 58]. In the survey by Gonzales and others 2 out of 21 patients with central pain for spinal cord compression had leptomeningeal cancer diffusion [65]. Chronic neuropathic pain after radiotherapy and/or surgical spinal cord tumor resection may affect several patients [70]. Interestingly, a direct association between intraoperative hypotension and postoperative steroids treatment with central neuropathic pain occurrence has been recently evidentiated [71].

In the Memorial Sloan-Kettering Cancer Center patients survey on central pain, 8 patients only out of 21 had a primitive medullary tumour: 5 out them were affected by a spinal cord ependymoma type, 1 by a spinal cord glioblastoma, 1 by an astrocytoma type and 1 by a neuroectodermal tumor [65]. Sensory abnormalities and a wide variability in pain evolution in the time are peculiar spinal cord central pain features, as well in brain tumours central pain [65, 72]. Pain qualities and its continuous rather than paroxysmal appearance are common in spinal neuropathic pain as in other central pain syndromes [72].

Spino—thalamic tract lesions only, thus involving anterolateral columns of the spinal cord, may generate central pain. In ventral spinal cord tumor lesions, pain and associated neurological deficits, such as thermal and pain insensitivity and paralyses below the cord damage, may develop suddenly as a result of ischemia in the Anterior Spinal Artery territories [68]. Neuropathic pain project to the trunk and lower limbs, and also to upper limbs in cervical neoplasms, with upper sensory level a few dermatomes under the cord lesion. When the cord damage prevails into a side, the Brown-Sequard syndrome features may be seen: neuropathic pain is distributed to the controlateral to the cord lesion side, under the cord damage level, and may associates with the homolateral lower limb paresis or hemiparesis, and with dissociated sensory loss, controlateral thermodolorific hypoesthesia and homolateral mechanical and kinaesthetic hypoesthesia. Central spinal cord tumours, as ependymoma, may interrupt spino-thalamic nerve fibres into their controlateral decussation, thus provoking suspended for a few dermatomes thermodolorific sensory loss and sometimes pain in the same regions.

12.6 Conclusions

Pain is a frequent complication of cancer and requires appropriate assessment and treatment. Pain due CNS tumours is usually different from pain due to other non-CNS tumors, and may have complex pathopysiology. Accurate diagnosis of the pain characteristics and cause is required to personalize treatment.

References

1. van den Beuken-van Everdingen MHJ, Hochstenbach LMJ, Joosten EAJ, Tjan-Heijnen VCG, Janssen DJA. Update on prevalence of pain in patients with cancer: systematic review and meta-analysis. J Pain Symptom Manag. 2016;51(6):1070–1090.e9.
2. Quill TE, Abernethy AP. Generalist plus specialist palliative care – creating a more sustainable model. N Engl J Med. 2013;368:1173–5.
3. Treede RD, Jensen TS, Campbell JN, Cruccu G, Dostrovsky JO, Griffin JW, et al. Neuropathic pain: redefinition and a grading system for clinical and research purposes. Neurology. 2008;70:1630–5.
4. Brunelli C, Bennett MI, Kaasa S, Fainsinger R, Sjøgren P, Mercadante S, et al. Classification of neuropathic pain in cancer patients: a Delphi expert survey report and EAPC/IASP proposal of an algorithm for diagnostic criteria. Pain. 2014;155:2707–13.
5. Finnerup NB, Haroutounian S, Kamerman P, Baron R, Bennett DL, Bouhassira D, et al. Neuropathic pain: an updated grading system for research and clinical practice. Pain. 2016;157:1599–606.
6. Finnerup NB. A review of central neuropathic pain states. Curr Opin Anaesthesiol. 2008;21:586–9.
7. Widerström-Noga E, Loeser JD, Jensen TS, Finnerup NB. AAPT diagnostic criteria for central neuropathic pain. J Pain. 2017;18:1417–26.

8. Watson JC, Sandroni P. Central neuropathic pain syndromes. Mayo Clin Proc. 2016;91:372–85.
9. Machelska H, Celik MÖ. Recent advances in understanding neuropathic pain: glia, sex differences, and epigenetics. F1000Res. 2016;5:2743–53.
10. Colloca L, Ludman T, Bouhassira D, Baron R, Dickenson AH, Yarnitsky D, et al. Neuropathic pain. Nat Rev Dis Primers. 2017;3:17002.
11. Dosenovic S, Jelicic Kadic A, Miljanovic M, Biocic M, Boric K, Cavar M, Markovina N, et al. Interventions for neuropathic pain: an overview of systematic reviews. Anesth Analg. 2017;125:643–52.
12. Dworkin RH, O'Connor AB, Kent J, Mackey SC, Raja SN, Stacey BR, et al. Interventional management of neuropathic pain: NeuPSIG recommendations. Pain. 2013;154:2249–61.
13. Finnerup NB, Attal N, Haroutounian S, McNicol E, Baron R, Dworkin RH, et al. Pharmacotherapy for neuropathic pain in adults: a systematic review and meta-analysis. Lancet Neurol. 2015;14:162–73.
14. Gilron I, Bailey JM, Tu D, Holden RR, Weaver DF, Houlden RL. Morphine, gabapentin, or their combination for neuropathic pain. N Engl J Med. 2005;352:1324–34.
15. Paice JA. Cancer pain management and the opioid crisis in America: how to preserve hard-earned gains in improving the quality of cancer pain management. Cancer. 2018;124(12):2491–7. https://doi.org/10.1002/cncr.31303.
16. Tamburin S, Lacerenza MR, Castelnuovo G, Agostini M, Paolucci S, Bartolo M, et al. Pharmacological and non-pharmacological strategies in the integrated treatment of pain in neurorehabilitation. Evidence and recommendations from the Italian Consensus Conference on Pain in Neurorehabilitation. Eur J Phys Rehabil Med. 2016;52:741–52.
17. Cragg JJ, Warner FM, Finnerup NB, Jensen MP, Mercier C, Richards JS, et al. Meta-analysis of placebo responses in central neuropathic pain: impact of subject, study, and pain characteristics. Pain. 2016;157:530–40.
18. Nees TA, Finnerup NB, Blesch A, Weidner N. Neuropathic pain after spinal cord injury: the impact of sensorimotor activity. Pain. 2017;158:371–6.
19. Cruccu G, Aziz TZ, Garcia-Larrea L, Hansson P, Jensen TS, Lefaucheur JP, Simpson BA, Taylor RS. EFNS guidelines on neurostimulation therapy for neuropathic pain. Eur J Neurol. 2007;14:952–7.
20. Leung A, Donohue M, Xu R, Lefaucheur JP, Khedr EM, Saitoh Y, et al. TMS for suppressing neuropathic pain: a meta-analysis. J Pain. 2009;10:1205–16.
21. Rintala DH, Holmes SA, Courtade D, Fiess RN, Tastard LV, Loubser PG. Comparison of the effectiveness of amitriptyline and gabapentin on chronic neuropathic pain in persons with spinal cord injury. Arch Phys Med Rehabil. 2007;88:1547–60.
22. Snedecor SJ, Sudharshan L, Cappelleri JC, Sadosky A, Desai P, Jalundhwala YJ, et al. Systematic review and comparison of pharmacologic therapies for neuropathic pain associated with spinal cord injury. J Pain Res. 2013;6:539–47.
23. Tzellos TG, Papazisis G, Amaniti E, Kouvelas D. Efficacy of pregabalin and gabapentin for neuropathic pain in spinal-cord injury: an evidence-based evaluation of the literature. Eur J Clin Pharmacol. 2008;64:851–8.
24. Vollmer TL, Robinson MJ, Risser RC, Malcolm SK. A randomized, double-blind, placebo-controlled trial of duloxetine for the treatment of pain in patients with multiple sclerosis. Pain Pract. 2014;14:732–44.
25. Vranken JH, Dijkgraaf MG, Kruis MR, van der Vegt MH, Hollmann MW, Heesen M. Pregabalin in patients with central neuropathic pain: a randomized, double-blind, placebo-controlled trial of a flexible-dose regimen. Pain. 2008;136:150–7.
26. Finnerup NB, Otto M, McQuay HJ, Jensen TS, Sindrup SH. Algorithm for neuropathic pain treatment: an evidence based proposal. Pain. 2005;118:289–305.
27. Dworkin RH, O'Connor AB, Backonja M, Farrar JT, Finnerup NB, Jensen TS, et al. Pharmacologic management of neuropathic pain: evidence-based recommendations. Pain. 2007;132:237–51.
28. Bennett MI, Rayment C, Hjermstad M, Aass N, Caraceni A, Kaasa S. Prevalence and aetiology of neuropathic pain in cancer patients: a systematic review. Pain. 2012;153:359–65.

29. Arthur J, Tanco K, Haider A, Maligi C, Park M, Liu D, Bruera E. Assessing the prognostic features of a pain classification system in advanced cancer patients. Support Care Cancer. 2017;25:2863–9.
30. Oh SY, Shin SW, Koh SJ, Bae SB, Chang H, Kim JH, et al. Multicenter, cross-sectional observational study of the impact of neuropathic pain on quality of life in cancer patients. Support Care Cancer. 2017;25:3759–67.
31. Torrance N, Ferguson JA, Afolabi E, Bennett MI, Serpell MG, Dunn KM, Smith BH. Neuropathic pain in the community: more under-treated than refractory? Pain. 2013;154:690–9.
32. Bennett MI, Laird B, van Litsenburg C, Nimour M. Pregabalin for the management of neuropathic pain in adults with cancer: a systematic review of the literature. Pain Med. 2013;14:1681–8.
33. Caraceni A, Zecca E, Bonezzi C, Arcuri E, Yaya Tur R, Maltoni M, et al. Gabapentin for neuropathic cancer pain: a randomized controlled trial from the Gabapentin Cancer Pain Study Group. J Clin Oncol. 2004;22:2909–17.
34. Kane CM, Mulvey MR, Wright S, Craigs C, Wright JM, Bennett MI. Opioids combined with antidepressants or antiepileptic drugs for cancer pain: systematic review and meta-analysis. Palliat Med. 2018;32:276–86.
35. Matsuoka H, Ishiki H, Iwase S, Koyama A, Kawaguchi T, Kizawa Y, et al. Study protocol for a multi-institutional, randomised, double-blinded, placebo-controlled phase III trial investigating additive efficacy of duloxetine for neuropathic cancer pain refractory to opioids and gabapentinoids: the DIRECT study. BMJ Open. 2017;7:e017280. https://doi.org/10.1136/bmjopen-2017-017280.
36. Caraceni A, Portenoy RK. An international survey of cancer pain characteristics and syndromes. Pain. 1999;82:263–74.
37. Koekkoek JA, Dirven I, Sizoo EM, Pasman HR, Heimans JJ, Postma TJ, et al. Symptoms and medication management in the end of life phase of high-grade glioma patients. J Neuro-Oncol. 2014;120:589–95.
38. Oberndorfer S, Lindeck-Pozza E, Lahrmann H, Struhal W, Hitzenberger P, Grisold W. The end-of-life hospital setting in patients with glioblastoma. J Palliat Med. 2008;11:26–30.
39. Pace A, Di Lorenzo C, Guariglia L, Jandolo B, Carapella CM, Pompili A. End of life issues in brain tumor patients. J Neuro-Oncol. 2009;91:39–43.
40. Bausewein C, Hau P, Borasio GD, Voltz R. How do patients with primary brain tumours die? Palliat Med. 2003;17:558–9.
41. Chen JY, Hovey E, Rosenthal M, Livingstone A, Simes J. Neuro-oncology practices in Australia: a Cooperative Group for Neuro-Oncology patterns of care study. Asia Pac J Clin Oncol. 2014;10:162–7.
42. Girvan AC, Carter GC, Li L, Kaltenboeck A, Ivanova J, Koh M, et al. Glioblastoma treatment patterns, survival, and healthcare resource use in real-world clinical practice in the USA. Drugs Context. 2015;4:212274.
43. Pace A, Dirven L, Koekkoek JAF, Golla H, Fleming J, Rudà R, et al. European Association for Neruro-Oncology (EANO) guidelines for palliative care in adults with glioma. Lancet Oncol. 2017;18:330–40.
44. Sizoo EM, Braam L, Postma TJ, Pasman HR, Heimans JJ, Klein M, et al. Symptoms and problems in the end-of-life phase of high-grade glioma patients. Neuro-Oncology. 2010;12:1162–6.
45. Thier K, Calabek B, Tinchon A, Grisold W, Oberndorfer S. The last 10 days of patients with glioblastoma: assessment of clinical signs and symptoms as well as treatment. Am J Hosp Palliat Care. 2016;33:985–8.
46. Wall M. Update on idiopathic intracranial hypertension. Neurol Clin. 2017;35:45–57.
47. Tsao MN. Brain metastases: advances over the decades. Ann Palliat Med. 2015;4:225–32.
48. Kaal EC, Vecht CJ. The management of brain edema in brain tumors. Curr Opin Oncol. 2004;16(6):593–600.
49. Ryken TC, McDermott M, Robinson PD, Ammirati M, Andrews DW, Asher AL, et al. The role of steroids in the management of brain metastases: a systematic review and evidence-based clinical practice guideline. J Neuro-Oncol. 2010;96:103–14.

50. Vecht CJ. Clinical management of brain metastasis. J Neurol. 1998;245:127–31.
51. Vecht CJ, Hovestadt A, Verbiest HB, Vliet JJ, Putten WL. Dose-effect relationship of dexamethasone on Karnofsky performance in metastatic brain tumors: a randomized study of doses of 4, 8, and 16 mg per day. Neurology. 1994;44:675–80.
52. Wolfson AH, Snodgrass SM, Schwade JG, Markoe AM, Landy H, Feun LG, et al. The role of steroids in the management of metastatic carcinoma to the brain. A pilot prospective trial. Am J Clin Oncol. 1994;17:234–8.
53. Ly KI, Wen PY. Clinical relevance of steroid use in neuro-oncology. Curr Neurol Neurosci Rep. 2017;17:13–6.
54. Wang N, Bertalan MS, Brastianos PK. Leptomeningeal metastasis from systemic cancer: review and update on management. Cancer Cytopathol. 2018;124:21–3.
55. Grisold W, Grisold A. Cancer around the brain. Neurooncol Pract. 2014;1:13–21.
56. Formaglio F, Caraceni A. Meningeal metastases: clinical aspects and diagnosis. Ital J Neurol Sci. 1998;19:133–49.
57. Van Horn A, Chamberlain MC. Neoplastic meningitis. J Support Oncol. 2012;10:45–53.
58. Reni M, Mazza E, Zanon S, Gatta G, Vecht CJ. Central nervous system gliomas. Crit Rev Oncol Hematol. 2017;113:213–23.
59. Matsuka Y, Fort ET, Merrill RL. Trigeminal neuralgia due to an acoustic neuroma in the cerebellopontine angle. J Orofac Pain. 2000;14:147–51.
60. Kotecha R, Kotecha R, Modugula S, Murphy ES, Jones M, Kotecha R, et al. Trigeminal neuralgia treated with stereotactic radiosurgery: the effect of dose escalation on pain control and treatment outcomes. Int J Radiat Oncol Biol Phys. 2016;96:142–8.
61. Zakrzewska JM, Linskey ME. Trigeminal Neuralgia. Am Fam Physician. 2016;94:133–5.
62. Cheek WR, Taveras JM. Thalamic tumors. J Neurosurg. 1966;24:505–13.
63. Gan YC, Choksey MS. Parafalcine meningioma presenting with facial pain: evidence for cortical theory or pain? Br J Neurosurg. 2001;15:350–2.
64. Patel RA, Chandler JP, Jain S, Gopalakrishnan M, Sachdev S. Dejerine-Roussy syndrome from thalamic metastasis treated with stereotactic radiosurgery. J Clin Neurosci. 2017;44:227–8.
65. Gonzales GR, Tuttle SL, Thaler H, Manfredi PL. Central pain in cancer patients. J Pain. 2003;4:351–4.
66. Putzke JD, Richards JS, Hicken BL, DeVivo MJ. Interference due to pain following spinal cord injury: important predictors and impact on quality of life. Pain. 2002;100:231–42.
67. Hatch MN, Cushing TR, Carlson GD, Chang EY. Neuropathic pain and SCI: identification and treatment strategies in the 21st century. J Neurol Sci. 2018;384:75–83.
68. DeAngelis LM, Posner JM. Epidural metastases. In: DeAngelis LM, Posner JM, editors. Neurologic complications of cancer. 2nd ed. Oxford: Oxford University Press; 2009. p. 197–227.
69. Helweg-Larsen S, Sørensen PS. Symptoms and signs in metastatic spinal cord compression: a study of progression from first symptom until diagnosis in 153 patients. Eur J Cancer. 1994;30:396–8.
70. Nakamura M, Tsuji O, Iwanami A, Tsuji T, Ishii K, Toyama Y, et al. Central neuropathic pain after surgical resection in patients with spinal intramedullary tumor. J Orthop Sci. 2012;17:352–7.
71. Onishi-Kato Y, Nakamura M, Iwanami A, Kato M, Suzuki T, Kosugi S, et al. Perioperative factors associated with chronic central pain after the resection of intramedullary spinal cord tumor. Clin J Pain. 2017;33:640–6.
72. Siddall PJ, McClelland JM, Rutkowski SB, Cousins MJ. A longitudinal study of the prevalence and characteristics of pain in the first 5 years following spinal cord injury. Pain. 2003;103:249–57.

Psycho-Oncology in Brain Tumour Patients

13

Alice Malabaila and Riccardo Torta

13.1 Psycho-Oncology

Since ancient times humans tried to find a link between psyche and disease; in modern times, the bio-psycho-social model is considered to be the foundation of psychosomatic medicine and the model to explain, as well as possible, the connection between mind and body.

Psycho-oncology is a multidisciplinary matter that studies the psychological, social and behavioural aspects of cancer and involves several health professionals, such as psychologists, psychiatrists, oncologists of various specialties, surgeons, radio- and chemotherapists, specialists in pain and rehabilitation therapy. The psycho-oncological care is comprehensive and goes from the psychological evaluation during the communication of the diagnosis to the rehabilitation phase or to the psycho-physic management of the terminal patient [1].

Psycho-oncology considers both the psychological responses of patients and their caregivers to cancer, during all the phases of the disease, and the psychological, behavioural and social aspects that may have repercussions on cancer.

Cancer is a disease that involves both the body and the mind.

13.1.1 Stress Reaction

Hans Selye, who pioneered research on biological effects of exposure to stressful stimuli with rats, provided one of the first definitions of stress [2]. He conceptualized the general adaptation syndrome that consists in the activation of the hypothalamic–pituitary–adrenal (HPA) axis with increased adrenocorticotropic (ACTH) and cortisone hormone scarring, atrophy of the thymus, spleen and other lymphoid tissue and

A. Malabaila (✉) · R. Torta
Clinical and Oncological Psychology, Department of Neuroscience, University of Turin, Turin, Italy

© Springer Nature Switzerland AG 2019
M. Bartolo et al. (eds.), *Neurorehabilitation in Neuro-Oncology*,
https://doi.org/10.1007/978-3-319-95684-8_13

gastric ulcerations. He described three stages: the first one consists in a brief alarm reaction, the second one in a prolonged period of resistance and the last one is over-tiredness and death [3]. Further studies were carried out by Lazarus who considered four concepts in the analysis of the stress process [4]: (1) a causal external or internal agent, which is the stressor; (2) an evaluation that discriminates what can be harmful and what not; (3) coping processes use to deal with stressful demands and (4) a complex pattern of effects on mind and body, which is the stress reaction.

Man, differently from rats, does not passively suffer an external stimulus, but, through a cognitive assessment, attributes a meaning: therefore, differentiated physiological responses result for each individual, due to exposure to the same stressor [5].

In psycho-oncology, the individual's response to the disease can be considered as a stress response involving psychological, social and relational aspects, which assumes a sense of threat to their own existence, integrity, identity and role [1]. The exposure to events that are significant emotional stressors for patient causes a series of cascade modifications involving the central nervous system (CNS), the peripheral nervous system (PNS), the endocrine system and the immune system. The importance of the relationship between stress, depression and hormonal changes was emphasized by Board [6] and Sachar [7].

When individuals are exposed to stress, the HPA axis and the sympathetic-adrenal-medullary (SAM) system can be activated commanding the secretion of corticosteroids and catecholamines; the chronic stimulation of the HPA axis is possibly associated with higher risk of developing cancer [8].

13.1.2 The Bio-Psycho-Social Model

The bio-psycho-social (BPS) model has ancient philosophical roots, which start from criticism to dichotomy between mind and body. Plato had already known the need for a global vision of man:

> For that is the biggest mistake in the treatment of disease, that mind and body are all too much separated, whereas they cannot be separated - however this is overlooked by Greek doctors… They should care for the whole, for there, where the whole is in a bad state, a part can never be healthy.
>
> —Plato, The Charmides

Plato's theorizations apply not only to physicians in ancient Greece but, in the same way, to contemporary medical practice including oncology [9].

Instead of these theories, Descartes conceptualized mind and matter as two great, mutually exclusive and mutually exhaustive divisions of the universe [10]. This vision was crucial to founding the basics of modern medicine.

In the twenty-first century, the biomedical model remains necessary, but it is no longer sufficient because it ignored the influence of the mind on the body. Consequently, the role of psychological factors in the onset and progress of disease and in the effects of the disease and its treatment on the patient's quality of life have been largely ignored or minimized [9]. This thought also involved oncology.

Fortunately, the situation has advanced in the past decades. Progresses in treatment have changed therapeutic strategies and have prolonged the lives of oncological patients, thereby focusing attention on the quality of life despite Cartesian dualism influences. This condition led to the emergence of two new medical disciplines: palliative medicine and psycho-oncology [11].

In this context of ideological innovation, great importance has had the Engel theory that was the first to discuss about a bio-psycho-social (BPS) approach to the disease [12]. The physical, emotional, cognitive, behavioural and social areas are included inside the BPS model. Engel theorized that biological, psychological (thoughts, emotions and behaviours) and social factors all together play a significant role in human functioning, in the context of the disease. Engel's studies focused to understand how psychological phenomena could influence physiology [13]. He espoused a dictum that is paradigmatic of the BPS model [14]:

> Science itself is a human activity; the lesson: that humanness and human phenomena cannot be excluded from science.
>
> —Engel

The words by which we identify different aspects of the disease are an example of the BPS model. The word "disease" is related to the biological area and means an abnormal and pathological condition that affects the organism. It's often construed as a medical condition, associated with specific symptoms and signs. The world "illness" represents the psychological aspects and identifies the subjective sense of feeling unwell, a person's perception of the disease. On the other hand, the world "sickness" is related to the social and cultural conception of health conditions that influence how the patient reacts.

Brain tumour is a serious and complex health condition that can have devastating physical, cognitive and psycho-social effects on patients and their caregivers.

Few studies have evaluated the influence of BPS factors on quality of life (QoL) in adults with a primary brain tumour [15]. Some research assessed the effects of both cognitive and psycho-social functioning in relation to QoL in this group of patients and we can affirm that these factors may partially explain the low QoL in neuro-oncological survivors.

Conversely, Ownsworth et al., in a BPS approach, examined the associations among quality of life, depression, performance status and fatigue and found that the relationship between pre-illness characteristics, neuropathological variables, psycho-social factors and quality of life was inconsistent [16].

Given the discrepancy of the results and the implications that such research could have in the clinical practice and, consequently, in the interventions offered to patients and their families, much attention to the methodology of the studies is needed.

13.2 Brain Tumour Patients

The patient affected by a cerebral tumour is a patient with peculiarities compared to patients with other oncological pathologies: the affected organ is the brain, the organ that manages emotions, thoughts, motivations, behaviours and actions. As a result, the symptoms that may appear in a neuro-oncological patient range from psychic disorders, cognitive deficits, temperamental changes, behavioural dysfunctions, motor and functional disorders that often lead to a reduced autonomy and independence of the subject.

Patients with cognitive deficits may have difficulty in several cognitive functions: they may have languages deficits in production, comprehension or para-verbal aspects or trouble in remembering and learning new information and they could also have executive dysfunctions, for example, in planning or organizing, problem solving, working memory or flexibility [17].

These impairments have a strong impact on patient's ability in daily life, in family, friends and professional context. The disease upsets the balance that the patient had previously built and so he/she needs for a new mental adjustment or coping [18].

The word "coping" means facing, holding head and struggling successfully. It indicates the cognitive, emotional and behavioural strategies implemented by an individual to manage a stressful situation as a disease; therefore, it represents the ability to face the problems and their emotional consequences [19]. This concept defines an adaptation process that keeps on for a long time throughout the disease, involving the patient's family, and is a flexible reaction to problematic life events that changes over time in relation to the situational context [20, 21].

The different behavioural patterns in relation to stressful events, characteristic of each individual, are defined as coping styles. This concept is crucial in oncology, because it represents an important parameter that can significantly influence the different psychological reactions and psycho-social adaptation to the disease, possible psychopathological complications, quality of life after diagnosis, adherence to treatments and, maybe, also the course of the disease itself [22].

Mental adjustment to cancer has been explored in a large body of the literature, Grassi et al. identified five coping styles: fighting spirit, hopelessness, fatalism, anxious preoccupation and avoidance. *Fighting spirit* is characterized by moderate levels of anxiety and depression; the patient tries to respond positively and constructively to the situation, maintaining a belief in internal control on the disease. *Hopelessness* is described with high levels of depression and anxiety, inability to implement cognitive strategies to accept the diagnosis, the belief of an external locus of control on the disease. Low levels of depression and anxiety, fatalistic attitude, belief in external control on the disease, the tendency to passivity and lack of opposition against the illness are typical of *fatalism*. Instead *anxious preoccupation* is characterized by anxious alarm response against the disease, excessive search for information and high levels of anxiety that affect the quality of life of the patient. At last, *avoidance* is identified as the absence of depression, anxiety and cognitive strategies, in the belief of a both internal and external control on the disease [22].

Heim et al. also studied coping in oncological patients and theorized a four-step model. According to this model, patient alternates four coping phases: the *cognitive phase* where the patient identifies some changes in physiological conditions and begins to analyse them, he is preoccupied with the disease and try to find the right definitions and estimations about the illness. In the *denial phase* the patient rejects the presence of the disease; this phase may have a favourable effect because it reduces anxiety, but it may interfere with getting treatment or disrupt the process of assimilating the stressful event. During the *anxiety phase* the patient shows apprehension, uncontrollable worry, agitation, panic attacks and sign of the autonomic arousal. Finally, the *depressive phase* is linked to the awareness of losses as part of the body or the role in family and society and the functional integrity [23, 24].

Patients affected by a brain cancer have limited options for improving quality of life during the disease, because learning to cope with such a debilitating disease can be difficult. According to Acquaye et al., being hopeful may be a significant factor in personal adjustments, but is plagued by illness-related uncertainty. In the initial stages of illness, hope should be an important theme, especially since it can play an essential role for neuro-oncological patients and their overall sense of well-being during the treatment [25]. The authors found that patients reporting more hope also suffered less of mood disturbances, furthermore patients with brain tumour recurrence reported lower hope and higher mood disturbance than those who were newly diagnosed or without recurrence. Targeted interventions are suggested to improve quality of life during the disease that may include measures to increase hope in order to facilitate positive coping strategies.

The neuro-oncological patient, as mentioned above, often develops disabilities in several areas that have a massive impact on quality of life and his/her functioning in everyday life. The use of functional coping strategies and the learning of new compensation cognitive strategies may increase the quality of life, the patient self-perception of functioning and, consequently, result in a mood improvement.

Functional coping leads to learn new compensation strategies and learning new compensations strategies makes a coping really functional. This process is only possible if patient is conscious of his/her deficit, but often neurological symptoms, as anosognosia or psychological defence as avoidance and denial, invalidate consciousness.

13.2.1 Psychological Disorders in Neuro-Oncology

The diagnosis of a brain cancer is an event that abruptly interrupts the person's path of life and breaks down the dimensions on which human existence is based. Changes resulting from the disease can lead to difficulties in daily lives, because of patient limitations, partial or total loss of autonomy, need for support and consequent dependence on others. Obviously, this status is often associated with important consequences on the psychological level.

Published studies have demonstrated that a substantial percentage of oncologic patients reports anxiety and depressive symptoms. McDaniel et al. found that up to one-half of oncological patients experience depressive symptoms [26]; furthermore, although not as extensively studied as depression in cancer populations, anxiety also has been shown to be prevalent among oncologic patients. In a study by Skarstein et al., using the hospital anxiety and depression scale (HADS) [27], 13% of 568 patients had a diagnosable anxiety [28].

It can be asserted that the anatomical, physiological, functional and emotional impact of a diagnosis of brain tumour can often induce anxious and depressive symptom. As observed, psychiatric symptoms often coexist and affect each other: depressive symptoms often accompany increased anxiety or irritability. Anxiety may result from situational fear related to diagnosis and prognosis or may be directly related to the effects of the tumour. Neurocognitive changes could moreover induce or worsen neuropsychiatric symptoms, as well as behavioural disturbances, in brain tumour patients.

According to Arnold et al., failing to adequately treat depression and other psychiatric symptoms in neuro-oncological patient populations can compromise and worsen overall health and quality of life [29]. Therefore, great importance needs to be given to the methodology used to survey the presence of mood disorders in these patients: Anderson et al. observed that the frequency of depressed patients with glioma ranged from 0 to 93% [30]. A further study, on a sample of 598 patients with high grade gliomas (HGG), found that clinicians reported depressive symptoms in 15% of patients, while 93% of patients attributed depressive symptom to themselves [31].

In the Rooney et al. review, examining 42 studies for a total of 4089 patients (90.3% with HGG and 9.7% with low grade gliomas–LGG), the different clinical variables associated with depression are analysed [32]. Among the variables associated with the patient, the female sex (only for patients with LGG), psychiatric disorders prior to the disease, physical dysfunctions and cognitive decline seem to have a positive association with the development of depression. From the analysis of variables associated with the disease, it emerges that localization of the tumour in the frontal lobe is more easily associated with clinical depression. Regarding treatments, corticosteroids seem to have a positive association with depression (depressive symptoms in 71.4% of patients treated with steroids, versus 44.3% of patients not treated), as well as radiotherapy, but only in the long period.

It can be asserted that being a female, having a lower grade tumour—maybe because at a minor cognitive deterioration corresponds a greater awareness of the disease—and having previous psychiatric disorders are predictive factors of anxiety development; the predictors of depression include being a female, having lower education, a lower grade tumour, history of psychiatric disorders and not being married [29].

Depressive disorder screening in patients with brain cancer should be routinely part of good clinical practice, because only identifying early the onset of psychic disturbance is possible a timely treatment that minimizes the possibility of chronicization and maximizes a functional coping to the disease. To this purpose, the self-assessed tools are of great importance, as they allow to easily select patients who may develop a psychiatric disorder. With this purpose, Rooney et al. validated three self-report psychological scales for depression—the distress thermometer (DT) [33], the subscale of depression from the hospital anxiety and depression scale (HADS-D) [27] and the patient health questionnaire–9 (PHQ-9) [34]—in a population of adults with gliomas. He concluded that HADS-D and PHQ-9 may be valid screening techniques for depression in brain cancer patients but alone they are not enough to identify depression; they could be used to screen patients with higher scores, which require further clinical evaluations [35].

Early prevention and identification of psychic disorders, realized through validated tools and clinical interviews, can only take place within a collaborative team in which health professionals aim for the bio-psycho-social patient's treatment. Recognizing psychic disturbances, such as anxiety and depression, can allow the team to improve the understanding of the symptoms and their causes, in order to better manage the patient and not solely his/her cancer.

13.3   Caregiver of Neuro-Oncological Patients

If the person affected by the disease is the main protagonist, the context in which he/she lives, especially the family, assumes an equally significant role. Cancer is a family traumatic event, a family disease that threatens the family unit and creates important changes in its structure and functioning [36]. Understanding the main characteristics of the family is necessary to provide more specific assistance and to manage the difficult situations that arise when the team relates to the family, as well as with the patient [22].

In this particular context, the diagnosis and treatment of a brain tumour are often associated with physical, emotional and social wellness interruption and represent a life-changing event for patients and their families [37, 38].

High levels of psychological distress were found among patients and caregivers, with both having high scores on anxiety and depression scales. Several studies reported that caregivers of patients with chronic illness in general, and with cancer in particular, have stress levels greater than those of the patients themselves [39]. Caregivers often report the lack of support in order to be prepared to cope with the difficulties of caring a patient with a brain tumour [40], and social support has been identified as a powerful factor increasing life satisfaction of caregivers [39, 41].

Patients and caregivers are exposed to physical and psycho-social stress that, if not properly managed, could lead to depressive symptoms [42]. Several studies have shown that psycho-education, skills training and therapeutic counselling of caregivers significantly increase self-efficacy and quality of life, reduce their burden and improve the ability to cope [43].

The time of diagnosis is a traumatic event for the caregiver, who experiences acute physiological reactions characterized by shock, with simultaneous feelings of anguish, anger and disbelief; moments of denial and rejection alternate at moments of despair, to which follow elaboration responses to adaptation and acceptance of the inevitability of events. During this period the caregiver and the patient's family can manifest very different defensive styles [44]: mechanisms of alteration of truth, determined by the need to maintain their own equilibrium and that of the patient, may be associated with mechanisms of hyper-involvement, marked anxiety and hyper-protection towards the patient; in other cases, distancing attitudes may prevail, in which removal mechanisms of the patient appear in the delegation of everything about the disease and therapy to places and people outside the family. The acceptance phase may help overcome the difficulties associated with the disease, which often leads to a new balance.

Furthermore, it is necessary to consider that the reactions just described may be present in the caregiver synchronously to that of the patient or at different times. In addition, often the disruptive effect of cancer highlights family related past problems, which cause the disorganization of the dynamics between the caregiver and the patient.

During the illness, the caregiver often experiences the loss of the patient's capabilities and the consequent change of his roles within the social, family and work environment; after becoming aware of this, the caregiver must therefore change his/her roles to compensate the dysfunctions of the patient.

13.4 Treatments

13.4.1 Psychotherapy

Psychotherapy is part of the patient's care and must be integrated into a context that involves specific interventions for different problems the patient and his family have to deal with [45, 46].

Psychotherapy in oncology, regardless of the specific psychological approach, aims to reduce or limit the level of emotional distress, promotes the development of more adaptive patterns of disease response, helps the patient understand the sense of the illness and integrates it into his/her own subjective experience and finally improves the quality of life.

In psycho-oncology, patients can be treated by several psychotherapeutic approaches: the most important of them are psychodynamic, cognitive-behavioural and psycho-educational interventions.

The psychodynamic therapy with oncological patients gains significant importance, although the confirmation of the results is complex. In this context the focus must be constantly on medical illness and quality of life and the therapist must pay attention to countertransference towards the patient [47]. This therapy should consider the meaning of the existence and the experience of the disease and, differently from psychotherapy with patients without life-threatening medical conditions, the therapist's purpose is to help the patient to live as satisfying as possible in the remaining time. For these reasons, the therapist usually is very active to lead the patient in a re-reading of his/her story, highlighting the strengths and goals achieved [48]. It's essential that the patient feels in control of his/her life facing it as the protagonist; this feeling for many patients results in a change of his/her own life and in a transformation of the relationships with others.

The cognitive-behavioural interventions seek the resolution of patient's problems by defining a specific focus. Therapy contemplates a leading and pedagogic role that helps the patient to examine the dysfunctional thoughts he/she has during the day, to analyse the emotions that arise from these thoughts, and, during therapy, to change the thoughts by contrasting them with more realistic alternatives. A further feature of this approach is the possibility of interventions with a limited number of sessions, qualifying it for the oncological context [49]. The cognitive-behavioural approach aims to encourage the expression of feelings, to increase the control over own life and an active participation in medical care, to help develop effective methods to manage cancer-related problems and to improve the communication between the patient and the caregiver. The therapy focuses on the subjective significance that cancer has for the patient and the coping style he/she is adopting.

Psycho-educational interventions are purposed to ensure greater knowledge about the disease and the therapies, to provide appropriate and realistic information supporting the resolution of practical psycho-social problems and to promote the patient adherence. Psycho-educational programs usually use educational material such as brochure, brief illustrative manuals and audio-visual supports.

In the neuro-oncological context, the choice of the psychotherapeutic approach is often dictated by the disease, its course and the residual cognitive abilities of the patient, frequently requiring a strictly limited in duration therapy and a lack of awareness as a consequence of the disease.

13.4.2 Psychopharmacology

The prescription of psychopharmacological drugs in patients with brain tumours mainly concerns benzodiazepines (BDZs), antipsychotics (APs) and antidepressants (ADs).

The spectrum of action of GABAergic compounds, such as BDZs, is mainly represented by anxiety and insomnia. The choice of a BDZ, in a patient with a brain tumour, shows the similar characteristics that in general population: particularly the consideration of which half-life (short and long acting BDZs) is more favourable for the patient and the kind of hepatic metabolism (it is better to use BDZs that are only glucurono-conjugate in order to avoid metabolic interferences). BDZ obviously can worsen the cognitive performance and the fatigue: so the use of this class has to be limited to the acute phase of anxiety and insomnia. In a chronic anxiety it is better to use antidepressants, particularly those with a more striking sedative activity.

The use of antipsychotics ranges over the old and new antipsychotic classes. Between the first generation (i.e. neuroleptics) it is better to avoid phenothiazines, because of the risk of induction of epileptic seizures. Haloperidol demonstrates a low risk on epileptic induction, but a higher risk of extrapyramidal side effects. For these problems usually, in the management of psychotic symptoms, delirium or agitation, atypical antipsychotic (AAPs) (e.g. risperidone, olanzapine, quetiapine) are preferred. Risperidone and olanzapine show a more incisive activity, quetiapine a more sedative one. Also with AAPs caution has to be used with clozapine, because this drug can favour the appearance of epileptic seizures, particularly in predisposed people as patients with brain tumours.

The use of antidepressants needs a more extensive discussion. The spectrum of AD's activity ranges over many clinical fields: chronic anxiety, chronic stress, mood depression and pain. So an antidepressant can act on several symptom clusters at the same time. Antidepressants actually have a broad range of potential neurological and general side effects that, conceivably, could cause harm to patients at increased risk of epilepsy, cognitive dysfunction and fatigue, such as patients with brain lesions [50]. Therefore the use of ADs in patients with brain tumours has to face with peculiar safety problems, such as the debated aspect of epileptogenesis, the interference with the tumour in itself, the worsening of cognitive symptoms and fatigue. Unlike other classes of drugs, antidepressants show a very differentiated intraclass profile, concerning such aspects that impose an accurate choice of a patient tailored approach.

Starting from the supposition that glioma stem cells (GSC) can have a relevant role in cancer progression, Bielecka-Wajdman et al. examined the evidence that some antidepressants (particularly imipramine and amitriptyline) can modulate plasticity, silence the GSC profile and partially reverse the malignant phenotype of GSM [51]. In the same way, Ma et al. found that a combined fluoxetine (an SSRI antidepressant) and temozolomide (TMZ) treatment showed a synergistic cytotoxic effect on the C6 glioma cells. The authors hypothesized that fluoxetine may sensitize glioma cells to TMZ, through activation of the CHOP-dependent apoptosis pathway [52]. Similarly, a previous study carried out from Liu et al. demonstrates that fluoxetine can induce apoptosis of glioma cells by evoking an AMPAR mediated calcium-dependent apoptosis [53]. Another mechanism of a possible anti-glioblastoma activity from antidepressants was studied by Hayashi et al. using fluvoxamine (another SSRI) that inhibits the human glioblastoma migration and invasion by disrupting actin polymerization in vitro [54].

Finally, from a clinical point of view, Pottegård et al. observed a protective effect of tricyclic antidepressants (TCAs) against gliomas in 3767 glioma cases and 75,340 population controls. The authors found that long-term use of TCAs was inversely associated with risk of glioma (OR 0.72, 95% CI: 0.41–1.25), while a similar pattern was not observed for the use of SSRIs [55].

All these studies are intriguing, but the transposition of in vitro studies to the clinical practice needs a larger number of in vivo controlled trials.

Another relevant problem that is subject for discussion from years is represented by the fact that the use of antidepressants could induce epileptic seizure in predisposed patients, included those with brain tumours. Actually such problem is also present, but in lesser extent, in the general population, or in patients with epilepsy associated with mood depression. In these cases, it is only an antidepressant overdose that is usually associated with an increased risk of epileptic seizures [56].

It is well known that epilepsy affects approximately 50% of patients with glioma, as an integral part of the illness, and practically all patients are at a generally increased risk of epilepsy throughout. The question therefore arises as to whether, in such a high-risk population, antidepressants could cause seizures also in therapeutic doses [57].

Alper et al. carried out a large meta-analysis of seizure risk in over 30,000 participants in the US Food and Drug Administration (FDA) antidepressant licencing trials. They found an increased risk of new-onset seizures for the antidepressants, particularly bupropion and clomipramine. Most antidepressants, however, showed no association with increased seizure risk, in therapeutic doses, and some were even associated with a reduced risk [58]. Also Ribot et al., in a retrospective observational study, pointed out that SSRIs or SNRIs did not appear to worsen seizure frequency, also in patients with frequent seizures. SSRIs and SNRIs may be even associated with a possible decrease in seizure frequency [59]. In this way, the study of the pharmacodynamic aspects of the administration of APs and ADs to patients with epilepsy can help to evaluate the importance of some mechanisms of action of several psychoactive drugs in relation to their pro- or anticonvulsant activity [60]. Obviously an evaluation bias is represented by the fact that no prospective trial has been carried out with the use of antidepressants within a high-risk group of patients with glioma. On the other hand, it is relevant to consider that also an untreated depression is itself a risk factor for epilepsy [61]. In this way the risk of seizure from ADs is a balance between the intrinsic epileptogenic activity from some compounds and the reduced risk achieved by the mood and stress improvement [62]. Anyway the potential risk of using antidepressants in glioma patients justifies prospective studies [63]. Another risk of harm, concerning the use of psychopharmacological drugs in patients with gliomas, lies in their potential effects on cognitive function [64].

Actually, nearly all glioma patients show some cognitive impairment that ranges in severity from subclinical to severe [65]. On this predisposing background antidepressants, particularly those with an intrinsic anticholinergic activity, such as TCAs, can worsen cognitive function in vulnerable individuals. As a matter of fact, the true impact of ADs in cognitive function in glioma patients is not clearly quantifiable because the cognitive impairment is not a univariate dimension, but several factors can contribute to it, for example, the presence/absence of mood depression that, in his turn, can be influenced by antidepressants. Cognitive dysfunction should be actually a part of the depressive syndrome. Retrospective data further suggest that selective serotonin reuptake inhibitor (SSRI) antidepressants may be safe in glioma. In one large case notes review ($n = 160$), there was no evidence of increased toxicity among patients with glioblastoma multiforme taking an SSRI [66].

A similar situation holds for fatigue that is reported by a clear majority of glioma patients and severely compromises the quality of life and the daily living. Obviously the causes of fatigue are multifactorial, including the effect of brain cancer in itself, radiotherapy, chemotherapy and mood depression [67]. But fatigue is also listed as a side effect of some antidepressants.

As a matter of fact, it is unclear whether antidepressants may improve or worsen fatigue in patients with glioma: there are currently no prospective data on their effect in a group as prone to fatigue as glioma patients. Yet it is possible that the successful treatment of depression could improve each of these outcomes.

Another remark is that different classes of ADs, acting on different neurotransmitters, can exert a different activity on fatigue: it is possible that ADs acting on norepinephrine and dopamine are more effective than serotonergic agents on the emotional component of fatigue [68].

References

1. Torta R, Mussa A. PsicOncologia. Il modello biopsicosociale. 2nd ed. Torino: Centro Scientifico Editore; 2007.
2. Selye H. A syndrome produced by diverse nocuous agents. J Neuropsychiatry Clin Neurosci. 1998;10(2):230–1.
3. Neylan TC. Hans Selye and the field of stress research. J Neuropsychiatry Clin Neurosci. 1998;10(2):230.
4. Lazarus RS. From psychological stress to the emotions: a history of changing outlooks. Annu Rev Psychol. 1993;44:1–21.
5. Fredrickson BL, Joiner T. Positive emotions trigger upward spirals toward emotional Well-being. Psychol Sci. 2002;13(2):172–5.
6. Board F, Persky H, Hamburg DA. Psychological stress and endocrine functions. Psychosom Med. 1956;18:324–33.
7. Sachar EJ, Hellman L, Roffwarg HP, Halpern FS, Fukushima DK, Gallagher TF. Disrupted 24-hour patterns of cortisol secretion in psychotic depression. Arch Gen Psychiatry. 1973;28(1):19–24.
8. Moreno-Villanueva M, Bürkle A. Stress hormone-mediated DNA damage response. Implications for cellular senescence and tumour progression. Curr Drug Targets. 2016;17(4):398–404.
9. Greer S. Healing the mind/body split: bringing the patient back into oncology. Integr Cancer Ther. 2003;2(1):5–12.
10. Descartes R. Meditations VI. In: Martin P, editor. The sickening mind. London: Flamingo; 1998.
11. Oken D. What to tell cancer patients: a study of medical attitudes. JAMA. 1961;175:1120–8.
12. Engel GL. The need for a new medical model: a challenge for biomedicine. Science. 1977;196:129–36.
13. Engel GL, Romano J. Delirium: II. Reversibility of the electroencephalogram with experimental procedures. Arch Neurol Psychiatr. 1944;51:378–92.
14. Engel GL. From biomedical to biopsychosocial: I. Being scientific in the human domain. Fam Syst Health. 1996;14:425–33.
15. Kangas M, Tate RL, Williams JR, Smee RI. The effects of radiotherapy on psychosocial and cognitive functioning in adults with a primary brain tumour: a prospective evaluation. Neuro-Oncology. 2012;14(12):1485–502.
16. Ownsworth T, Hawkes A, Steginga S, Walker D, Shum D. A biopsychosocial perspective on adjustment and quality of life following brain tumour: a systematic evaluation of the literature. Disabil Rehabil. 2009;31(13):1038–55.
17. van Kessel E, Baumfalk AE, van Zandvoort MJE, Robe PA, Snijders TJ. Tumor-related neurocognitive dysfunction in patients with diffuse glioma: a systematic review of neurocognitive functioning prior to anti-tumour treatment. J Neuro-Oncol. 2017;134(1):9–18.
18. Saria MG, Courchesne N, Evangelista L, Carter J, MacManus DA, Gorman MK, et al. Cognitive dysfunction in patients with brain metastases: influences on caregiver resilience and coping. Support Care Cancer. 2017;25(4):1247–56.
19. Stone AA, Neale JM. New measure of daily coping: development and preliminary results. J Pers Soc Psychol. 1984;46(4):892–906.
20. Folkman S, Lazarus RS. If it changes it must be a process: study of emotion and coping during three stages of a college examination. J Pers Soc Psychol. 1985;48(1):150–70.
21. Zani B, Cicognani E. Le vie del benessere. Eventi di vita e strategie di coping. 6th ed. Roma: Carocci Editore; 2008.
22. Grassi L, Biondi M, Costantini A. Manuale pratico di psiconcologia. Roma: Il Pensiero Scientifico Editore; 2009.
23. Heim E, Augustiny KF, Schaffner L, Valach L. Coping with breast cancer over time and situation. J Psychosom Res. 1993;37(5):523–42.

24. Heim E, Valach L, Schaffner L. Coping and psychosocial adaptation: longitudinal effects over time and stages in breast cancer. Psychosom Med. 1997;59(4):408–18.

25. Acquaye AA, Lin L, Vera-Bolanos E, Gilbert MR, Armstrong TS. Hope and mood changes throughout the primary brain tumour illness trajectory. Neuro-Oncology. 2016;18(1): 119–25.

26. McDaniel JS, Musselman DL, Porter MR, Reed DA, Nemeroff CB. Depression in patients with cancer. Diagnosis, biology, and treatment. Arch Gen Psychiatry. 1995;52(2): 89–99.

27. Zigmond AS, Snaith RP. The hospital anxiety and depression scale. Acta Psychiatr Scand. 1983;67:361–70.

28. Skarstein J, Aass N, Fossa SD, Skovlund E, Dahl AA. Anxiety and depression in cancer patients: relation between the Hospital Anxiety and Depression Scale and the European Organization for Research and Treatment of Cancer Core Quality of Life Questionnaire. J Psychosom Res. 2000;49(1):27–34.

29. Arnold SD, Forman LM, Brigidi BD, Carter KE, Schweitzer HA, Quinn HE, et al. Evaluation and characterization of generalized anxiety and depression in patients with primary brain tumours. Neuro-Oncology. 2008;10(2):171–81.

30. Anderson SI, Taylor R, Whittle IR. Mood disorders in patients after treatment for primary intracranial tumours. Br J Neurosurg. 1999;13(5):480–5.

31. Litofsky NS, Farace E, Anderson F Jr, Meyers CA, Huang W, Laws ER Jr. Depression in patients with high-grade glioma: results of the Glioma outcomes project. Neurosurgery. 2004;54(2):358–66.

32. Rooney AG, Carson A, Grant R. Depression in cerebral glioma patients: a systematic review of observational studies. J Natl Cancer Inst. 2011;103(1):61–76.

33. National Comprehensive Cancer Network. NCCN clinical practice guidelines in oncology: distress management. 2nd ed. Fort Washington: NCCN; 2009.

34. Kroenke K, Spitzer R, Williams J. The PHQ-9: validity of a brief depression severity measure. J Gen Intern Med. 2001;16(9):606–13.

35. Rooney AG, McNamara S, Mackinnon M, Fraser M, Rampling R, Carson A, et al. Screening for major depressive disorder in adults with cerebral glioma: an initial validation of 3 self-report instruments. Neuro-Oncology. 2013;15(1):122–9.

36. Baider L, Cooper CL, De-Nour AK. Cancer and the family. 2nd ed. New York: Wiley; 2000.

37. McCarter H, Furlong W, Whitton AC, Feeny D, DePauw S, Willan AR, Barr RD. Health status measurements at diagnosis as predictors of survival among adults with brain tumours. J Clin Oncol. 2006;24:3636–43.

38. Brown PD, Decker PA, Rummans TA, Clark MM, Frost MH, Ballman KV, Arusell RM, Buckner JC. A prospective study of quality of life in adults with newly diagnosed high-grade gliomas: comparison of patient and caregiver ratings of quality of life. Am J Clin Oncol. 2008;31(2):163–8.

39. Ergh TC, Hanks RA, Rapport LJ, Coleman RD. Social support moderates caregiver life satisfaction following traumatic brain injury. J Clin Exp Neuropsychol. 2003;25(8):1090–101.

40. Sherwood PR, Given BA, Doorenbos AZ, Given CW. Forgotten voices: lessons from bereaved caregivers of persons with a brain tumour. Int J Palliat Nurs. 2004;10:67–75.

41. Horowitz S, Passik SD, Malkin MG. In sickness and in health: a group intervention for spouses caring for patients with brain tumours. J Psychosoc Oncol. 1996;14:43–56.

42. Litofsky NS, Resnick AG. The relationship between depression and brain tumours. J Neuro-Oncol. 2009;94:153–61.

43. Northouse LL, Katapodi MC, Song L, Zhang L, Mood D. Interventions with family caregivers of cancer patients. CA Cancer J Clin. 2010;60:317–39.

44. Invernizzi G, Bressi C, Comazzi AM. La famiglia del malato neoplastico. Padova: Piccin; 1992.

45. Bloch S, Kissane D. Psychotherapies in psycho-oncology. An exciting new challenge. Br J Psychiatry. 2000;177:112–6.

46. Cunningham AJ. Adjuvant psychological therapy for cancer patients: putting it on the same footing as adjunctive medical therapies. Psycho-Oncology. 2000;9:367–71.
47. Straker N. Psychodynamic psychotherapy for cancer patients. J Psychother Pract Res. 1998;7:1–9.
48. LeShan L. Cancers a turning point. New York: Penguin Books; 1990.
49. Moorey S, Greer S. Psychological therapy for patients with cancer. A new approach. Oxford: Heinemann Medical Books; 1989.
50. Rooney AG, Brown PD, Reijneveld JC, Grant R. Depression in glioma: a primer for clinicians and researchers. J Neurol Neurosurg Psychiatry. 2014;85(2):230–5.
51. Bielecka-Wajdman AM, Lesiak M, Ludyga T, Sieroń A, Obuchowicz E. Reversing glioma malignancy: a new look at the role of antidepressant drugs as adjuvant therapy for glioblastoma multiforme. Cancer Chemother Pharmacol. 2017;79(6):1249–56.
52. Ma J, Yang YR, Chen W, Chen MH, Wang H, Wang XD, Sun LL, Wang FZ, Wang DC. Fluoxetine synergizes with temozolomide to induce the CHOP-dependent endoplasmic reticulum stress-related apoptosis pathway in glioma cells. Oncol Rep. 2016;36(2):676–84.
53. Liu KH, Yang ST, Lin YK, Lin JW, Lee YH, Wang JY, Hu CJ, Lin EY, Chen SM, Then CK, Shen SC. Fluoxetine, an antidepressant, suppresses glioblastoma by evoking AMPAR-mediated calcium-dependent apoptosis. Oncotarget. 2015;6(7):5088–101.
54. Hayashi K, Michiue H, Yamada H, Takata K, Nakayama H, Wei FY, Fujimura A, Tazawa H, Asai A, Ogo N, Miyachi H, Nishiki T, Tomizawa K, Takei K, Matsui H. Fluvoxamine, an antidepressant, inhibits human glioblastoma invasion by disrupting actin polymerization. Sci Rep. 2016;6:1–12.
55. Pottegård A, García Rodríguez LA, Rasmussen L, Damkier P, Friis S, Gaist D. Use of tricyclic antidepressants and risk of glioma: a nationwide case-control study. Br J Cancer. 2016;114(11):1265–8.
56. Judge BS, Rentmeester LL. Antidepressant overdose-induced seizures. Neurol Clin. 2011;29:565–80.
57. Gross A, Devinsky O, Westbrook LE, et al. Psychotropic medication use in patients with epilepsy: effect on seizure frequency. J Neuropsychiatry Clin Neurosci. 2000;12:458–64.
58. Alper K, Schwartz KA, Kolts RL, Khan A. Seizure incidence in psychopharmacological clinical trials: an analysis of Food and Drug Administration (FDA) summary basis of approval reports. Biol Psychiatry. 2007;62:345–54.
59. Ribot R, Ouyang B, Kanner AM. The impact of antidepressants on seizure frequency and depressive and anxiety disorders of patients with epilepsy: is it worth investigating? Epilepsy Behav. 2017;70:5–9.
60. Torta R, Monaco F. Atypical antipsychotics and serotoninergic antidepressants in patients with epilepsy: pharmacodynamic considerations. Epilepsia. 2002;43:8–13.
61. Kanner AM. Depression in epilepsy: a complex reaction with unexpected consequences. Curr Opin Neurol. 2008;21:190–4.
62. Hesdorffer DC, Hauser WA, Olafsson E, Ludvigsson P, Kjartansson O. Depression and suicide attempt as risk factors for incident unprovoked seizures. Ann Neurol. 2006;59:35–41.
63. Rooney A, Grant R. SSRIs may (or may not) be a safe treatment for depression in GBM. Am J Clin Oncol. 2012;35:100.
64. Mendlewicz J, Lecrubier Y. Antidepressant selection: proceedings from a TCA/SSRI consensus conference. Acta Psychiatr Scand Suppl. 2000;403:5–8.
65. Klein M, Taphoorn MJ, Heimans JJ, van der Ploeg HM, Vandertop WP, Smit EF, Leenstra S, Tulleken CA, Boogerd W, Belderbos JS, Cleijne W, Aaronson NK. Neurobehavioral status and health-related quality of life in newly diagnosed high-grade glioma patients. J Clin Oncol. 2001;19(20):4037–47.

66. Caudill JS, Brown PD, Cerhan JH, Rummans TA. Selective serotonin reuptake inhibitors, glioblastoma multiforme, and impact on toxicities and overall survival: the mayo clinic experience. Am J Clin Oncol. 2011;34(4):385–7.
67. Valko PO, Siddique A, Linsenmeier C, Zaugg K, Held U, Hofer S. Prevalence and predictors of fatigue in glioblastoma: a prospective study. Neuro-Oncology. 2015;17(2):274–81.
68. Morrow GR, Hickok JT, Roscoe JA, Raubertas RF, Andrews PL, Flynn PJ, Hynes HE, Banerjee TK, Kirshner JJ, King DK. Differential effects of paroxetine on fatigue and depression: a randomized, double-blind trial from the University of Rochester Cancer Center Community Clinical Oncology Program. J Clin Oncol. 2003;21(24):4635–41.

Neuro-Oncology Nursing

14

Ingela Oberg

14.1 Introduction

Neuro-oncology nurses act as patient advocates, signposting for advice, information and support. They liaise with general practitioners (GP's) and community care teams, and support relatives and carers; they ensure patients have an understanding of their diagnosis and prognosis, whilst trying to ensure they still maintain a degree of hope and supporting them through end-of-life decisions and care; they talk them through treatment options, side effects and intended benefits and they hold treatment clinics and follow-up clinics; they arrange admissions and discharges to aid patient flow and they undertake nurse-led research to improve standards of patient care. Neuro-oncology nurses teach junior doctors and graduate nurses about the specifics of neuro-oncology nursing and they run support groups. In short, neuro-oncology nurses are the lynchpin that holds the service together, and they are their consultant's right-hand (wo)man.

But despite the diverse and autonomous nature of their work, there are no formal training requirements to become a neuro-oncology nurse—in the United Kingdom (UK) for example, there are no specific qualifications apart from holding relevant experience in the chosen field. It is a role most nurses 'slip into', and despite the high turnover of patients and short life expectancy of those with high-grade gliomas, it can be a truly rewarding job.

This chapter will explore some of the reasoning behind this and how the role of specialist nursing has developed and evolved in the UK, along with some of the core skills and daily requirements of this role.

I. Oberg (✉)
Department of Neurosurgery, Addenbrooke's Hospital, CUH Foundation Trust,
Cambridge, UK
e-mail: ingela.oberg@addenbrookes.nhs.uk

© Springer Nature Switzerland AG 2019
M. Bartolo et al. (eds.), *Neurorehabilitation in Neuro-Oncology*,
https://doi.org/10.1007/978-3-319-95684-8_14

14.2   Background

In 2006, the UK saw the launch of the 'Improving Outcomes Guidance' (IOG) for people with brain and other central nervous system tumours. For the first time, this document detailed the composition of teams required to run an effective, multidisciplinary team. Furthermore, this document indicated who were the so-called core members and set out minimum standards to be adhered to, such as rate of attendance of core members and key skills of each role [1].

In 2008, the 'cancer reform strategy' came into force which built on the specifics of the IOG and provided a 5-year forward plan for upgrading, and significantly overhauling, all cancer services. As part of both these documents, particular importance was given to the role of specialist nurses: '*Commissioners ...should give particular consideration to the role of Clinical Nurse Specialists, who play a critical role in cancer care*', followed by '*Priority will be given to ensuring there is adequate provision of Clinical Nurse Specialists*' [2].

In reality, what this meant was that suddenly the nursing work-force was being invested in, and by 2009, every single neurosurgical centre in the UK had at least one neuro-oncology specialist nurse as part of their team. It had and continues to have a profound effect. General ward-based nursing has over the decades become less patient facing and more managerial—flowcharts and assessment scores have to be filled in, along with undertaking clinical audits, administering drugs, doing ward rounds and documenting outcomes and clinical plans. This leaves nurses very little time to care, and with the introduction of clinical nurse specialists (CNSs), this suddenly changed. The specialist nurses were able to support the ward-based nurses, taking some of the patient facing tasks away from them, providing specialist information and knowledge right at the patient's bedside. CNSs were able to offer advice on wound care, post-operative follow-up, treatment choices and disease trajectories; they go through information leaflets and liaise with primary, secondary and tertiary care providers and make onward referrals as required.

Specialist nurses know their patients better than anyone and this symbiotic relationship between ward-based nurses and CNSs continues to thrive in the UK. Some CNSs have undertaken specialist generic training such as nurse prescribing courses or clinical assessment modules, meaning they undertake tasks similar to that of doctors and can prescribe patients medication and provide nurse-led discharges. Furthermore, many of the larger UK hospitals have allowed CNSs to undergo radiology training to gain a clinical understanding of radiation risks and intended benefits of various scans, enabling them to order CT (computed tomography) and MRI (magnetic resonance imaging) scans on behalf of their consultants.

It's a win–win situation: the patient and their carers have a single point of contact both in hospital and once discharged home; specialist nurses are cheaper to employ than senior doctors and they free up vital nursing (and to some extent medical) time and help alleviate bed capacity issues and aid patient flow on the wards.

14.3   Triaging Multidisciplinary Team Meetings

Most cancer care services around the world now work within multidisciplinary teams (MDTs), and brain cancer is no exception despite being a relatively small service in comparison to the 'big four' groups incorporating lung, breast, colorectal and prostate cancers.

The aim of an MDT is to increase the effectiveness between health care teams, hopefully producing more positive outcomes. But, this effectiveness is wholly dependent on the MDT meeting running as smoothly as possible; although an MDT coordinator is pivotal in ensuring medical reports and images are available, (s)he normally has very limited clinical knowledge and would not possess the required skills to triage any referrals as being either premature or very urgent [1, 3].

Historically, this triaging of referrals has been undertaken by a neurosurgical registrar, who would advise the referring teams and clinicians about required scans and medications and arrange for urgent transfer across if required. In some centres, however, triaging of MDT referrals has been taken over by an experienced neuro-oncology nurse, providing continuity and access for the regions referring centres to a single point of contact. It has had a positive effect not only on the quality of cases presented but also on overall cancer waiting times (time from initial referral to treatment), which are nationally audited.

In the process, the neuro-oncology nurses gain in-depth knowledge about neuroimaging and can become quite apt at distinguishing durally based metastasis from meningioma's, or a centrally restricted diffusion (on diffusion weighted imaging) pointing towards a cerebral abscess. However, the purpose of taking on this role is not solely to enhance individual learning, but predominantly to help reduce the amount of MDT rediscussions occurring (mainly due to incomplete set of images or lacking information regarding any pertinent medical history), which subsequently causes inevitable delays to the patient's treatments—be it surgical interventions, oncology treatments or palliative care.

Imaging and clinical history of the patient being referred is reviewed beforehand, and the referring hospitals are often contacted directly regarding any discrepancies such as type of previous malignancies (if applicable), treatments given and treatment intent, as well as overall expected survival from a primary disease perspective. Having an updated performance status prior to MDT (if they have been commenced on high-dose dexamethasone, for example) is also of great importance as it helps to establish if symptoms have resolved on steroids, in which case surgery may be of added importance. Finally, a direct phone call prompts the referring teams to ensure a contrast enhanced MRI and full staging CT chest, abdomen and pelvis (if clinically indicated) are made available for discussion as minimum requirements [4].

Within some UK neuro-oncology services, if all required imaging has already been made available, and the MRI is in keeping with a high-grade glioma, the patient is pre-booked into a consultant-led outpatient clinic as part of the triaging process, prior to the MDT discussion by the CNS. This avoids another week's delay, and minimised distress to the patients who would otherwise have to wait another week prior to receiving any specific answers around treatment decisions. If imaging is consistent with either an abscess or primary lymphoma of the brain, an urgent inpatient transfer is arranged by the CNS in conjunction with the on-call neurosurgical consultant for an expedited diagnostic biopsy. These are often done prior to the MDT discussion as they are dealt with as clinical emergencies.

Thankfully, the era when patients were admitted to hospital following identification of a brain tumour, occupying a hospital bed until they were operated on is not a common undertaking any more. As regional neurosurgical centres cover large geographical areas, there is simply not the available bed capacity for a patient to 'block' a bed if they are otherwise well, in order to await surgery. The patients are given relevant information leaflets regarding their condition such as brain tumour booklets, driving regulations and steroids, they are shown their scans so they know what the relevant concerns are, given the CNSs contact details, and are discharged home with an appointment to attend the very next outpatient neuro-oncology clinic under the auspices of a consultant neurosurgeon [5]. A pre-surgical stealth MRI (a surgical neuro-navigation scan) is ordered by the CNS which the patient can attend in conjunction with their outpatient clinic (or surgical pre-admission) appointment. The money saved in discharging the patient prior to surgery (i.e. the amount of inpatient bed days saved) can then be reinvested into obtaining updated imaging for surgical planning purposes, which in turn helps to increase patient safety prior to and during surgery [5].

Needless to say, if patients are deemed unsafe for discharge or require a care package (with district/community nurses coming in to the patients' home, for example), then they will likely remain inpatients until deemed safe for discharge or until surgery has been undertaken.

14.4   Neuro-Rehabilitation

In the UK, neuro-rehabilitation specifically aimed at brain tumour patients is a very scarce resource. There are lots of rehabilitation centres available for stroke patients or trauma patients, but not for those diagnosed with a malignant glioma, or indeed any cancerous brain tumour. Historically, their disease trajectory has been so poor that it has been felt to be a wasted resource, with patients not surviving long enough to benefit from rehabilitation and they would not see the benefits of reaching their maximal potential in terms of mobility or cognition [6].

However, it must be considered that rehabilitation is not only about having access to specialist inpatient facilities. Rehabilitation is an everyday process and it encompasses several different aspects and disciplines within neuro-oncology which will be explored in further detail below: occupational therapy (OT), physiotherapists and speech/language teams (SLT) to name a few as well as every day nursing care. Nurses caring for neurosurgical patients undertake a pivotal role within rehabilitation: daily tasks such as washing, dressing, maintaining hygiene needs and assessing pressure sores; keeping the patient pain free and mobile, monitoring oral intake and fluid output—are all essential elements of neuro-rehabilitation [6]. The overall aim of rehabilitation is to maximise an individual's potential, enabling and supporting them to recover or adjust to their new situation, and helping them to live as full and active lives as possible [7].

Physiotherapists (Physio's) provide rehabilitation through movement and exercise, manual therapy, education and advice. Loss of muscle strength and use, loss of sensation, impaired balance and coordination, and changes in muscular tone are frequently seen in people with brain tumours. Rehabilitation by the physiotherapist focuses on retraining and establishing functional strategies for impairments based on the patient's goals, their prognosis and their stage of illness [7].

Encouraging the patient to get out of bed and mobilise, with help if required, is pivotal to help redress the aforementioned balance. Getting out of bed and getting dressed has more benefits than simply keeping muscle tone supple. Being mobile reduces the risk of developing venous-thromboembolisms (VTE) and helps minimise surgical complications such as chest infections [6]. It makes the patient feel more 'human' and less of a patient, and it encourages independence and recovery. The quicker the patients can demonstrate they are able to look after their own care needs, the quicker they can anticipate leaving hospital. Patients recover quicker at home, in familiar surroundings and are less at risk of picking up nosocomial infections.

Occupational therapists (OT) in the UK (there are practical differences depending on which country OTs practice in) will look at what tools and equipment the patient may require both in hospital but more importantly at home to help them maintain their independence. Given a certain task, they will assess the patient's cognitive abilities of planning, organising, remembering location of items, safety awareness, completion of the required task and how the patients problem solve. In addition, motor processes are assessed (such as how they reach into cupboards, and how they balance), and based on these findings an occupational therapist can extrapolate what their individual function is likely to be at home for the patient [8].

The term 'occupation' refers to practical and purposeful activities that allow people to live independently and have a sense of identity such as essential day-to-day tasks including self-care, work or leisure. OTs aim to prevent further disability, facilitate recovery, promote health and independent function and enable individuals to overcome barriers that prevent them from doing the activities (or occupations) that matter to them. Items such as grab rails to help get in and out of the bath, kitchen equipment for safe handling of hot food are examples of things OTs can help with [8].

Communication and swallowing difficulties are assessed, diagnosed and treated by a speech and language therapist (SLT)—they aim to optimise a person's ability to communicate effectively and eat and drink as safely as possible whilst maintaining quality of life throughout all stages of the illness [7].

Whilst having access to specialist inpatient rehabilitation is fantastic for those patients with more complex recovery needs, such as those recovering from supplementary motor syndrome, or those who had post-surgical complications such as ischaemic stroke, one needs to bear in mind that rehabilitation can and should occur as an everyday activity to help promote independence. Specialist inpatient rehabilitation remains available for those patients (in particular those with low-grade gliomas with a favourable long-term outlook) whose rehabilitation needs go beyond the everyday facilities provided on the neuro-surgical ward by the nurses, OTs, physio's and SLT specialist teams.

14.5 Discharge Planning

Certainly, in the UK, it is very common for patients to live in two storey houses, with upstairs bathrooms and bedrooms. For a patient with limited neurological recovery, with say for instance a right-sided hemiparesis, this can prove very difficult to manage. They will need to try and navigate up the stairs with their (predominantly) dominant side severely weakened and many patients end up living in temporary downstairs accommodation with a commode for their toileting needs, a quick wash in the kitchen sink, and sleeping on the downstairs sofa bed… far from ideal!

Prior to discharge home from hospital, patients will therefore need to undergo a full assessment by the physiotherapists as well as the OTs. The physiotherapists will actually determine when the patient is deemed safe for discharge, and can overrule a consultant if patient safety may otherwise be compromised. They will undertake mobility assessments and ensure patients can manage at least one flight of stairs independently prior to discharge home [8]. In many instances, this may require the instalment of another hand rail (or bannister), so the patient has one on either side of the stairs for stability and support.

The role of the CNS here is one of advice to the patient, their carer and the allied health professional (AHP) teams of OTs and physiotherapists. The AHPs will likely not have met the patient prior to surgery, so they will be unaware if they had already managed well at home with a long-term disability, like a continuing mild hemiparesis or foot drop for example, prior to their admission for surgery. In many instances, the patients' weakness may have improved after surgery, but the physiotherapists will likely see their current situation as their baseline status (as they will not have assessed them previously) and may determine they are unsafe for discharge. To help patient flow and prevent unnecessary delays to their discharge planning, it is therefore imperative for the CNS to communicate effectively with the AHPs about their patient's pre-surgical state and overall treatment intent [9–11]. Likewise, patients and carers obtaining practical advice on how to manage situations at home can be of real benefit, and can help instil a sense of confidence about the post-discharge phase [9]. For instance, consider telling the patient who is still a bit unsteady on their feet to do what small children do in stairs: climb up the stairs with both feel on one step before taking the next step, and 'bum-shuffling' down the steps if required. As their strength and stamina gradually returns, so too will their mobility and ability to manage stairs without untoward risks.

The OT will also need to assess the patient to ascertain what equipment and tools they need at home to remain mobile and independent. In most cases, the OTs perform what we refer to as a "kitchen assessment". This is to ensure they have no short-term memory impairment that may affect their safety, such as leaving the gas (cooker) on without igniting it; managing to make a cup of tea or coffee without scalding oneself, safe handling of kitchen knives, etc. OTs can order in items such as raised toilet seats, shower stools and bath grab rails, easy-to-use kitchen equipment such as jar openers to tripods and Zimmer frames for mobility purposes and even hospital beds for home if required [8].

For patients unable to go home, who are rapidly deteriorating and who are nearing the end of their life, a process known as 'fast track discharge planning' can be instigated [12]. Please see below Sect. 14.7 on 'Supporting End-of-Life Care' for more details on this.

14.6   The Clinically Deteriorating Patient

Either pre- or post-operatively, one of the major risk factors of neuro-oncology is the potential for patients to deteriorate rather suddenly. Glioma's have a propensity to bleed due to the weakened blood vessels caused by the breach of the blood–brain barrier (BBB)

[4]. Increased intracranial pressure (ICP), oedema and tumour infiltration can cause significant neurological decline [4], and managing a patient who is deteriorating at home prior to surgery can be very difficult. However, admitting a patient into hospital to simply await surgery a week or two later is also risky as it is acknowledged that the patients are at increased risk of picking up nosocomial infections the longer they remain inpatients. Any infection would delay the onset of treatment, which can ultimately have dire consequences for the patient and may even result in premature death. A GP may never have come across a glioma patient before, and quite often they ring the neuro-oncology specialist nurses for advice and reassurance—this requires a degree of autonomous decision-making from the CNS in order to best advise the GP on the required next steps, such as medication titration and side effects, or even required emergency admissions.

In some situations, this involves treating the cause of deterioration (e.g. treat seizures; increase dexamethasone dose if worsening weakness or other lateralising neurology)—in other instances, this requires prompt clinical review and re-scanning to see if the tumour has progressed or bled. Should the latter be the case, the benefits of intended neurosurgery need to be carefully explored and discussed with the patient and their carer, as it may offer very little benefits to them.

From a nursing perspective, the more common scenarios involving deteriorating patients are around post-operative neurosurgical care. For example, ensuring the patient is mobilised within a day following surgery to prevent the onset of VTEs, and ensuring the right manual handling equipment is available, to help mobilise the patient and maintain their independence as much as possible.

As the post-operative swelling manifests itself following neurosurgery, some decline in the patient's neurological function would be expected, especially if surgery was undertaken around the left fronto-temporal area involving (in most right-handed patients) their speech and language centre. The patient may start to slur their words or develop dysphasia and/or aphasia (difficulty in forming or comprehending the spoken word) a day or so following surgery. Over the course of 3–4 days however, this should recover if the patient's intraoperative speech mapping was intact (following awake surgery) and the post-operative MRI scan showed no evidence of restricted diffusion, ischaemia or stroke. It is important to remember that post-surgical MRIs should ideally be obtained within 72 h following surgery to prevent blood degradation products from obscuring any residual tumour mass as blood also shows up as enhancement after this time frame, making it difficult to distinguish between blood and enhancing tumour [4, 5]. Should the former issues around stroke be identified, a referral to an inpatient-based neuro-rehabilitation service would be required (pending a favourable overall prognosis) to see if targeted rehabilitation therapy aiding neuroplasticity may recover some neurological function given time [6].

Any issues with dysphasia or aphasia and/or dysphagia (inability to swallow) require a prompt referral by the ward nurse or CNS to the SLT teams to undertake a full assessment of their speech deficits and to ensure a full swallow assessment is undertaken in order to ensure the patient is not silently aspirating for example; as well as being able to provide them with adequate aids, communication tools and resources should this be required. If swallowing problems have been identified, then a further referral by the CNS or nursing team will need to be made to a dietitian, who in turn can advise on the requirements of special diets such as thickened liquids to help prevent aspiration and choking [7].

To assist the nurses (and doctors) in identifying the clinically deteriorating patient, various tools and assessment scores can be used and documented. The most common one being the Glasgow coma scale (GCS, see image below)—this is a score that is predominantly used within neurosurgical settings as it assesses a patient's level of consciousness and is very applicable for the head injured patient for example [13, 14].

The GCS (and its use) is comprised of three components: eyes, voice (verbal) and motor function. The combined score out of 15 indicates their level of consciousness, with 15/15 meaning the patient is orientated to time, person and place and can open eyes spontaneously and follow motor commands without any weaknesses. A patient with a GCS of 13 or lower requires prompt senior review and anyone with a GCS of 8 or below will most likely require intubation to protect their airways and an intensive care bed for close monitoring [13, 14].

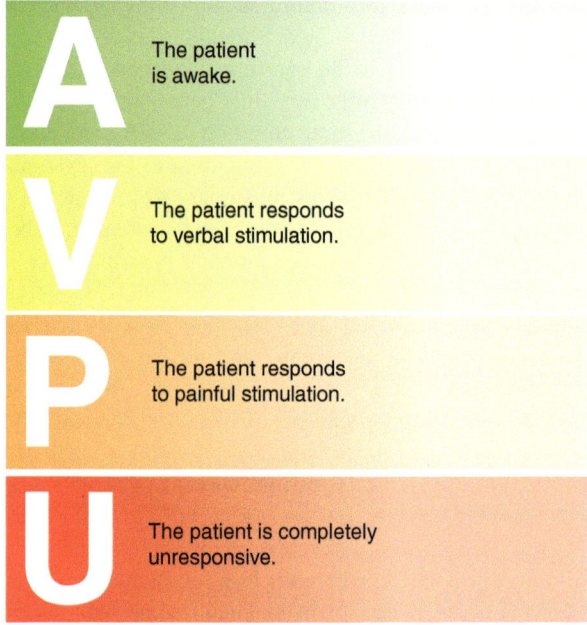

Image below shows the components of the AVPU Score. Image reproduced from firstaidforfree. com.

On the general wards and in settings outside of neurosurgery, another useful tool is the AVPU score (see above diagram), similar to GCS but deemed by many to be more versatile and a simplified version to use than the GCS.

A = Alert, V = Voice, P = Painful stimuli and U = unresponsive. It is also colour coded like a traffic light, so as you go from green down to the red category, this is a visual prompt that the situation, and more importantly the patient, is deteriorating [13, 14].

Depending on their level of alertness, it also indicates their level of consciousness—from a neuro-oncology perspective, anyone with a deteriorating AVPU score (or indeed GCS) needs to have an urgent assessment by a senior clinician. Some hospitals have access to critical care outreach teams which are a specialist team of nurses and doctors helping to support wards and the clinically deteriorating patient with the aim of keeping them safe and out of critical care if at all possible [13, 14].

Whilst a senior review is underway, the specialist nurse should ensure a full septic screen including blood cultures, urine cultures and blood tests (such as electrolyte levels) are obtained to rule out (or indeed in) metabolic and/or infectious reasons for the clinical deterioration. An urgent CT head with contrast to examine the cause for decline, such as a bleed into the tumour bed, stroke or ischaemia, subdural or extradural haematoma (also known as epidural bleeds) and/or infection will also need to be obtained.

Glasgow Coma Scale

BEHAVIOR	RESPONSE	SCORE
Eye opening response	Spontaneously	4
	To speech	3
	To pain	2
	No response	1
Best verbal response	Oriented to time, place, and person	5
	Confused	4
	Inappropriate words	3
	Incomprehensible sounds	2
	No response	1
Best motor response	Obeys commands	6
	Moves to localized pain	5
	Flexion withdrawal from pain	4
	Abnormal flexion (decorticate)	3
	Abnormal extension (decerebrate)	2
	No response	1
Total score:	*Best response*	15
	Comatose client	8 or less
	Totally unresponsive	3

Image below shows the Glasgow Coma Scale. Copied from firstaidforfree.com.

14.7   Supporting End-of-Life Care

Nurses and health care professionals want to do everything possible to ensure patients have the best quality (as well as quantity) of life; it is part of the Hippocratic Oath to do no harm. It can however be difficult at times to accept when 'the end of the line' in regard to treatment options having been exhausted. When that time comes, nurses need to support and enable their patients and their loved ones, to experience the best end-of-life care possible. In many circumstances, the patient remains in hospital due to their continuing complex care needs. In the UK, there has been great emphasis in trying to improve seamless transitions from hospital to community-based services, and this has led to something known as 'fast track discharge' services.

If a patient is nearing the end of their life, a fast track assessment can be implemented whereby the local health authority pays for continuing health care provisions in the community, providing an appropriate care and support package, sometimes as quickly as within 48 h of receiving the application. This enables the patient to live out the remainder of their days at home (or in an appropriate setting like a hospice), with provided care according to their level of need [12].

Sometimes, particularly with malignant gliomas, a patient's rapid disease progression and subsequent neurological decline lends itself to natural decisions about what is often the only way forward—palliation and end-of-life care. In other circumstances, there may be treatment options available, but the patient chooses not to pursue them, as the below case highlights:

Adrian (not his real name) was a 52-year-old gentleman who was radiologically diagnosed with a suspected glioblastoma (GBM). He had a teenage daughter (age 15) and he was the main carer for his wife who was wheelchair bound by multiple sclerosis (MS). He was self-employed and they had a mortgage on their house. He also had a personal life insurance which in his case meant if he was diagnosed with a terminal diagnosis and had <12 months to live, his life insurance policy would pay out and additionally their mortgage would be paid off in full.

Subsequently, following radiological diagnosis of his tumour, Adrian opted for a biopsy only for diagnostic purposes so he could confirm the diagnosis of a GBM to his insurers. Despite being suitable for 5-ALA (fluorescent) guided resection of the tumour and the full 'Stupp protocol' for post-operative treatments, he chose to decline everything to ensure his family were looked after following his death [15]. From his perspective, he was given a terminal diagnosis whichever way he looked at it—if he declined all treatment, his family could live mortgage free and his wife could afford carers to help with her MS needs following his life insurance pay out. If he chose to accept treatment, this may mean his survival statistics rose to beyond a year, in which case his insurance may not pay out, and that was a risk he was not willing to take—his main and only concern was to ensure his family were taken care of after his passing.

His specialist nurse found this a very hard decision to support clinically—she felt angry that a patient had to make such drastic choices and effectively end his life prematurely by actively declining treatment and robbing him of the quality time he could have had with his family, creating precious memories for his daughter. It felt like a systematic betrayal. Counterarguments were presented to him where letters of support were promised regarding the very varied statistics, providing evidence that ultimately, he still had a terminal diagnosis with a very bleak outlook… This was to no avail—he had made his mind up, with immense support and love from his family who attended clinic alongside him. The CNS was visibly moved, but had to respect his decisions and choices and felt it was one of the greatest acts of selfless love she had ever witnessed.

14.8 Breaking Bad News

Another cornerstone of specialist nursing practice is providing clear, effective communication, be it verbal or written. Whether nurses are consciously aware of it or not, they undertake this core element daily—in communicating with peers, patients and relatives to name but a few. How *approachable* they are deemed to be depends not only on their verbal skills but also on their non-verbal cues [16]. Within this daily element of communication also lies the ability of how to break bad news, albeit in a good way—is there such a thing?

There are several communication skills frameworks that can be adhered to, and shortly after the introduction of the IOG, it was imperative anyone undertaking patient facing tasks within cancer care undertook specialist communication skills training [1]. This was predominantly to help one reflect on one's own personal communication style and how this may be perceived by others, to encourage self-reflection and adaptation of communication styles.

Many consultants see their own patients in a clinic setting (away from busy, non-confidential ward areas) to relay the diagnosis to them as part of the doctor–patient relationship. But in equally as many circumstances, clinic is overbooked and running late, meaning often the specialist nurses end up seeing the patients who return for pathology results, to help lessen their wait and keep clinic running as smoothly as possible.

Whichever communication framework is chosen, it is important to use plain language that is easily understood, and to avoid too much medical jargon or terminologies that can be confusing or misleading [16]. Ascertain what they are aware of regarding their situation—ask for example, if they (and anyone accompanying them) have fully understood the rationale for why they were offered a biopsy over a full resection. This either leads on to the next steps or one would need to go back to the beginning and explain why a certain approach was favoured over another. Ensure there are plenty of pauses for information to sink in, allow time for questions from everyone present and ensure written information is given in manageable 'chunks' [9, 10].

Do not refrain from using the correct terminology either. Some clinicians and nurses skim past the word 'cancer' and 'incurable' when it comes to breaking bad news around malignant gliomas. These words *can* be said in a soft, empathic way.

Words such as malignancy, 'needs further treatment', radical intent, palliative chemotherapy or simply referring to the WHO grading are used instead, which can cause confusion and uncertainties around the diagnosis [2, 9]. Results have previously been relayed literally as short as: '*You have a grade 4 glioma that has been resected. This is a GBM as we suspected. The oncologists will see you tomorrow to discuss further treatments that you will need; likely a combination of chemotherapy and radiotherapy. OK? Any questions?*'

Where do you start with this? Firstly, no—it's not OK! How could one be certain if the patient knew what a grade 4 glioma was and what it means to them in regards to not only prognosis but quality of life? Or what the difference is between a resection and debulking? From a patient's perspective, if the entire tumour has successfully been removed, why is chemotherapy and radiotherapy required? Is the patient aware this is a non-curable, progressive disease that will come back in a matter of (several) months if in keeping with a GBM? Have they been reassured that none of this is their fault and that this is not the type of cancer that can be inherited (or indeed passed down generations) as far as modern science can predict? Have they left with a degree of hope that although they can't be cured, they are being offered vital treatment—who knows what breakthroughs may lie around the corner? If they ask about prognosis, to remind them that a prognosis is just an average—people are individuals and prognosis today (with the clinical era of molecular markers) depends on so much more than simply a tumour grade [9, 10]. Bear in mind please that often it's the relatives that ask about prognosis over the patient themselves—should this be the case, please establish whether this is something the patient wishes to know; if not, then the patient's wishes should be adhered to at this stage, and this information should not be divulged.

Have they started to cry? It may sound odd, but often patients who seem overly optimistic and accepting of their diagnosis are in a bit of denial—those patients (and relatives) who start to cry seem to comprehend and grasp the severity of the situation and understand this is a non-curable diagnosis (in terms of gliomas) that will significantly shorten the patient's life expectancy. As hard as it sometimes is to do in a busy clinic setting, give them time to grieve: offer them some tissues and a comforting hug if appropriate. Show them empathy and consider offering them a quiet room where they can have some time alone as a family, prior to heading back out through the busy waiting area and back home—perhaps even offer them a hot drink? Go back in after 5–10 min to see if they have any further questions before moving on to the next patient.

Breaking bad news can be complex and time consuming, but it should not be difficult. Let the patient and their carers set the pace and let their questions guide the discussions along the correct path and everything else should fall into place; most patients are very humble in return. Patients have often stated nurses have a very difficult job, shortly after being informed they have an incurable cancer. Patients often acknowledge that nurses break news in a very genteel and sympathetic way, but also in a manner which enables them to completely understand their diagnosis, treatment options and subsequent prognosis.

14.9   Patient Advocacy/Mental Capacity

In the UK Nursing and Midwifery Council's (our governing body) code of conduct booklet, it clearly states that: "*…You make sure that those receiving care are treated with respect, that their rights are upheld and that any discriminatory attitudes and behaviours towards those receiving care are challenged*" [17].

Most nurses can likely recall a time when they did not agree with the doctor regarding a recommended treatment choice or how a particular situation was handled. There have been times when personality clashes and communication styles have differed vastly between consultants and patients, requiring a CNS to interject to try and calm fraught situations down. It is very easy for feelings to become tense when patients are faced with situations outside of their control.

Challenging colleagues to maintain their professionalism and high standards of communication is thankfully not something that needs to be done with any recurring regularity, but more challenging is to ensure the patient and their carers have the same mutual respect for these invisible boundaries towards one another and those helping to care for them. This is even more important should the patient have a cognitive issue which puts his/her ability to make autonomous decisions at risk. In such situations, it is pertinent a more in-depth professional assessment is carried out to assess if the patient formally lacks capacity to make decisions or not. This assessment needs to be conducted by a doctor, but undoubtedly arranged by the CNS, as a patient advocate.

In more severe cases, lack of capacity can also lead to a situation where the patient in question is deemed vulnerable and needs to have their needs and best wishes safeguarded from those around him—in the UK, this complex process is called 'safeguarding of vulnerable adults' (SOVA) and can involve court applications to safeguard their finances amongst other things [18]. As the patients nursing advocate, CNSs have a substantial role within this process to ensure overall patient safety and wellbeing. All hospitals have an adult (and paediatric) safeguarding team to contact for information, advice and support.

Example Mr. Jones (pseudonym) was a 49-year-old married man, separated from his wife but not yet legally divorced. She was still living in the marital home, he had moved out into rented accommodation. They had no children and he himself was an only child. Both his parents were dead—his mother, who he had been very close to, died the previous year following a cancer diagnosis; his father had passed away from a heart attack over a decade previously.

Mr. Jones had become withdrawn and depressed and did not look after himself very well—he had become very unkempt and risked losing both his job (he simply did not show up to work) and his apartment due to rental and bill arrears. A close friend of his felt all this was very out of character for him (despite his recent grief over losing his mother to whom he was very close) and eventually she managed to persuade the GP to admit him to hospital for investigations into possible early onset dementia. A CT head showed an enormous bi-frontal meningioma (around 8 cm) with significant mass effect and midline shift, minimal oedema, causing frontal lobe syndrome. He was transferred across to a neurosurgical unit and given a date for urgent surgical resection. As he was unable to look after himself, he was kept as an inpatient and was formally deemed to lack mental capacity for any decision-making.

His estranged wife contacted the CNSs, asking for a headed letter from the hospital stating that his brain tumour did not affect his capacity to sign the divorce papers. She felt she had waited long enough for the divorce proceedings and wanted nothing more to do with him. She did not want to be 'lumbered' with any legal responsibility to look after him after surgery and wanted to put their house on the market and move on with her life.

In one way, her reaction was understandable, but in another way very alarming. The size and location of his tumour is exactly what has caused him to lack insight or have capacity to make *any* decisions of any sort. Who is to say she would not sell the house and keep all the money herself, without his knowledge or consent? Although they remain married, they are separated and judging by her reaction towards him (even when knowing of his brain tumour diagnosis), they did not appear amicable in any way. It would be doubtful whether Mr. Jones would want her as his formal next-of-kin had he had capacity to make his own decisions, in which case his CNSs are limited to what they can tell her from a patient confidentiality perspective.

She was informed he did not currently possess formal capacity to make ANY decisions and that whilst understanding of her frustrations and situation, it was not something he could currently control. His specialist nurses would hence not be in a position to supply her with her requested letter or information. She was reassured however that she would be under no obligation (legal or otherwise), to care for him after discharge. Due to her persistent and increasingly irate nature of phone calls, advice was sought from the internal adult safeguarding team who agreed that his overall needs required safeguarding—he was assessed by the safeguarding team and duly appointed a temporary legal guardian.

Resulting from this legal guardian appointment, both his job and apartment (and his marital home!) were secured, as the guardians were able to provide evidence to the various tribunal bodies (employment, rental, banks, etc.) and courts of his medical condition and the proven effects it had on his cognition—his rental arrears and bills were cancelled and he underwent post-operative neuro-rehabilitation with good effect.

Only through the CNS thinking beyond Mr. Jones' immediate care needs and thinking of how the whole situation may affect him in the long-term was a potential crisis avoided. The nurse acted as a patient advocate and ensured (with the appropriate help and support) that both Mr. Jones' job, apartment and marital house were still available to him upon recovery and following discharge from hospital. Furthermore, his finances were protected until such time he was deemed able to have capacity one again. Sometimes, especially with patients who are cognitively affected by the presence of a brain tumour, the CNS is required to think of situations outside of the hospital setting to ensure the patient is protected and all aspects of their best interest are adhered to.

14.10 Nurse-Led Clinics

Depending on the previous levels of experience, a lot of neuro-oncology nurses undertake specialist nurse-led clinics for patient follow-up and support. The types of clinics offered may vary depending on whether the CNS covers neurosurgery or oncology solely, or whether they are in a combined role covering all aspects of patient's surgical and oncological needs.

From a neurosurgical perspective, follow-up clinics are offered for those patients on a pre- or post-operative surveillance course. These could be meningioma patients on imaging surveillance, or low-grade glioma patients who have been operated on, who also remain under surveillance. There is more to these clinics than simply relaying the results of the patient's surveillance MRI results: a nurse-led clinic also offers advice on post-operative side effects and treatments, medication side effects, work-related issues, fatigue management, family stresses and issues, support groups, financial advice, driving restrictions, travel advice and epilepsy management. They are very comprehensive clinics that offer a holistic approach to individualised patient care [10, 11, 19].

In oncology, the same approach remains, but nurses also offer treatment clinics for those patients undergoing (or completed) oncology treatments such as radiotherapy or chemotherapy. They monitor side effects and management of such; they assess full blood profiles and adjust chemotherapy doses (with their clinicians) accordingly, depending on the extent of bone marrow suppression and other factors such as white blood counts and neutrophils. The CNSs offer advice on side effects (including adverse reactions and toxicity) and monitor patients for signs of recurrence with regular MRI scans. Nurse-led clinics in oncology offer counselling services and signposting to other palliative care services and community facilities such as hospices and day respite centres [10, 19].

14.11 Conclusion

Specialist neuro-oncology nurses (whether neurosurgical, oncological or both) become the patients, family and carers life-line. The specialist nurses become the first line of defence for patients and families to utilise: relatives often ring 'their CNS' for complex clinical advice, seeking (re)assurance in instances where they need to call an ambulance immediately. Relatives have phoned for advice whilst abroad on holiday as their loved one has suffered a new-onset seizure; there have been instances where patients call their specialist nursing teams only to hand the phone over to the ambulance paramedics who are with them needing to speak to someone who is aware of their clinical situation.

Neuro-oncology nurses are often referred to as 'key workers' and it's easy to see why—they are the key to their patient's wellbeing, and the ripple effect spreads far and wide, from the hospital into the community and beyond. But, it is because of this key relationship that neuro-oncology nursing is such a niche cornerstone of specialist nursing, so special, and so very vital.

The role of specialist nursing is bound to become increasingly important within the health care setting given the context of the ever-increasing need to achieve better individualised management of patients, utilising scarce resources, and the need for reduced inpatient stay.

References

1. National Institute for Clinical Health and Excellence. Guidance on cancer services – improving outcomes for people with brain and other CNS tumours. The manual. Chapter 2. London: NICE; 2006.
2. Department of Health (DH). Cancer reform strategy. London; Dec 2017.
3. Taylor C, Munro A, Glynne-Jones R, et al. Multidisciplinary team working in cancer: what is the evidence? BMJ. 2010;340:c951. https://doi.org/10.1136/bmj.c951.
4. Weller M, Bent MV, Tonn JC, Stupp R, Preusser M, Cohen-Jonathan-Moyal E, et al. European Association for Neuro-Oncology (EANO) guideline on the diagnosis and treatment of adult astrocytic and oligodendroglial gliomas. Lancet Oncol. 2017;18(6):e315–29. https://doi.org/10.1016/s1470-2045(17)30194-8.
5. Guilfoyle MR, Weerakkody RA, Oswal A, et al. Implementation of neuro-oncology service reconfiguration in accordance with NICE guidance provides enhanced clinical care for patients with glioblastoma multiforme. Br J Cancer. 2011;104(12):1810–5.
6. Bartolo M, Zucchella C, Pace A, Lanzetta G, Vecchione C, Bartolo M, et al. Early rehabilitation after surgery improves functional outcome in inpatients with brain tumours. J Neurooncol. 2012;107(3):537–44.
7. National Cancer Action Team, NHS England. Rehabilitation Care Pathway - Brain CNS. 2009.
8. Pergolotti M, Williams GR, Campbell C, et al. Occupational therapy for adults with cancer: why it matters. Oncologist. 2016;21(3):314–9.
9. Cavers D, Hacking B, Erridge S, Morris P, Kendall M, Murray S. Adjustment and support needs of glioma patients and their relatives: serial interviews. Psycho-Oncology. 2012;22(6):1299–305.
10. Molassiotis A, Wilson B, Brunton L, Chaudhary H, Gattamaneni R, McBain C. Symptom experience in patients with primary brain tumours: a longitudinal exploratory study. Eur J Oncol Nurs. 2010;14(5):410–6.
11. Rooney AG, Netten A, McNamara S, Erridge S, Peoples S, Whittle I, et al. Assessment of a brain-tumour-specific patient concerns inventory in the neuro-oncology clinic. Support Care Cancer. 2014;22(4):1059–69.
12. NHS continuing healthcare: https://www.nhs.uk/conditions/social-care-and-support/nhs-continuing-care/. Accessed 02 Feb 2018.
13. Jevon P. *Neurological Assessment Part 1 – assessing level of consciousness.* Nurs Times. 2008;104(27):26–7.
14. Teasdale G, Allen D, Brennan P, McElhinney E, Mackinnon L. The Glasgow coma scale: an update after 40 years. Nurs Times. 2014;110:12–6.
15. Stupp R, Mason WP, Van Den Bent MJ, et al. Radiotherapy plus concomitant and adjuvant temozolo- mide for glioblastoma. N Engl J Med. 2005;352:987–96.
16. Stanfield RB, editor. The art of focused conversation: 100 ways to access group wisdom in the workplace. Toronto: The Canadian Institute of Cultural Affairs; 1997.
17. Nursing and Midwifery Council. The code: professional standards of practice and behaviour for nurses and midwives. London: NMC; 2015.
18. Mental Capacity Act: https://www.legislation.gov.uk/ukpga/2005/9/contents. 2005. Accessed 02 Feb 2017.
19. Loftus LA, Weston V. The development of nurse-led clinics in cancer care. J Clin Nurs. 2001;10(2):215–20.

Improving Patient's Functioning and Well-Being with Neurorehabilitation

15

Quirien Oort, Linda Dirven, and Martin J. B. Taphoorn

There are two main types of brain tumours: primary and secondary brain tumours [1]. Primary brain tumours originate from cellular abnormalities in brain tissue or in the tissues surrounding the brain. The most prevalent type of primary brain tumours in adults are meningiomas. Meningiomas are tumours that arise in the meninges, the layers of tissue that surround the outer part of the brain and spinal cord. Regarding tumours that originate in the brain itself, in childhood the majority of tumours that arise from brain tissue are neuronal tumours, while in adults the far majority originate from glial cells and are called gliomas, such as astrocytomas, oligodendrogliomas, glioblastomas and ependymomas [2]. Secondary brain tumours, also known as metastatic brain tumours or brain metastases, originate from tumours outside the central nervous system that have metastasized to the brain. In adults, metastatic brain tumours are even more common than primary brain tumours [2]. Brain tumours can be either malignant, including gliomas, primary central nervous system lymphomas (PCNSL) and brain metastases, or benign, such as the majority of meningiomas.

The overall symptom burden and disability in patients with brain tumours are significant [3–5]. Brain tumour patients may suffer from a variety of tumour-induced neurological symptoms including seizures, focal neurological deficits, cognitive deficits and behavioural and personality changes, in addition to more general cancer-related and treatment-induced symptoms such as nausea and vomiting, depression, anxiety and fatigue. These symptoms can have substantial negative

Q. Oort
Department of Neurology and Brain Tumor Center Amsterdam, Amsterdam University Medical Centers (VUmc), Amsterdam, The Netherlands

L. Dirven
Department of Neurology, Leiden University Medical Center, Leiden, The Netherlands

M. J. B. Taphoorn (✉)
Department of Neurology, Leiden University Medical Center, Leiden, The Netherlands
Department of Neurology, Haaglanden Medical Center, The Hague, The Netherlands
e-mail: m.taphoorn@haaglandenmc.nl; m.j.b.taphoorn@lumc.nl

© Springer Nature Switzerland AG 2019
M. Bartolo et al. (eds.), *Neurorehabilitation in Neuro-Oncology*,
https://doi.org/10.1007/978-3-319-95684-8_15

impact on the patient's activities in daily life and his/her social interactions, as well as the patient's health-related quality of life (HRQoL) [6–10].

The prognosis of brain tumour patients may range from only several months (e.g. brain metastases) to more than 20 years (e.g. low-grade gliomas or meningiomas), and depends on tumour characteristics (histopathology and grade, cytogenetic abnormalities) and patient factors such as age and clinical condition [11]. There is a variety of treatment options for brain tumour patients. Currently, anti-tumour treatment consists of surgery (resection or biopsy for diagnostic reasons), radiotherapy and/or systemic chemotherapy, depending on the type and location of the tumour. Other more recently developed interventions include targeted treatment and immunotherapy [12–18]. In addition, supportive treatments (e.g. anti-epileptic drugs and corticosteroids) are administered to relieve symptoms [19–26].

Given the progressive and incurable nature of most gliomas and brain metastases, treatment is intended not merely to prolong life, but also to relieve the patient's symptoms and maintain or improve the patient's functioning, as well as to preserve patient's HRQoL as much and as long as possible. Apart from incurable brain tumours, also benign brain tumours may lead to longstanding decrease in functioning and well-being, be it due to the tumour or its treatment. Although anti-tumour treatment may result in improved functioning, neurorehabilitation can be seen as an additional supportive treatment option to maintain or improve functioning and well-being during the disease trajectory. Neurorehabilitation offers a variety of therapies that focus on helping patients with neurological diseases to overcome their disabilities by improving and/or preserving specific aspects of patients' functioning. These therapies include developing motor, communication and cognitive skills, coping with psychological problems and educating daily life functioning and community reintegration. By improving and/or preserving functional abilities and educating on how to cope and adjust to more permanent functional deficiencies, neurorehabilitation ultimately aims to improve the patient's HRQoL.

This chapter will focus on the role of neurorehabilitation in improving brain tumour patients' functioning. First, we will discuss how patients' functioning is defined and can be measured. Next, we will focus on neurorehabilitation treatment options, taking into account their impact on the different levels of functioning.

15.1 Levels of (Dys)function

Health is not only defined as physical well-being. In 1948, the World Health Organization (WHO) defined health as "*a state of complete physical, mental and social well-being and not merely the absence of disease or infirmity*" [27]. The WHO International Classification of Functioning, Disability and Health (ICF) describes changes in health and health-related domains on three levels of human functioning: (1) body, (2) person and (3) society. For these three levels, respectively, changes in health can manifest as (a) impairments, (b) activity limitations and (c) participation restrictions.

Impairments are losses or abnormalities of body functions or structures and reflect the basic level of well-being [28]. As mentioned earlier, brain tumour patients may suffer from a wide range of impairments, including physical and cognitive impairments [6–10].

As a result of these *impairments,* persons might be constraint in their ability to perform activities of daily living (ADL). This is referred to as *activity limitations* [28–30]. ADL can be categorized in basic activities of daily living (BADL) and instrumental activities of daily living (IADL). BADL include basic skills such as walking and taking care of one's self [31]. IADL, on the other hand, include skills required for autonomous functioning like driving, handling finances and the ability to use a computer or smartphone [31, 32].

Activity limitations, in turn, may result in problems at the highest level, the societal level. Dysfunction on this level is referred to as *participation restrictions* [28–30]. Whereas *activity limitations* refer to problems with specific activities, *participation restrictions* reflect the interference the bodily *impairments* and *activity limitations* have on a person's ability to fulfil a certain role at work or school, in the home or during community or leisure activities. The WHO ICF states: *"Activity limitations are difficulties an individual may have in executing activities. Participation restrictions are problems an individual may have in involvement in life situations"* [29, 30].

As an example, a brain tumour patient with severe memory and concentration problems (*impairment*) is no longer able to work (*activity limitations*), and is therefore restricted in his/her ability to be an active member of the working society (*participation restriction*). Therefore, functional decline or disabilities on a basic level of functioning can have an extensive negative impact on higher levels of functioning and well-being.

15.2 Value of Functional Assessments in Research and Clinical Practice

Assessing patients' level of functioning is valuable in both clinical research and clinical practice. In clinical drug trials, outcome measures reflecting the patients' functioning are used to determine the net clinical benefit of a treatment strategy, in conjunction with traditional outcome measures such as overall and progression-free survival and objective response rate on imaging. The net clinical benefit is determined by how a patient "feels, functions, or survives" [33, 34]. Historically, overall survival has been the favoured primary endpoint in clinical trials, as it is generally viewed as the ultimate objective and a reliable measurement of treatment effect. However, patient-centred outcome measures are increasingly implemented as secondary outcome measures to determine the net clinical benefit [33, 34]. In contrast to clinical drug trials, outcome measures in neurorehabilitation trials reflecting the patients' functioning are usually the primary endpoint. The focus of rehabilitative treatment could be on a single or multiple domains, such as physical, cognitive or emotional functioning, activities of daily living, or social or vocational skills.

In clinical practice, assessing the level of functioning is particularly useful. Foremost, functional assessments are implemented to assess individual patient's present level of functioning and at multiple intervals to monitor for potentially foreseen and unforeseen functional decline during the course of disease and/or treatments [35]. Outcomes on functional assessments can have several applications. Functional outcomes may be used, for example, to determine if the patient's physical state is well enough to undergo or continue certain treatments (e.g. patients with Karnofsky performance status (KPS) scores >70 [36]), if measures need to be undertaken to avoid any (further) decline (e.g. physical therapy to avoid muscle atrophy), if alterations need to be made to the treatment regimen to better manage symptoms (e.g. adjusting anti-epileptic drug or dose) or if treatment has been or continues to be effective (e.g. functional improvements due to tumour response). Furthermore, functional outcomes on each level of well-being can facilitate the patient–physician communication and can be applied in shared decision-making regarding treatment options. Especially the functional assessments of the higher-order level of functioning (i.e. participation restrictions) can make the physician aware of potential problems beyond the purely physical or cognitive symptoms and may improve the patient's overall functioning and well-being [35].

15.3   Measuring (Dys)function

The US Food and Drug Administration (FDA) categorized patient-centred outcome measures, referred to as clinical outcome assessments (COAs), into four subtypes based on the source of information: patient-reported outcome (PRO) measures, observer-reported outcome (ObsRO) measures, clinician-reported outcome (ClinRO) measures and performance outcome (PerfO) measures [37]. ClinRO measures are measurements based on the evaluation of health care professionals, while PROs directly reflect the patient's perspective [38]. Although the consensus is that patients are the best source to rate their functioning and well-being [39], there are situations where patients may not be the most reliable source. In that case, ObsRO measures may be useful. Proxy ratings should be considered as a potentially appropriate alternative in neuro-oncology because proxies might better judge the patients' functioning in those situations where patients are cognitively impaired or have a very poor health status. Lastly, PerfO measures assess patient's (physical or neurocognitive) functioning based on their performance on a task and are, unlike the other outcome measures, objective measurements. PerfOs have the benefit of having good face validity and reproducibility, are sensitive to change over time and may detect functional limitations before it is reflected in the self-reported questionnaires (PROs) [40]. However, they are typically more expensive, time consuming and burdensome for patients. Furthermore, a recent systematic review found moderate to large correlation coefficients between the self-reported and performance-based assessment within the same domain of disability [41].

The development of measurement tools evaluating levels of functioning mirrors the evolution of the concept of dysfunction. At first, measurement tools were developed that mainly focused on assessing impairments (physical capabilities and sensory abilities), shifting to an increase in the development of tools assessing self-care abilities (e.g. BADL and IADL) and more recently towards social participation (fulfilment of social roles) [42–44]. Since (dys)function is a broad multi-dimensional concept, it can be challenging to measure this entire concept accurately.

In neuro-oncology, several COAs are used to assess the different levels of functioning. First, dysfunction on the *impairment* level is commonly assessed using PROs. This includes assessment of physical symptoms (e.g. visual analogue scale (VAS) for pain and fatigue), subjective cognitive complaints (e.g. functional assessment of cancer therapy-cognition (FACT-Cog)) and psychological problems (e.g. hospital anxiety and depression scale (HADS)). In addition, many HRQoL questionnaires comprise items on impairments, including items on sensory disorders, trouble sleeping, appetite loss, constipation, motor dysfunction, dyspnoea and seizures (e.g. European Organization for Research and Treatment for Cancer (EORTC), Quality of Life Questionnaire Core 30 (QLQ-C30) and the brain cancer module, the QLQ-BN20). Although more common in paediatric brain tumour patient research [45–47], proxy ratings (ObsRO) are also used to assess symptoms, cognitive functioning or behavioural changes in adults with brain tumours [48]. There are also several ClinROs that measure on the *impairment* level. The neurologic assessment in neuro-oncology (NANO) scale [49], for instance, evaluates brain tumour patients on nine relevant neurologic domains (symptoms and cognitive skills). Although performance status scales, such as the Eastern Cooperative Oncology Group Performance Status (ECOG), WHO performance status and the KPS scale, are often seen as measures of *impairment*, they also reflect aspects of *activity limitations*. PerfO measures assessing on the *impairment* level can focus on physical impairment, such as a neurological examination (i.e. physical and sensory tests to examine physical or sensory impairments) or cognition, typically assessed with a neuropsychological test battery. Neuropsychological tests assess impairments regarding many different cognitive domains, for example, memory (e.g. Hopkins verbal learning test-revised (HVLT-R); assessing direct free recall, delayed free recall and recognition), attention (e.g. D2 test of attention, selective and sustained attention and visual scanning speed), executive functioning (e.g. Delis-Kaplan executive function system (D-KEFS)), visuospatial constructional ability (e.g. Rey complex figure test and recognition trial (RCFT)) or language (e.g. Boston naming test).

Dysfunction on the level of *activity limitations* is typically assessed with BADL and IADL scales. Most commonly used BADL scales in neuro-oncology are the Barthel index (BI) and the Katz index of activities of daily living (Katz ADL). The BI and Katz ADL were originally developed as ClinROs [50–53]. However, nowadays BADL as well as IADLs can be assessed either by a health care professional, a proxy or by the patients themselves [32, 44, 54–57]. The functional independence measure and functional activity measure (FIM–FAM) is also commonly implemented as an ADL scoring system to assess the effectiveness of a rehabilitation program. This measure includes items with regard to both BADL and IADL, and is administered as a ClinRO. Assessing IADL can be particularly valuable in brain tumour patients, since cognitive decline is presumed to negatively impact their abilities to perform IADL. IADL involves higher-order activities *"with little automated skills for which multiple cognitive processes are necessary"* [58] and is therefore more sensitive to early effects of cognitive decline when compared to BADL [56,

59, 60]. However, unlike BADL, IADL is not commonly measured as a separate construct in neuro-oncological research. In some rare cases, the Lawton and Brody instrumental activities of daily living scale is used to assess IADL [61, 62]. Currently, a brain tumour-specific instrumental ADL measure is being developed as a PRO as well as an ObsRO [63], facilitating use in clinical trials and clinical practice. BADL and IADL can also be measured using PerfOs, such as the physical performance test (PPT) [64] and direct assessment of functional status (DAFS) [56], yet these are not commonly used in neuro-oncology.

To the best of our knowledge, there are no measures available for use in neuro-oncology that assesses functioning at the level of *participation restriction* only. HRQOL questionnaires cover some items on *participation restriction*, but they do not capture the full extent of potential issues on this level of functioning. The EORTC QLQ-C30 and QLQ-BN20 questionnaires, for example, contain items on the interference of the patient's physical condition or medical treatment with their family life or social activities. The FACT-general and brain module contains similar items, such as having trouble meeting the needs of the family, and being bothered by the drop in contribution to the family. A questionnaire such as the social role participation questionnaire (SRPQ) [65] (developed for patients with arthritis), focusing on participation restrictions only, could perhaps be useful in neuro-oncology to better assess functioning on this level. The SRPQ is a broad instrument assessing the influence of health on 11 specific social role domains and one "general participation" item. Patients rate (a) how important the social roles are to them, (b) their satisfaction with the amount time spent in that particular social role and (c) their ability to participate in that role in the way they want (i.e. role performance) on a 5-point Likert scale. As with the brain tumour-specific IADL, the development of a brain tumour-specific questionnaire on participation restrictions or social roles should be considered.

15.4 Neurorehabilitative Interventions

Neurorehabilitation can be implemented to address patients' various dysfunctions associated with the treatment or disease, and may contribute to maintaining and improving HRQoL. Neurorehabilitation considers physical, psychological and social aspects of the patient's well-being and, therefore, requires a multidisciplinary team care, including psychologists, nurses and rehabilitation specialists, to obtain optimal results. Despite the fact that rehabilitation is commonly being practiced in clinical settings, it has not been extensively recognized in cancer care. In recent years, however, the increase in the number of long-term survivors due to advances in cancer care has led to an increased interest in cancer rehabilitation [66]. The type of neurorehabilitative treatment is often determined by several factors, including the patient's diagnosis, received treatment and their anticipated survival. Although this suggests that neurorehabilitation programs should be different for the various types of brain tumour patients, several studies have indicated that rehabilitation provides significant functional gains in patients with

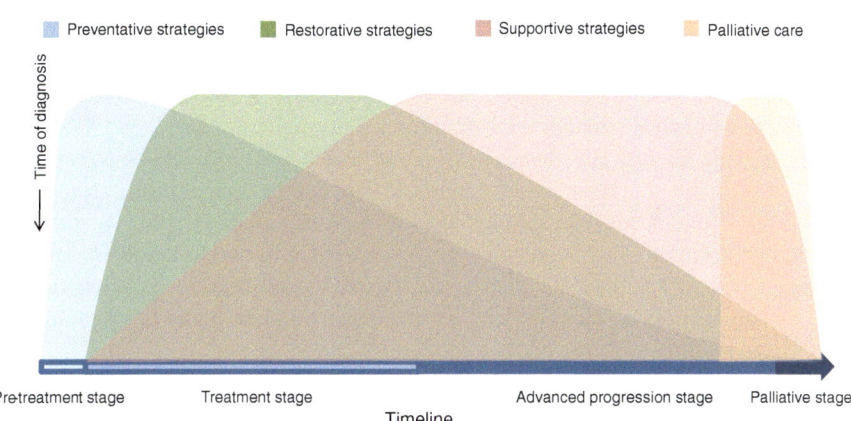

Fig. 15.1 Schematic depiction of the adaptive rehabilitation strategies during the stages of functional progression

brain tumours irrespective of tumour type, location of lesion or the presence of metastases during inpatient rehabilitation [67–73].

Several neurorehabilitative interventions are available for brain tumour patients. However, the potential effects of rehabilitation on the patients functioning may vary in the different phases of the disease. Therefore, the so-called adaptive rehabilitation program for patients with cancer described by Dietz may also be useful for brain tumour patients. This program consists of four categories: prevention, restoration, support and palliation [74]. Adaptive rehabilitation reflects the stages of functional progression, from the time of diagnosis until end of life, and introduces the relevant intervention strategies for these stages (Fig. 15.1).

Neurorehabilitation at the time of diagnosis and prior to treatment mainly consists of preventative strategies. In this phase, the focus lies on education and early intervention to abate the effects of the tumour and prevent functional loss [75]. As mentioned earlier, baseline levels of function (i.e. impairments, activity limitations and participation restrictions) can be assessed prior to treatment and monitored during the course of the disease. Preventative strategies can be implemented to retain patients' functioning and to prevent occurrence of impairments during the course of disease or during treatment [74, 76, 77]. For example, rehabilitation could be focused on maintaining a good physical condition [78] and making certain decisions to change lifestyle prior to treatment (e.g. quit smoking [79]) that may decrease the impact of potential adverse outcomes of treatment. Physical therapy can be implemented to prevent (further) physical decline. Another form of a preventative strategy is psychological support, which can be introduced after receiving the diagnosis or prior to or during treatment. By informing (newly) diagnosed patients about what may be expected with regard to the effects (e.g. physical, emotional, cognitive, behavioural) of having a brain tumour and undergoing treatment, and addressing patients' present and future concerns, (further) psychological distress may be reduced or prevented.

During the treatment stage, preventative, restorative and supportive strategies can be implemented. One such preventative strategy is part of physical therapy, and includes early postoperative ambulation and improving physical functions. It is known that physical strength tends to diminish during treatment due to fatigue and other adverse effects. However, physical and muscle strength can be enhanced by physical therapy to prevent disuse syndrome (e.g. contractures, muscle atrophy, loss of muscle strength and decubitus due to decline in mobility) [66]. Directly after treatment, restorative strategies may be implemented to maximize the recovery of patients' level of functioning either to levels prior to treatment or regaining maximal functional recovery in patients with more extensive impairments of functioning or decreased abilities [74, 76, 77].

There are various restorative strategies that can be implemented during the treatment stage, both physical and cognitive. The physical restorative strategy during this stage aims to restore the patient's balance, walking ability and general mobility. One study showed that brain tumour patients receiving comprehensive individualized multidisciplinary rehabilitation significantly improved on the FIM-mobility subscale (i.e. 13 out of 18 FIM items, excluding the items on communication and social cognition) at 3 months post-treatment follow-up compared to the waitlist control group; however, this effect was no longer present after 6-month follow-up [80]. Another study showed that brain tumour patients made significant improvements in their FIM scores from admission to discharge [81]. Although the length of rehabilitation was not a significant independent predictor of high or low FIM gain for patients with brain tumours, patients with brain metastases and glioblastoma who had the highest increase in functional gains were also the ones who had the longest survival time.

An example of a restorative strategy with regard to cognition is cognitive rehabilitation. Cognitive rehabilitation depends on the principles of neural plasticity of the brain. Neural plasticity refers to the brains capability to reorganize itself by neurons changing in structure and function and forming new neural connections [82]. It allows neurons to compensate for brain injuries and diseases, and mediates in the acquisition of knowledge and skills. Cognitive rehabilitation offers exercises aimed at improving various domains of cognition such as attention, memory, language and executive/control functions. Although cognitive deficits are characteristic for brain tumour patients, only few published studies have examined the potential benefits of cognitive rehabilitation in this patient population. One of these studies evaluated a multifaceted cognitive rehabilitation program (CRP), a computer-based attention retraining and compensatory skills training of attention, memory and executive functioning in patients with different types of brain tumours [83]. Patients were randomized to the intervention group or the waiting-list control group. The effect of CRP was evaluated by administering a battery of neuropsychological tests and self-report questionnaires at baseline, which was directly after the cognitive rehabilitation for the intervention group and at an equivalent time point for the control group, and at the 6-month follow-up. The study revealed less cognitive complaints immediately post-treatment and significant better scores on several neuropsychological tests in the intervention group: on four out of the seven individual attention tests (effect sizes ranged from 0.23 to 0.55) and two of the three individual verbal memory tests (effect sizes, 0.48 and 0.43). Moreover, patients in the intervention group reported less mental fatigue at the 6-month follow-up measurement. Although few studies have been conducted to evaluate the effects of neurocognitive rehabilitation, and though it is usually not integrated into the routine care of patients with brain tumours, neurocognitive training is feasible and might be able to induce improvements in cognitive skills. To help patients to manage the effects of their neurocognitive impairments better, neurocognitive rehabilitation should occur in parallel with medical management to treat fatigue, behaviour, memory, mood and the management of drugs that may be associated with neurocognitive side effects (e.g. anti-epileptic drugs) [84].

Although preventative and restorative strategies predominantly focus on the improvements gained on the *impairment* level of functioning, it is expected that this has an indirect positive impact on activities in everyday life. This is evident from a meta-analysis revealing a statistically significant effect of inpatient physical rehabilitation on functional improvement for both the Barthel index (an average of +44% score change from admission until discharge) and the functional independence measurement (FIM) scores (an average of +23% score change from admission until discharge), resulting in an overall average increase of 36% in independence [85]. In a recent study by Han et al. [86] brain tumour patients received conventional rehabilitation. This conventional rehabilitation therapy included physical therapy by neuro-developmental treatment (NDT)-certified therapists for one hour per day, neuromuscular electrical stimulation therapy, aerobic exercise, occupational therapy for stretching and strengthening of the upper extremity, and task-oriented therapy for ADL, fine motor training and sensory motor recovery. Computerized or focused cognitive training of neuropsychological deficits was not included. The combination of the physical restorative strategies and supportive strategies in this conventional therapy induced significant physical and cognitive (Korean versions of the motricity index (K-MI) and mini mental status examination (K-MMSE)) improvements in both benign and malignant brain tumour patients, as well as improved functioning in activities of daily living (Korean version of the modified BI (K-MBI)). In addition, results demonstrated that aspects of motor and cognitive dysfunction predicted lower levels of ADL function, before and after rehabilitation [86].

For some brain tumour patients, supportive care in the form of occupational therapy can be relevant in the treatment stage following initial treatment. One aspect of occupational therapy is professional integration, i.e., helping patients return to work to some extent. During prevocational therapy, the job reinstatement possibilities for brain tumour patients vary extremely depending on the tumour type and clinical condition. Even for brain tumour patients with more favourable prognosis, whom might benefit from this training, it is imperative to help develop a realistic view of their working potential. Some patients might have to come to grips with the realization that a return to work might not mean returning to their former employment position and/or not in the same capacity.

During prevocational training, work simulations can be implemented to teach and reinforce the use of compensatory strategies. These may include using a daily planner to maintain daily schedules or using written checklists for operating equipment (e.g. computers). In addition, education on the reorganization of the workspace and structuring/organizing the work day can allow successful completion of tasks which would otherwise be too challenging. The therapist could also encourage patients to resume or assume the role of homemaker or volunteer, or help develop a structured routine for leisure/avocational activities [87]. One study reported favourable participation outcomes (community independence and employment) after outpatient multidisciplinary rehabilitation in people with brain tumours [73].

However, most supportive interventions are designed to teach patients to accommodate to their disabilities and to minimize debilitating changes from ongoing disease. As the disease progresses and patients develop more permanent disabilities, the predominant focus shifts even more from the prevention and restoration of impairments towards higher levels of functioning in order to maintain a decent level of independence. In the advanced stage of the disease, the purpose of supportive strategies is to maintain a level self-care and independence using education and guidance (e.g. educating self-care strategies and skills and assisting with the use of supportive medical devices). Patients are assisted in learning how to cope and adjust to the disabilities, and are educated in the use of medical devices (e.g. learning to adjust to prosthetic devices or wheelchair) [74, 76, 77]. Occupational therapy may also focus on maximizing a person's independence with regard to daily functioning [87]. For example, *activity limitations* (i.e. BADL and IADL) could be improved by addressing problems regarding self-care, functional mobility, meal preparation, money management, driving and leisure activities due to physical and/or cognitive disabilities [87, 88]. Also, occupational therapy in the form of community reintegration training can be implemented to enhance the level of *participation restrictions,* by learning patients to reintegrate into the community despite their disabilities. Community living skills are essential to be a productive participant in society. Community reintegration training includes planning and participating in community-based activities. Tasks learned or re-learned in the clinic can be practiced in a more natural context during community reintegration activities.

Neuro-palliative rehabilitation is at the interface between rehabilitation and palliative care and focuses on symptom management and interventions to maximize HRQoL during the terminal stages of the disease. In this phase, the intent is to make patients feel as comfortable as possible, either physically, psychologically and/or socially, and respect their wishes. Palliative care may, for example, focus on symptom relieve (e.g. pain control), psychological support and reducing the chances of adverse effects of being bedridden, such as contractures and pressure ulcers, by using heat, (re-)positioning of the body, breathing assistance and relaxation, and with the use of low-frequency electromagnetic therapy equipment or with the use of assistive devices [74, 76, 77].

15.5 Conclusion and Future Perspectives

In conclusion, patients with brain tumours can have impairments on all levels of functioning, which may negatively affect their overall HRQoL. Neurorehabilitation can improve functioning on all levels of functioning, using different types of interventions which depend on the stage of the disease. Although several tools exist to assess functioning and well-being, there is still a need for brain tumour-specific tools on all levels of functioning, especially the higher-order levels of functioning. Moreover, there is a need for more empirical studies evaluating neurorehabilitative interventions in brain tumour patients using these functional assessment tools. By optimally assessing functioning and adequately addressing functional decline at the right moment with the right treatments and interventions, patient's HRQoL can subsequently be improved.

Developments have been made in the field of neurorehabilitation as a result of the emergence of new technological advances. In the past years, there has been a growing interest in e-health, i.e., digitized assessment tools and therapies. Several studies have been published recently regarding the development and testing of computerized neuropsychological test (CNT) batteries, virtual reality training tools and online/app-based rehabilitation [89–95]. However, the current emphasis is on preserving physical and cognitive functioning. Further well-designed studies in different brain tumour patient populations are needed to investigate how these e-health tools may help improve the patients' functioning and well-being on higher levels (I-ADL and societal participation).

References

1. Buckner JC, et al. Central nervous system tumors. Mayo Clin Proc. 2007;82(10):1271–86.
2. The American Cancer Society medical. Cancer.org.
3. Davies E, Clarke C, Hopkins A. Malignant cerebral glioma--I: survival, disability, and morbidity after radiotherapy. BMJ. 1996;313(7071):1507–12.
4. Osoba D, et al. Effect of disease burden on health-related quality of life in patients with malignant gliomas. Neuro-Oncology. 2000;2(4):221–8.
5. Taphoorn MJ, et al. Cognitive functions and quality of life in patients with low-grade gliomas: the impact of radiotherapy. Ann Neurol. 1994;36(1):48–54. https://doi.org/10.1002/ana.410360111.
6. Bennett SR, et al. Investigating the impact of headaches on the quality of life of patients with glioblastoma multiforme: a qualitative study. BMJ Open. 2016;6(11):e011616.
7. Boele FW, et al. The association between cognitive functioning and health-related quality of life in low-grade glioma patients. Neurooncol Pract. 2014;1(2):40–6.
8. Gazzotti MR, et al. Quality of life and physical limitations in primary brain tumor patients. Qual Life Res. 2011;20(10):1639–43.
9. Klein M, et al. Epilepsy in low-grade gliomas: the impact on cognitive function and quality of life. Ann Neurol. 2003;54(4):514–20.
10. Li J, et al. Relationship between neurocognitive function and quality of life after whole-brain radiotherapy in patients with brain metastasis. Int J Radiat Oncol Biol Phys. 2008;71(1):64–70.
11. Porter KR, et al. Conditional survival of all primary brain tumor patients by age, behavior, and histology. Neuroepidemiology. 2011;36(4):230–9. https://doi.org/10.1159/000327752.

12. Ahluwalia MS, Winkler F. Targeted and immunotherapeutic approaches in brain metastases. Am Soc Clin Oncol Educ Book. 2015;35:67–74.
13. Doorduijn JK, et al. Treatment of secondary central nervous system lymphoma with intrathecal rituximab, high-dose methotrexate, and R-DHAP followed by autologous stem cell transplantation: results of the HOVON 80 phase 2 study. Hematol Oncol. 2016;35(4):497–503. 17(10).
14. McArthur GA, et al. Vemurafenib in metastatic melanoma patients with brain metastases: an open-label, single-arm, phase 2, multicentre study. Ann Oncol. 2017;28(3):634–41. https://doi.org/10.1093/annonc/mdw641.
15. Neagu MR, Reardon DA. An update on the role of immunotherapy and vaccine strategies for primary brain tumors. Curr Treat Options in Oncol. 2015;16(11):54. https://doi.org/10.1007/s11864-015-0371-3.
16. Reardon DA, et al. Efficacy and safety results of ABT-414 in combination with radiation and temozolomide in newly diagnosed glioblastoma. Neuro-Oncology. 2017;19(7):965–75. https://doi.org/10.1093/neuonc/now257.
17. Schuster J, et al. A phase II, multicenter trial of rindopepimut (CDX-110) in newly diagnosed glioblastoma: the ACT III study. Neuro-Oncology. 2015;17(6):854–61. https://doi.org/10.1093/neuonc/nou348.
18. Sperduto PW, et al. A phase 3 trial of whole brain radiation therapy and stereotactic radiosurgery alone versus WBRT and SRS with temozolomide or erlotinib for non-small cell lung cancer and 1 to 3 brain metastases: Radiation Therapy Oncology Group 0320. Int J Radiat Oncol Biol Phys. 2013;85(5):1312–8. https://doi.org/10.1016/j.ijrobp.2012.11.042.
19. Baumert BG, et al. Temozolomide chemotherapy versus radiotherapy in high-risk low-grade glioma (EORTC 22033-26033): a randomised, open-label, phase 3 intergroup study. Lancet Oncol. 2016;17(11):1521–32.
20. Buckner JC, et al. Radiation plus Procarbazine, CCNU, and Vincristine in low-grade glioma. N Engl J Med. 2016;374(14):1344–55.
21. Goldbrunner R, et al. EANO guidelines for the diagnosis and treatment of meningiomas. Lancet Oncol. 2016;17(9):e383–91.
22. Lippitz B, et al. Stereotactic radiosurgery in the treatment of brain metastases: the current evidence. Cancer Treat Rev. 2014;40(1):48–59.
23. Stupp R, et al. Radiotherapy plus concomitant and adjuvant temozolomide for glioblastoma. N Engl J Med. 2005;352(10):987–96.
24. Thiel E, et al. High-dose methotrexate with or without whole brain radiotherapy for primary CNS lymphoma (G-PCNSL-SG-1): a phase 3, randomised, non-inferiority trial. Lancet Oncol. 2010;11(11):1036–47.
25. van den Bent MJ, et al. Adjuvant procarbazine, lomustine, and vincristine chemotherapy in newly diagnosed anaplastic oligodendroglioma: long-term follow-up of EORTC brain tumor group study 26951. J Clin Oncol. 2013;31(3):344–50.
26. Wick W, et al. NOA-04 randomized phase III trial of sequential radiochemotherapy of anaplastic glioma with procarbazine, lomustine, and vincristine or temozolomide. J Clin Oncol. 2009;27(35):5874–80.
27. WHO constitution. Geneva: WHO; 1948.
28. Towards a common language for functioning, disability and health ICF. World Health Organization; 2002.
29. ICF CHECKLIST Version 2.1a, Clinician form for international classification of functioning, disability and health. World Health Organization; 2003.
30. World Health Organisation. International classification of functioning, disability and health: ICF. Geneva: World Health Organisation; 2001.
31. Lawton MP, Brody EM. Assessment of older people: self-maintaining and instrumental activities of daily living. Gerontologist. 1969;9(3):179–86.
32. Overdorp EJ, et al. The combined effect of neuropsychological and neuropathological deficits on instrumental activities of daily living in older adults: a systematic review. Neuropsychol Rev. 2016;26(1):92–106. https://doi.org/10.1007/s11065-015-9312-y.

33. Clinical outcome assessment (COA): glossary of terms. US Food and Drug Administration.
34. Helfer JL, et al. Report of the jumpstarting brain tumor drug development coalition and FDA clinical trials clinical outcome assessment endpoints workshop (October 15, 2014, Bethesda MD). Neuro-Oncology. 2016;18(Suppl 2):ii26–36.
35. Dirven L, et al. Health related quality of life in brain tumor patients: as an endpoint in clinical trials and its value in clinical care. Expert Rev Qual Life Cancer Care. 2016;1(1):37–44.
36. Gaspar L, et al. Recursive partitioning analysis (RPA) of prognostic factors in three Radiation Therapy Oncology Group (RTOG) brain metastases trials. Int J Radiat Oncol Biol Phys. 1997;37(4):745–51.
37. Clinical Outcome Assessment Qualification Program. US Food and Drug Administration.
38. Dirven L, Armstrong TS, Taphoorn MJ. Health-related quality of life and other clinical outcome assessments in brain tumor patients: challenges in the design, conduct and interpretation of clinical trials. Neurooncol Pract. 2015;2(1):2–5.
39. Fayers P, Machin D. Quality of life. Assessment, analysis and interpretation. Chichester: John Wiley and Sons; 2000.
40. Rozzini R, et al. The effect of chronic diseases on physical function. Comparison between activities of daily living scales and the physical performance test. Age Ageing. 1997;26(4):281–7.
41. Coman L, Richardson J. Relationship between self-report and performance measures of function: a systematic review. Can J Aging. 2006;25(3):253–70.
42. Gill TM. Assessment of function and disability in longitudinal studies. J Am Geriatr Soc. 2010;58(Suppl 2):S308–12. https://doi.org/10.1111/j.1532-5415.2010.02914.x.
43. McDowell I. Measuring health: a guide to rating scales and questionnaires. 3rd ed. New York: Oxford University Press; 2006.
44. Yang M, Ding X, Dong B. The measurement of disability in the elderly: a systematic review of self-reported questionnaires. J Am Med Dir Assoc. 2014;15(2):150.e1–9. https://doi.org/10.1016/j.jamda.2013.10.004. Epub 2013 Dec 4.
45. Barakat LP, et al. Health-related quality of life of adolescent and young adult survivors of childhood brain tumors. Psychooncology. 2015;24(7):804–11. https://doi.org/10.1002/pon.3649. Epub 2014 Aug 11.
46. Gregg N, et al. Neurobehavioural changes in patients following brain tumour: patients and relatives perspective. Support Care Cancer. 2014;22(11):2965–72. https://doi.org/10.1007/s00520-014-2291-3. Epub 2014 May 28.
47. Hocking MC, et al. Neurocognitive and family functioning and quality of life among young adult survivors of childhood brain tumors. Clin Neuropsychol. 2011;25(6):942–62. https://doi.org/10.1080/13854046.2011.580284. Epub 2011 Jul 04.
48. Simpson GK, et al. Frequency, clinical correlates, and ratings of behavioral changes in primary brain tumor patients: a preliminary investigation. Front Oncol. 2015;5:78. https://doi.org/10.3389/fonc.2015.00078.
49. Nayak L, et al. The Neurologic Assessment in Neuro-Oncology (NANO) scale: a tool to assess neurologic function for integration into the Response Assessment in Neuro-Oncology (RANO) criteria. Neuro-Oncology. 2017;19(5):625–35. https://doi.org/10.1093/neuonc/nox029.
50. Brorsson B, Asberg KH. Katz index of independence in ADL. Reliability and validity in short-term care. Scand J Rehabil Med. 1984;16(3):125–32.
51. Katz S. Assessing self-maintenance: activities of daily living, mobility, and instrumental activities of daily living. J Am Geriatr Soc. 1983;31(12):721–7.
52. Mahoney FI, Barthel DW. Functional Evaluation: The Barthel Index. Md State Med J. 1965;14:61–5.
53. Granger CV, Albrecht GL, Hamilton BB. Outcome of comprehensive medical rehabilitation: measurement by PULSES profile and the Barthel Index. Arch Phys Med Rehabil. 1979;60(4):145–54.
54. Collin C, et al. The Barthel ADL Index: a reliability study. Int Disabil Stud. 1988;10(2):61–3.
55. Hartigan I, O'Mahony D. The Barthel Index: comparing inter-rater reliability between nurses and doctors in an older adult rehabilitation unit. Appl Nurs Res. 2011;24(1):e1–7. https://doi.org/10.1016/j.apnr.2009.11.002.

56. Jekel K, et al. Mild cognitive impairment and deficits in instrumental activities of daily living: a systematic review. Alzheimers Res Ther. 2015;7(1):17. https://doi.org/10.1186/s13195-015-0099-0.

57. Wyller TB, Sveen U, Bautz-Holter E. The Barthel ADL index one year after stroke: comparison between relatives' and occupational therapist's scores. Age Ageing. 1995;24(5):398–401.

58. Sikkes SA, et al. A new informant-based questionnaire for instrumental activities of daily living in dementia. Alzheimers Dement. 2012;8(6):536–43. https://doi.org/10.1016/j.jalz.2011.08.006.

59. Ahn IS, et al. Impairment of instrumental activities of daily living in patients with mild cognitive impairment. Psychiatry Investig. 2009;6(3):180–4. https://doi.org/10.4306/pi.2009.6.3.180.

60. Reppermund S, et al. The relationship of neuropsychological function to instrumental activities of daily living in mild cognitive impairment. Int J Geriatr Psychiatry. 2011;26(8):843–52. https://doi.org/10.1002/gps.2612.

61. Sabater S, et al. Predicting compliance and survival in palliative whole-brain radiotherapy for brain metastases. Clin Transl Oncol. 2012;14(1):43–9. (1699-3055 (Electronic)).

62. Wong GKC, Wong R, Poon WS. Cognitive outcomes and activity of daily living for neurosurgical patients with intrinsic brain lesions: a 1-year prevalence study. Hong Kong J Occup Ther. 2011;21(1):27–32.

63. Oort Q, et al. Development of a questionnaire measuring instrumental activities of daily living (IADL) in patients with brain tumors: a pilot study. J Neuro-Oncol. 2017;132(1):145–53. https://doi.org/10.1007/s11060-016-2352-1.

64. Terret C, et al. Karnofsky Performance Scale (KPS) or Physical Performance Test (PPT)? That is the question. Crit Rev Oncol Hematol. 2011;77(2):142–7. https://doi.org/10.1016/j.critrevonc.2010.01.015.

65. Gignac MA, et al. Understanding social role participation: what matters to people with arthritis? J Rheumatol. 2008;35(8):1655–63.

66. Okamura H. Importance of rehabilitation in cancer treatment and palliative medicine. Jpn J Clin Oncol. 2011;41(6):733–8.

67. Fu JB, et al. Comparison of functional outcomes in low- and high-grade astrocytoma rehabilitation inpatients. Am J Phys Med Rehabil. 2010;89(3):205–12. https://doi.org/10.1097/PHM.0b013e3181ca2306.

68. Marciniak CM, et al. Functional outcomes of persons with brain tumors after inpatient rehabilitation. Arch Phys Med Rehabil. 2001;82(4):457–63.

69. O'Dell MW, et al. Functional outcome of inpatient rehabilitation in persons with brain tumors. Arch Phys Med Rehabil. 1998;79(12):1530–4.

70. Greenberg E, Treger I, Ring H. Rehabilitation outcomes in patients with brain tumors and acute stroke: comparative study of inpatient rehabilitation. Am J Phys Med Rehabil. 2006;85(7):568–73.

71. Huang ME, Wartella JE, Kreutzer JS. Functional outcomes and quality of life in patients with brain tumors: a preliminary report. Arch Phys Med Rehabil. 2001;82(11):1540–6.

72. Mukand JA, et al. Incidence of neurologic deficits and rehabilitation of patients with brain tumors. Am J Phys Med Rehabil. 2001;80(5):346–50.

73. Sherer M, Meyers CA, Bergloff P. Efficacy of postacute brain injury rehabilitation for patients with primary malignant brain tumors. Cancer. 1997;80(2):250–7.

74. Dietz JH Jr. Adaptive rehabilitation in cancer: a program to improve quality of survival. Postgrad Med. 1980;68(1):145–7.

75. Ching W, Luhmann M. Neuro-oncologic physical therapy for the older person. Topics Geriatr Rehabil. 2011;27(3):184–92.

76. Dietz JH Jr. Rehabilitation of the cancer patient. Med Clin North Am. 1969;53(3):607–24.

77. Moroz A, Flanagan SR, Zaretsky H. Medical aspects of disability for the rehabilitation professional. 5th ed. New York: Springer; 2016.

78. Ruden E, et al. Exercise behavior, functional capacity, and survival in adults with malignant recurrent glioma. J Clin Oncol. 2011;29(21):2918–23. https://doi.org/10.1200/JCO.2011.34.9852.

79. Lau D, et al. Cigarette smoking: a risk factor for postoperative morbidity and 1-year mortality following craniotomy for tumor resection. J Neurosurg. 2012;116(6):1204–14. https://doi.org/10.3171/2012.3.JNS111783.
80. Khan F, et al. Effectiveness of integrated multidisciplinary rehabilitation in primary brain cancer survivors in an Australian community cohort: a controlled clinical trial. J Rehabil Med. 2014;46(8):754–60. https://doi.org/10.2340/16501977-1840.
81. Tang V, et al. Rehabilitation in primary and metastatic brain tumours: impact of functional outcomes on survival. J Neurol. 2008;255(6):820–7. https://doi.org/10.1007/s00415-008-0695-z.
82. Raskin SA. Neuroplasticity and rehabilitation. New York: Guilford Publications; 2011.
83. Gehring K, et al. Cognitive rehabilitation in patients with gliomas: a randomized, controlled trial. J Clin Oncol. 2009;27(22):3712–22. https://doi.org/10.1200/JCO.2008.20.5765.
84. Day J, et al. Neurocognitive deficits and neurocognitive rehabilitation in adult brain tumors. Curr Treat Options Neurol. 2016;18(5):22.
85. Formica V, et al. Rehabilitation in neuro-oncology: a meta-analysis of published data and a mono-institutional experience. Integr Cancer Ther. 2011;10(2):119–26. https://doi.org/10.1177/1534735410392575.
86. Han EY, et al. Functional improvement after 4-week rehabilitation therapy and effects of attention deficit in brain tumor patients: comparison with subacute stroke patients. Ann Rehabil Med. 2015;39(4):560–9. https://doi.org/10.5535/arm.2015.39.4.560.
87. Kearney P, et al. The role of the occupational therapist on the neuro-rehabilitation team. In: Elbaum J, Benson DM, editors. Acquired brain injury: an integrative neuro-rehabilitation approach. New York: Springer; 2007. p. 215–37.
88. Creek J. The core concepts of occupational therapy: A dynamic framework for practice. London: Jessica Kingsley Publishers; 2010.
89. Yang S, et al. Effect of virtual reality on cognitive dysfunction in patients with brain tumor. Ann Rehabil Med. 2014;38(6):726–33. https://doi.org/10.5535/arm.2014.38.6.726.
90. Gualtieri CT, Johnson LG. Reliability and validity of a computerized neurocognitive test battery, CNS Vital Signs. Arch Clin Neuropsychol. 2006;21(7):623–43.
91. Gualtieri CT, Johnson LG. A computerized test battery sensitive to mild and severe brain injury. Medscape J Med. 2008;10(4):90.
92. van der Linden SD, et al. Home-based cognitive rehabilitation in brain tumor patients: Feasibility of the evidence-based ReMind program. J Int Neuropsychol Soc. 2016;22(2):83.
93. Meskal I, et al. Cognitive improvement in meningioma patients after surgery: clinical relevance of computerized testing. J Neuro-Oncol. 2015;121(3):617–25. https://doi.org/10.1007/s11060-014-1679-8.
94. Yang S, Chun MH, Son YR. Effect of virtual reality on cognitive dysfunction in patients with brain tumor. Ann Rehabil Med. 2014;38(6):726–33. https://doi.org/10.5535/arm.2014.38.6.726.
95. Yoon J, et al. Effect of virtual reality-based rehabilitation on upper-extremity function in patients with brain tumor: controlled trial. Am J Phys Med Rehabil. 2015;94(6):449–59. https://doi.org/10.1097/PHM.0000000000000192.

Palliative Care and Palliative Rehabilitation: Approaches to the End-of-Life

Andrea Pace and Veronica Villani

16.1 Introduction

The concept of palliative care is an emerging field in neuro-oncology. The WHO definition of palliative care (PC) affirms that "palliative care is an approach that improves the quality of life of patients and their families facing the problem associated with life-threatening illness, through the prevention and relief of suffering by means of early identification and impeccable assessment and treatment of pain and other problems, physical, psychosocial and spiritual" (www.who.int/cancer/palliative/definition/en/).

However, brain tumour (BT) patients are different respect from other cancer patients because of trajectory of the disease, short life expectancy and complexity of palliative care needs due to specific symptoms related to neurological deterioration and therefore they require a specific and appropriate palliative care approach especially in the last stage of disease when incidence of neurological symptoms and psychosocial troubles becomes higher [1].

Despite the advance in treatment options has lengthened the life expectancy, BT patients suffer significant functional and psychosocial impairments that limit daily activity and quality of life.

During the course of the disease, BT patients present with multiple neurological deficits that can be due either to primary tumour effects and/or the adverse effects of oncologic treatment [2–5]. The localization of the tumour leads to several neurological symptoms including focal symptoms (hemiparesis, seizures and speech difficulties) and neurocognitive deficits (aphasia, impaired attention, concentration difficulty, reduced short-term memory and behaviour changes). One study found that 75.4% of BT patients presented more than three concurrent deficits, and 39.2% had more than five [6].

A. Pace (✉) · V. Villani
Neurooncology Unit, IRCCS Regina Elena National Cancer Institute, Rome, Italy
e-mail: andrea.pace@ifo.gov.it

© Springer Nature Switzerland AG 2019
M. Bartolo et al. (eds.), *Neurorehabilitation in Neuro-Oncology*,
https://doi.org/10.1007/978-3-319-95684-8_16

There is a large consensus on the need to improve the quality of palliative and supportive care for neuro-oncological patients. However, several papers have reported a lack of knowledge and of evidence-based guidelines about supportive care in BTs and confirm that there is a great need for education in palliative care and end-of-life decision-making in neuro-oncology setting [7, 8].

In this chapter, we will address palliative care issues in BT patients at the end-of-life (EoL) and the role of palliative rehabilitation interventions in advanced stage of disease.

16.2   Palliative Care Issues in Brain Tumour Patients

To date, palliative care in neuro-oncologic patients and the ongoing needs for care from discharge to the terminal phase of disease are not well documented. Literature data reported this to be a heterogeneous group of patients with complex needs [9].

Care needs increase in the last stage of disease with a high incidence of neurological symptoms and psychosocial problems often inducing caregivers and/or family members to hospitalize the patient [1]. The main goal of palliative care in neuro-oncology is the control of symptoms during the course of disease and particularly in advanced stage and at the end of life. Malignant BT patients at the end of life require specific palliative interventions, with a multidisciplinary approach performed by a well-trained neuro-oncological team, for the control of pain, confusion, agitation, delirium or seizures management with the aim to allow the patient to experience a peaceful death [10].

Table 16.1 reports the symptoms observed in the last weeks/months of life of BT patients in recent studies (Table 16.1) [10–14]. A recent study showed that in the last

Table 16.1 Symptoms in brain tumour patients at the end of life reported in the literature

Symptoms	Sizoo et al. [11]	Pace et al. [10]	Faithfull et al. [12]	Koekkoek et al. [13]	Oberndorfer et al. [14]
Drowsiness, loss of consciousness	87	85		75	90
Seizures/epilepsy	45	30	56	25.9	48
Cognitive/psychological cognitive deficits/ memory loss confusion	33		39	44.7	
Anxiety/depression	29				
Agitation/delirium/ confusion		15	31	45	
Dysphagia nausea/ vomiting	71	85	10	24.5	79
Headache	33	36	62	34.6	38
Dyspnoea/death rattle / pneumonia	16	12			
Fatigue	25		44		

stage of disease of BT patients disease-specific symptoms such as somnolence, focal neurological deficits, cognitive disturbances and dysphagia are more prevalent respect from non-disease-specific symptoms [13].

Considering that randomized controlled trials are difficult to conduct in the palliative care setting and are sometimes unethical, alternative research methodologies need to be utilized, including qualitative studies, observational studies and expert opinion recommendations.

Recently, the European Association of Neuro-Oncology (EANO) guidelines on palliative care in neuro-oncology have underscored the need to establish the best methods to provide palliative care and to develop and assess adequate supportive care interventions [15]. EANO guidelines provided a systematic review of the available scientific literature integrated with expert opinions and formulated the best possible evidence-based recommendations for the palliative care of adult patients with glioma, particularly in the end-of-life phase.

One of the most important issues in palliative care is the timing of delivery. Recent randomized controlled trials have documented the significant benefits of early provision of palliative care to cancer patients [16]. Early integration of palliative care, compared with normal care, is related to significant improvement of quality of life, better symptom control, reduction of health expenditures and in some cases also an improvement of survival. However, at present the majority of BT patients receive palliative care interventions only in the last weeks or days before death [17].

Palliative care should not be considered to be synonymous with end-of-life care. The modern concept of palliative care highlights the importance of early integration of palliative care with oncological treatments. Several authors have proposed that for patients with cancer, palliative care should start early in the course of disease and should be delivered along the entire disease trajectory from diagnosis and initial tumour treatment until death [18].

The identification of the beginning of the dying phase is crucial to avoid suboptimal care. Palliative care goal at the EOL phase should be primarily aimed at reducing symptom burden while maintaining quality of life as long as possible without inappropriate prolongation of life. However, there is currently no validated instrument for determining the beginning of the dying phase and no common definition of end of life does exist.

Recently, pathways that can support clinicians in the process of identifying the beginning of the dying phase have been developed in cancer patients and in patients affected by neurological degenerative diseases [19, 20]. The knowledge of early predictors of end-of-life stage and the assessment for changes in signs and symptoms that may suggest a person is dying may help clinicians to plan and deliver appropriate care that integrates active and palliative management.

In general cancer populations several symptoms have been identified as potential predictors of entering in the last stage of disease: changes in breathing, general deterioration, lowering of consciousness, caregivers' clinical judgement and lowered oral intake [21].

In patients with progressive neurological disease several trigger symptoms have been suggested for the recognition of end of life such as swallowing problems, recurring infections, marked decline in functional status, first episode of aspiration pneumonia, cognitive difficulties, weight loss and significant complex symptoms [20]. There is evidence that these triggers may help in the recognition of the end of life and that early recognition of the final stages can be useful in allowing the focus of care to be clarified and a palliative care approach initiated.

Nevertheless, several studies showed that end-of-life phase of brain tumour patients is quite different respect from the expected trajectory observed in general cancer population [22]. Additionally, disease history and needs of care in the last stage of BT patients have few similarities with other progressive neurologic diseases.

Most of symptoms observed in BT patients approaching death occur in the last month of life and do not allow to plan in advance the appropriate end-of-life care. The cluster of symptoms observed at the EoL in BT show that the decline in physical and cognitive functions is rapid in the last 4–6 weeks before death and it is difficult to identify trigger symptoms as early predictor of EoL stage [23].

Moreover, disease trajectory of BT appears to be very different respect from the pathway of general cancer population and from neuro-degenerative diseases, and is characterized by fluctuating episodes of neurological deterioration often followed by period of improvement or stability.

Despite the emerging evidence of the positive effects of PC and hospice, the neuro-oncology community still have difficulty to apply models of care based on triggered, targeted interventions that result in high-quality, cost-effective, patient-centred and coordinated care.

Recent data reported that BT hospice enrollment was generally late: 22.5% of patients entered hospice within 7 days of death, 35% within 14 days and 59.4% entered within 30 days of death [24, 25].

The finding that hospice referral in BT patients is predominantly late suggests that a substantial proportion of BT patients in the later stages of disease does not receive appropriate palliative care.

Therefore, it is important to promote models of care that should incorporate earlier palliative care referral, to facilitate the timing provision of adequate supportive and palliative care in BT patients and their families.

16.3 End-of-Life Issues/Treatment Decisions

BT patients who are approaching the EoL need high-quality of care that support them to live as well as possible until death, and to die with dignity.

Neuro-oncologists dedicate most of their effort to offer active treatment against the tumour but, according to several authors, they are not well trained to give adequate care to patients who have progressive disease and no other oncologic treatment options available [7]. Little is known about symptoms and needs of BT patients at the end of their life, and too many patients do not receive adequate palliative care so that the burden of care often falls to patients' families [26, 27]. Recent studies reported that BT patients at the end of life present a high incidence of distressing symptoms that may influence the quality of life during the process of dying [4, 11]. In order to allow the patient to experience a peaceful death, specific palliative interventions are requested for the control of pain, confusion, agitation, delirium or seizures [11]. The main goals of palliative care and end-of-life care in BTs patients are to offer adequate symptom control, relief of suffering, to avoid inappropriate prolongation of dying and to support the psychological and spiritual needs of patients and families. The lack of control of symptoms, in patients not included in palliative care programs, often lead to re-hospitalization with an increase in health system economic costs and a worsening of patient's quality of life [27].

However, there is an increasing attention to palliative care and end-of-life issues in neuro-oncology. In the last stage of disease BT patients present both complex needs similar to the general cancer population, and severe symptoms due to the growing tumour, to treatment side effects, and specific problems that require adequate management from a multidisciplinary neuro-oncology team.

Recently, several studies have explored the supportive care needs of BT patient in the last stage of disease. One study reported in a population of 231 BT patients assisted at home until death with a neuro-oncological palliative home-care program, a high incidence of distressing symptoms influencing the quality of life during the last stage of disease and during the process of dying [2]. Most frequent symptoms observed in the last 4 weeks of life were epilepsy (30%), headache (36%), drowsiness (85%), dysphagia (85%), death rattle (12%), agitation and delirium (15%). Two other papers reported similar data about end-of-life symptoms in BT [4, 11]. In a little series of BT patients dying in hospital an Austrian group described the symptoms in the last weeks of life reporting that most frequent clinical symptoms were decreased vigilance, fever, dysphagia, seizures and pain [4]. In the study of Sizoo et al. the clinical records of 55 patients death for high-grade glioma were retrospectively examined: the majority of the patients experienced loss of consciousness and difficulty with swallowing, often arising in the week before death. Seizures occurred in nearly half of the patients in the end-of-life phase and in one-third of the patients in the week before dying [11].

A recent review on BT EoL symptoms confirmed that drowsiness and loss of consciousness was the most common symptom (90%) and focal neurological deficits (3–62%), seizures (3–56%), dysphagia (7–85%) and headaches (4–62%) were also frequent [28].

Other common symptoms reported in the end-of-life phase were progressive neurological deficits, incontinence, progressive cognitive deficits and headache. However, although an increasing number of researches on the palliative care needs of patients with BT have been recently conducted, symptoms before death have been described in small, retrospective and single-site studies and in different setting of care [11].

Given the paucity of Class I literature data on supportive care issues in BT, it is difficult to draw guidelines and treatment recommendations for the treatment of the more frequent symptoms; however, recent studies may help to optimize the quality of care in the management of BT patients at the EoL [15].

16.3.1 End-of-Life Treatment Decision-Making Process

EoL treatment decisions in neuro-oncology present unique features and require specific approaches concerning the decisions relating to medical treatment, including withdrawing–withholding of nutrition and hydration of patients in prolonged vegetative state, withholding of steroid treatment and palliative sedation [2, 4, 5].

The most challenging treatment decisions at the EoL in BT patients are generally about withdrawing or withholding a treatment when it has the potential to prolong the patient's life. This may concern treatments such as artificial nutrition and hydration and steroid treatment.

Withholding is a planned decision not to undertake symptomatic therapies that were otherwise warranted; withdrawal is the discontinuation of symptomatic treatments that have been started. Terminal sedation is defined as the pharmacologically induced reduction of vigilance up to the point of the complete loss of consciousness with the aim of reducing or abolishing the perception of symptoms that would otherwise be intolerable ("refractory symptoms"). Few data are available on end-of-life decision-making process in BTs patients. The process of treatment decision-making in the terminal stage of brain tumour patients is often complicated by the presence of cognitive problems that may affect patients' competence to express treatment preferences [5]. Recent studies highlight that participation in EoL decision-making is only possible with advanced care planning [15].

A recent European study evaluating the EoL decision-making process in three European countries revealed that only 40% of competent patients are involved in EoL treatment decisions; fewer than 7% express their wishes in advance and more than 50% of decisions are made without involving the patients or their families [29]. However, considering that the large majority of BT patients become incompetent in participating to share treatment decisions, it is of outstanding importance to plan EoL treatment decisions in advance, discussing, when possible, also with families. The aim is to obtain a consensus about the withholding–withdrawing decisions between all participants, respecting both patients and families values.

There are wide disparities in the provision of palliative care in different countries. To receive good palliative care during the course of disease and particularly at the end of life is a human right and the access to the right care should be facilitated for every patient.

The relationship between palliative care and health-related QOL in advanced stage of disease of BT patients has been poorly evaluated; however, there is growing concern about the quality of care given at the end of life in these patients. Palliative care is now understood as an approach to care concerned with caring for the whole person faced with a range of physical, psychological and social needs. Studies reported that administrative data, and particularly hospital re-admission rate in the last stage of disease, may be considered a potential indicator of quality of EoL care [30]. However, prospective studies specifically addressing palliative care and EoL issues in BT patients are lacking. Nevertheless, there is a great need for education in palliative care and end-of-life care for brain tumour. A better knowledge of clinical and ethical issues could help to improve the educational training and quality of care of neuro-oncology services [7]. Palliative programs and home-care models of assistance may represent an alternative to in-hospital care for the management of patients with brain tumour and may improve the quality of care, especially in the last stage of disease. Neuro-oncological literature in recent years highlights the need to improve the approach to palliative care in brain tumour patients and to identify delivery models to better answer patients' and caregivers' needs. Recently, simultaneous care model based on early provision of supportive and palliative care interventions during the course of disease has been proposed, with proactive support for patients and their families at illness transition points such as diagnosis, conclusion of radiotherapy, tumour recurrence, deterioration to death and following death [18].

16.4   Ethical Concerns

In the recent years, patient autonomy has become an important issue and cancer patients express wish to be involved in treatment decisions. However, the high symptom burden of patients with brain tumours affects their quality of life as well as their ability to make treatment decisions. It is therefore warranted to involve patients with high-grade glioma in treatment decision-making early in the course of disease, with a focus on end-of-life care and advance care planning. Research in other cancers has shown that the early involvement of specialty palliative care improves quality of life and caregiver satisfaction [31].

Some studies have reported that capacity to make decisions relating to medical treatment is impaired in up to half of patients with malignant glioma [32, 33]. A study evaluating the medical decision-making capacity (MDC) in malignant glioma patients showed that more than 50% of patients have a compromised MDC compared to controls [32]. Also, this study investigated the relationship between cognitive functioning and consent capacity suggesting a correlation between medical capacity impairment and cognitive impairment.

The reduced medical capacity of brain tumour patients has relevant implications in different settings; it may influence the capacity to consent to medical treatment in the early stage of disease, the capacity to consent to clinical trial enrollment and most important from an ethical point of view, in the process of end-of-life treatment decisions. These patients have difficulty in understanding the treatment situation, choices, and risks and benefits associated with the choices, and providing a rational reason for their decision.

Changes in cognition often occur as a consequence of brain tumours and their treatment, including surgical resection, which has implications for decision-making capacity. From an ethical perspective, patients lacking capacity need to be protected, and an evidence-based approach to determine capacity is essential [34].

At present, there is a lack of consensus on the most effective process for assessing capacity in brain tumour patients. However, there does seem to be agreement that cognitive changes are associated with difficulties in making decisions [35]. Neuropsychological assessment is considered to be the "gold standard" for assessing cognitive functioning and decision-making in patients with a brain tumour, particularly as there is high heterogeneity in the cognitive profiles of these patients.

Considering that the large majority of brain tumour patients lose the competence to participate in a shared decision-making process, it is of outstanding importance to plan in advance treatment decisions about nutrition and hydration, discussing them with families and with patients, when it is possible. To discuss end-of-life issues with BT patients becomes progressively more difficult during the course of their disease because of cognitive disturbances, confusion and decreasing consciousness. According to a recent review of supportive care in neuro-oncology only a little proportion of BT patients had established advance directives about end-of-life treatment, and progressive neurological deficits and loss of consciousness often meant that decisions had to be made on their behalf [5]. A study exploring the decision-making process in the end-of-life phase of high-grade glioma patients reported that the physician did not discuss EoL treatment decisions preferences in 40% of patients. Since most cancer patients wish to be involved in decision-making at the end-of-life, the results of this study underscore that EoL decision-making process for BT patients warrants improvement and timely organization of advance care planning could contribute to improve end-of-life decision-making [5].

As the "shared decision" taken together by physicians, nurses and the patient's family may be the best approach to end-of-life decisions, common guidelines are needed.

Making decisions regarding medical treatment is often difficult, and such is especially true when the patient's capacity to participate is questionable or even impossible. In such cases, it is important to carefully seek to assess the patient's competence and decision-making capacity and, if necessary, empower a suitable surrogate to act on his or her behalf.

16.5 Caregivers' Perspective at the End of Life

Very little is known about quality of life and well-being in caregivers of patients with brain tumours. Usually, carers' own needs are neglected because the focus is on the patients. Recent publication reports that in the context of this severe and often devastating disease, the caregivers burden of suffering and despair is often neglected, suggesting a more global and comprehensive approach, possibly with pharmacological and psychological support, to the care of the affected family [36]. The severity of symptoms is not only detrimental to patients' quality of life but also affects carers, who present high levels of distress, depression and significant reduction in their quality of life [8]. Two studies recently surveyed relatives of deceased BT patients with the aim to explore the caregivers' perspective. In the Dutch study relatives were asked to fill a questionnaire detecting several aspects, including quality of care and quality of death [37]. The results of this study indicate that, in the perception of their relatives, one quarter of patients did not die with dignity and most important aspect related to good quality of care were the place of death and the satisfaction with health care providers of EoL care. In a similar study performed on

52 caregivers of deceased GBM, more frequent complains reported by relatives were low quality of life, burnout, financial difficulties and perception of insufficient information [38].

Several programs of caregivers support with family consultation, internet-based or telephone support groups have been recently suggested as methods for supporting caregivers' emotional needs [8]. More recently Philip et al. have proposed a collaborative framework of supportive and palliative care for patients with high-grade glioma and their caregivers based on the early integration of palliative care approach into neuro-oncology disease trajectory [18].

16.6   Palliative Rehabilitation in BT Patients

The role of rehabilitation in BT patients has been investigated in few studies [39, 40]. Many authors have reported that BT patients may benefit from inpatient rehabilitation and outpatient rehabilitation interventions. Nevertheless, a significant effect of rehabilitation therapies has been demonstrated mainly in acute inpatient rehabilitation with comparable functional gain in respect to other models of neurologic disability such as stroke or traumatic brain injury [39]. However, given the positive impact of rehabilitation interventions on functional outcome and patients' quality of life, there is an increasing consensus about the need to improve strategies for physical and cognitive disability management in BT patients. In general, rehabilitation in the early stages of disease aims at restoring function during or after cancer therapy, while in the advanced stages it is important for maintaining patients' independence and quality of life [41].

Although previous studies have demonstrated the efficacy of rehabilitation programs for brain tumour patients and the positive impact on quality of life in the early stage of disease, the role of rehabilitation in the last stage of disease of BT patients has not been adequately demonstrated. Qualitative data reflect the importance of physiotherapy from a patients' perspective within a palliative care setting [42]. According to the literature data rehabilitation for cancer patients is expected to be an important means of supporting the hopes of patients and their families, and attempting to maintain and improve patients' quality of life. Several studies supported the utilization of rehabilitation throughout the entire phase from the time of diagnosis to the terminal stage, with the aim to involve psychosocial aspects as well as physical aspects [43].

Rehabilitation should be included in the management of BT patients as important part of palliative care given that its positive effect is not limited to functional outcome but strongly influences patients' quality of life facilitating symptoms' palliation, prevention of complications and improvement in mobility and daily living activities.

Rehabilitation approach should not be related only to physiotherapy, and the goal of rehabilitation intervention is not only to achieve maximal functional recovery in patients who have progressive impairments of functions and decreased abilities.

Rehabilitation in palliative care context can be defined as multi-professional intervention to treat and manage the person holistically in the context of their impairments, function and adaptation to environmental disability, with the aim to improve experience of living with, functioning and societal participation [44].

Rehabilitation definition includes different models according to the clinical context and aims of interventions:

Restorative rehabilitation is aimed to obtain the maximal recovery of function in patients with remaining function and ability.

Supportive rehabilitation is aimed mainly to maintain patient autonomy and self-care ability and mobility for patients whose impairments of function and declining abilities are progressing using methods that are effective (e.g. guidance with regard to self-help devices, self-care and more skillful ways of doing things). Also includes preventing disuse, such as contractures, muscle atrophy, loss of muscle strength and decubitus.

Palliative rehabilitation enables patients in the terminal stage to lead a high QOL physically, psychologically and socially, while respecting their wishes. Rehabilitation intervention in this setting is designed to relieve symptoms, such as pain, dyspnoea and oedema and to prevent contractures and decubitus, correct positioning, breathing assistance, relaxation or the use of assistive devices [44].

Particularly important, in palliative care setting, is the role of education for patients and families about maintaining independence and quality of life, mobility training, correct patients' mobilization and supervising the patient in an appropriate program to prevent physical decline and complications. Also, rehabilitation interventions are aimed to prevent contractures, muscle atrophy, loss of muscle strength and decubitus. Qualitative data reflect the importance of physiotherapy from a patients' perspective within a palliative care setting [42]. In addition, it is now widely agreed that high-quality treatment and holistic palliative care approach towards the end of life should include rehabilitation interventions to optimize patients' autonomy and quality of life.

References

1. Catt S, Chalmers A, Fallowfield L. Psychosocial and supportive-care needs in high-grade glioma. Lancet Oncol. 2008;9(9):884–91.
2. Pace A, Di Lorenzo C, Guariglia L, Jandolo B, Carapella CM, Pompili A. End of life issues in brain tumor patients. J Neuro-Oncol. 2009;91(1):39–43.
3. Davies E, Higginson IJ. Communication, information and support for adults with malignant cerebral glioma: a systematic literature review. Support Care Cancer. 2003;11:21–9.
4. Oberndorfer S, Lindeck-Pozza E, Lahrmann H, Struhal W, Hitzenberger P, Grisold W. The end of life hospital setting in patients with glioblastoma. J Palliat Med. 2008;11:26–30.
5. Sizoo EM, Pasman HR, Buttolo J, Heimans JJ, Klein M, Deliens L, Reijneveld JC, Taphoorn MJ. Decision-making in the end-of-life phase of high-grade glioma patients. Eur J Cancer. 2012;48(2):226–32.
6. Mukand JA, Blackinton DD, Crincoli MG, Lee JJ, Santos BB. Incidence of neurological deficits and rehabilitation of patients with brain tumours. Am J Rehabil Med. 2001;80:346–50.

7. Carver AC, Vickrey BG, Bernat JL, Keran C, Ringel SP, Foley KM. End-of-life care. A survey of US neurologists' attitudes, behavior and knowledge. Neurology. 1999;53:284–93.
8. Ford E, Catt S, Chalmers A, Fallowfield L. Systematic review of supportive care needs in patients with primary malignant brain tumors. Neuro-Oncology. 2012;14(4):392–404.
9. Ostgathe C, Gaertner J, Kotterba M, et al. Hospice and Palliative Care Evaluation (HOPE) Working Group in Germany. Differential palliative care issues in patients with primary and secondary brain tumours. Support Care Cancer. 2010;18(9):1157–63. https://doi.org/10.1007/s00520-009-0735-y. Epub 2009 Sep 8.
10. Pace A, Di Lorenzo C, Guariglia L, et al. End of life issues in brain tumor patients. J Neuro-Oncol. 2009;91(1):39–43.
11. Sizoo EM, Braam L, Postma TJ, et al. Symptoms and problems in the end-of-life phase of high-grade glioma patients. Neuro-Oncology. 2010;12(11):1162–6.
12. Faithfull S, Cook K, Lucas C. Palliative care of patients with a primary malignant brain tumour: case review of service use and support pro- vided. Palliat Med. 2005;19(7):545–50.
13. Koekkoek JA, Dirven L, Sizoo EM, et al. Symptoms and medication management in the end of life phase of high-grade glioma patients. J Neuro-Oncol. 2014;120:589–95.
14. Oberndorfer S, Lindeck-Pozza E, Lahrmann H, et al. The end of life hospital setting in patients with glioblastoma. J Palliat Med. 2008;11:26–30.
15. Pace A, Dirven L, Koekkoek JAF, Golla H, Fleming J, Rudà R, Marosi C, Le Rhun E, Grant R, Oliver K, Oberg I, Bulbeck HJ, Rooney AG, Henriksson R, Pasman HRW, Oberndorfer S, Weller M, Taphoorn MJB. European Association of Neuro-Oncology palliative care task force. European Association for Neuro-Oncology (EANO) guidelines for palliative care in adults with glioma. Lancet Oncol. 2017;18(6):e330–40.
16. Temel JS, Greer JA, Muzikansky A, Gallagher ER, Admane S, Jackson VA, Dahlin CM, Blinderman CD, Jacobsen J, Pirl WF, Billings JA, Lynch TJ. Early palliative care for patients with metastatic non–small-cell lung cancer. N Engl J Med. 2010;363(8):733–42. 19.
17. Walbert T, Pace A. End-of-life care in patients with primary malignant brain tumors: early is better. Neuro-Oncology. 2016;18(1):7–8.
18. Philip J, Collins A, Brand C, et al. A proposed framework of supportive and palliative care for people with high grade glioma. Neuro-Oncology. 2017;20(3):391–9. https://doi.org/10.1093/neuonc/nox140.
19. Oliver D. Palliative care for people with progressive neurological disease: what is the role? J Palliat Care. 2014;30(4):298–301.
20. Hussain J, Adams D, Allgar V, Campbell C. Triggers in advanced neurological conditions: prediction and management of the terminal phase. BMJ Support Palliat Care. 2014;4(1):30–7.
21. Eychmüller S, Domeisen Benedetti F, Latten R, et al. "Diagnosing dying" in cancer patients – a systematic literature review. Eur J Palliat Care. 2013;20:292–6.
22. Philip J, Collins A, Brand CA, Gold M, Moore G, Sundararajan V, Murphy MA, Lethborg C. Health care professionals' perspectives of living and dying with primary malignant glioma: implications for a unique cancer trajectory. Palliat Support Care. 2015;13(6):1519–27.
23. Pace A, Benincasa D, Villani V. Trigger symptoms at the end of life in brain tumor patients. WFNO Magazine. 2016;1(3):74–8.
24. Dover LL, Dulaney CR, Williams CP, Fiveash JB, Jackson BE, Warren PP, Kvale EA, Boggs DH, Rocque GB. Hospice care, cancer-directed therapy, and Medicare expenditures among older patients dying with malignant brain tumors. Neuro-Oncology. 2017;20(7):986–93. https://doi.org/10.1093/neuonc/nox220.
25. Diamond EL, Russell D, Kryza-Lacombe M, Bowles KH, Applebaum AJ, Dennis J, DeAngelis LM, Prigerson HG. Rates and risks for late referral to hospice in patients with primary malignant brain tumors. Neuro-Oncology. 2016;18(1):78–86.
26. Batchelor TT, Byrne TN. Supportive care of brain tumor patients. Hematol Oncol Clin North Am. 2006;20(6):1337–61.
27. Pace A, Metro G, Fabi A. Supportive care in neurooncology. Curr Opin Oncol. 2010 Nov;22(6):621–6.

28. Walbert T, Khan M. End-of-life symptoms and care in patients with primary malignant brain tumors: a systematic literature review. J Neuro-Oncol. 2014;117(2):217–24.
29. Koekkoek JA, Dirven L, Reijneveld JC, et al. End of life care in high-grade glioma patients in three European countries: a comparative study. J Neuro-Oncol. 2014;120:303–10.
30. Earle CC, Park ER, Lai B, Weeks JC, Ayanian JZ, Block S. Identifying potential indicators of the quality of end-of-life cancer care from administrative data. J Clin Oncol. 2003;21(6):1133–8. Review.
31. McDonald J, Swami N, Hannon B, et al. Impact of early palliative care on caregivers of patients with advanced cancer: cluster randomised trial. Ann Oncol. 2017;28(1):163–8.
32. Triebel KL, Martin RC, Nabors LB, Marson DC. Medical decision-making capacity in patients with malignant glioma. Neurology. 2009;73:2086–92.
33. Marson DC, Martin RC, Triebel KL, Nabors LB. Capacity to consent to research participation in adults with malignant glioma. J Clin Oncol. 2010;28:3844–50.
34. Kim SY, Marson DC. Assessing decisional capacity in patients with brain tumors. Neurology. 2014;83(6):482–3.
35. Dwan TM, Ownsworth T, Chambers S, Walker DG, Shum DH. Neuropsychological assessment of individuals with brain tumor: comparison of approaches used in the classification of impairment. Front Oncol. 2015;5:56.
36. Finocchiaro CY, Petruzzi A, Lamperti E, Botturi A, Gaviani P, Silvani A, Sarno L, Salmaggi A. The burden of brain tumor: a single-institution study on psychological patterns in caregivers. J Neuro-Oncol. 2012;107(1):175–81.
37. Sizoo EM, Taphoorn MJ, Uitdehaag B, Heimans JJ, Deliens L, Reijneveld JC, Pasman HR. The end-of-life phase of high-grade glioma patients: dying with dignity? Oncologist. 2013;18(2):198–203.
38. Flechl B, Ackerl M, Sax C, Oberndorfer S, Calabek B, Sizoo E, Reijneveld J, Crevenna R, Keilani M, Gaiger A, Dieckmann K, Preusser M, Taphoorn MJ, Marosi C. The caregivers' perspective on the end-of-life phase of glioblastoma patients. J Neuro-Oncol. 2013;112(3):403–11.
39. Huang ME, Wartella JE, Kreutzer JS. Functional outcome and quality of life in patients with brain tumor: a preliminary report. Arch Phys Med Rehabil. 2001;82(11):1540–6.
40. Bartolo M, Zucchella C, Pace A, Lanzetta G, Vecchione C, Bartolo M, Grillea G, Serrao M, Pierelli F, Tassorelli C, Sandrini G. Early rehabilitation after surgery improves functional outcome in brain tumors inpatients. J Neuro-Oncol. 2012;107(3):537–44. IF 3.115.
41. Santiago-Palma J, Payne R. Palliative care and rehabilitation. Cancer. 2001;92:1049–52.
42. Dahlin Y, Heiwe S. Patients' experiences of physical therapy within palliative cancer care. J Palliat Care. 2009;25(1):12–20. PubMed PMID: 19445338.
43. Hansen A, Rosenbek Minet LK, Søgaard K, Jarden JO. The effect of an interdisciplinary rehabilitation intervention comparing HRQoL, symptom burden and physical function among patients with primary glioma: an RCT study protocol. BMJ Open. 2014;4(10):e005490.
44. Barawid E, Covarrubias N, Tribuzio B, Liao S. The benefits of rehabilitation for palliative care patients. Am J Hosp Palliat Care. 2015;32(1):34–43. https://doi.org/10.1177/1049909113514474.

Surviving a Brain Tumour Diagnosis and Living Life Well: The Importance of Patient-Centred Care

17

Kathy Oliver and Helen Bulbeck

17.1 Background

Your loved one is diagnosed with a brain tumour. Suddenly, the world you have inhabited until now comes crashing down around you within a matter of minutes. You feel like you are standing on the edge of a huge precipice, about to be pushed off without a parachute. And then you're falling…falling fast. You don't speak the language of medicine. You don't know how to get from A to B. You have no map, no compass to guide you. You are filled with fear and dread of the unknown road ahead.

(A brain tumour caregiver)

The diagnosis of a brain tumour is one of the most shocking pieces of news that people can receive. Brain tumours know no geographic boundaries. They strike people of all ages with equal ferocity—from tiny babies to the elderly. They intersect three major disease areas:

- they are a rare disease [1]
- they are a progressive neurological disease, resulting in significant physical and cognitive deficit
- and brain tumours are, of course, a cancer, with the most malignant types such as glioblastoma, resulting in survival times ranging from 6 to 21 months [2].

Brain tumours remain one of the most intransigent of all cancers with a 5-year survival rate for glioblastoma, for example, of just 5.5% [3]. Little progress in improving survival has been made in the last 30 years because the treatment of brain tumours involves unique challenges not associated with other cancers, not least of

K. Oliver (✉)
International Brain Tumour Alliance (IBTA), Tadworth, UK
e-mail: kathy@theibta.org

H. Bulbeck
Brainstrust - the brain cancer people, Cowes, UK

© Springer Nature Switzerland AG 2019
M. Bartolo et al. (eds.), *Neurorehabilitation in Neuro-Oncology*,
https://doi.org/10.1007/978-3-319-95684-8_17

which is the ability of effective therapies to successfully cross the blood brain barrier.

Brain tumours are also the biggest cancer killer of children and adults under 40 years old [4]. Additionally, brain tumours are responsible for the highest number of per person life years lost—approximately 20—of any cancer [5].

Against this stark background, and given the devastating impact that a brain tumour diagnosis has on a person's everyday lived experiences, maintaining a good quality of life is absolutely crucial. Lehman et al. [6] highlighted that there is a need for rehabilitation in 80% of central nervous system tumours, in comparison to 60% in bone, prostate and bladder cancer. Mukand [7] identified the following neurological complications in brain tumour inpatients:

- cognitive deficits 80%
- weakness 78%
- visual-perceptual deficit 53%
- sensory loss 38%
- bowel/bladder dysfunction 37%
- cranial nerve palsy 29%
- dysarthria 27%
- dysphagia 26%
- aphasia 24%
- ataxia 20%
- diplopia 10%

Seventy-five percent of inpatients will have three or more of these neurological complications; 39% will have five or more.

Key to achieving a good quality of life while living with a brain tumour is a comprehensive, sustained rehabilitation programme, tailored to each patient's needs, goals and personal preferences.

Services offering rehabilitation across a wide spectrum of activities (work, leisure, interpersonal relationships, physical exercise, emotional resilience) should be delivered by a multidisciplinary team and form the backbone of a comprehensive survivorship plan for each brain tumour patient. It goes without saying that such a plan should also be relevant to the caregivers of these patients because a brain tumour diagnosis deeply affects not only the patient but also the family and friends of that patient.

Pivotal to such a survivorship plan is an understanding by researchers, healthcare professionals, regulatory bodies and others of what really matters to patients and what is of value to them. In other words, the patient perspective must be completely integral to the way brain tumour care—including rehabilitation—is planned, delivered and evaluated.

This kind of approach is central for the patient to successfully live well with and beyond a brain tumour diagnosis and demands not only a focus on the costs of delivery but on the outcomes that need to be achieved so that what patients value is at the core of treatment pathways.

17.2   Defining Patient Value

A recent review [8] on "Patient Value: Perspectives from the Advocacy Community" highlighted that value frameworks (such as those developed by ASCO, ESMO, NCCN and others) which are used to determine the value of medicines, need to reflect what matters most to patients.

The review found that: "It is difficult to define one single homogeneous set of patient values as these are shaped by social, religious and cultural factors, and health-care environment, as well as many factors such as age, gender, education, family and friends and personal finances" [9]. Nevertheless, despite varying opinions on what constitutes value, perspectives across a wide range of patients, caregivers and patient advocates need to be considered.

The value review concluded that: "Patient input is necessary to define the response to the full range of outcomes that patients may experience, whether this is at an aggregated level or a personal level, rather than the limited set of outcomes considered relevant by researchers. The patient perspective cannot be inferred by expert panels, but needs to be provided by patients and advocacy groups" [9].

17.3   Building a Framework for Survivorship and Rehabilitation in Brain Tumour Care: Some Definitions

For the purposes of this chapter, we have adopted the definition of survivorship used in the European Commission's Cancer Control Joint Action (CANCON). This was an EU Member State effort to "harmonise the way we fight cancer in Europe…" and to "reduce the cancer burden in the EU by creating a European Guide on Quality Improvement in Comprehensive Cancer Control." CANCON succeeded the first Joint Action on cancer, called the European Partnership Action Against Cancer—EPAAC. The CANCON definition of "survivorship" is *anyone with a diagnosis of cancer and who is still alive*" [10].

Additionally, the definition of "rehabilitation" for this chapter is based on that provided by the UK National Institute for Health and Care Excellence (NICE). NICE's guidance for *Improving Supportive and Palliative Care for Adults with Cancer* defines rehabilitation as the "*attempts to maximise patients' ability to function, to promote their independence and to help them adapt to their condition. It offers a major route to improving their quality of life, no matter how long or short the timescale. It aims to maximise dignity and reduce the extent to which cancer interferes with an individual's physical, psychosocial and economic functioning*" [11].

Many experts in the field of cancer rehabilitation also acknowledge that rehabilitation can be *preventive, restorative, supportive and palliative*.

When it comes to building a framework for survivorship and rehabilitation for brain tumour patients, considerations pertaining to health-related quality of life (HRQoL) are crucial. There are varying definitions of HRQoL [12]. But for the purposes of this chapter, HRQoL as described by the European Organisation for Research and Treatment of Cancer (EORTC) covers *"the subjective perceptions of the positive and negative aspects of cancer patients' symptoms, including physical, emotional, social, and cognitive functions and, importantly, disease symptoms and side effects of treatment"* [13].

17.4   What Brain Tumour Patients and Caregivers Say

Based on two important, patient-advocacy group-led research projects in the UK, we know that there can be significant gaps for brain tumour patients in accessing neuro-rehabilitation and neuro-psychosocial support [14, 15].

Sometimes, patients and caregivers simply don't know what services are available to them because they have not been provided with a care or survivorship plan once discharged from hospital.

The brainstrust paper *"Quality of Life: what the brain cancer community needs"* [16] states: *"Carers and patients don't understand the purpose of neuro-rehabilitation or how the emphasis is placed on restoring maximum independence with activities of daily living, mobility, cognition and communication. Rehabilitation interventions can be applied in all stages of the disease, although rehabilitation goals change as the stage of illness advances."*

Sometimes rehabilitation facilities don't exist in a particular geographic area, necessitating the patient to travel to another city or region. Sometimes, this *"isn't just a resource issue, but also an attitude of mind of all involved"* [17]. This, according to brainstrust, can be related to a clinical mindset that *"once the patient is through a particular phase of their care pathway, they are no longer [the doctor's] problem. And again, once discharged home, the secondary care team assumes that the primary care team will pick up the support and rehabilitation. This is not always the case, particularly if the caregiver and patient don't know what to ask for, who to ask or where to go"* [16].

In the UK, the National Cancer Patient Experience Survey, which is conducted every year, highlighted in the 2016 survey [18] the fact that only:

- twenty-six percent of people with a brain tumour received a care plan
- forty percent felt supported by their GP
- forty-two percent felt happy with the provision of care and support post treatment

Unfortunately, these statistics represented a decline from the results in the 2015 National Cancer Patient Experience Survey.

In 2015, The Brain Tumour Charity (TBTC) released a report called "Losing Myself: the Reality of Life with a Brain Tumour" [15]. The report was the result of an initial survey involving 1,004 people between 13 February and 13 March that year. Following the survey, face-to-face, in-depth interviews were held with 15 people, and an additional 25 people kept reflective diaries over the course of a week.

The resultant report highlighted levels of access to neuro-rehabilitation in the United Kingdom. Of the 1,004 survey responders, 52% had access to physiotherapy, 50% had access to occupational therapy and 43% had seen a psychologist. Only 25% of those surveyed had accessed speech and language therapy.

The report further found that the main difficulties regarding access to rehabilitation were finding these services in the first place, long waiting lists and poor communication between healthcare professionals and patients. The report also found that "*people with a high grade brain tumour are significantly more likely than those with a low grade brain tumour to have had access to speech and language therapy, occupational therapy and physiotherapy*" [15].

If these shortcomings are occurring in an advanced society like the United Kingdom, it would not be unreasonable to assume that in developing areas of Europe and the rest of the world, access to rehabilitation and survivorship plans is either very low or totally non-existent. Brain tumour patients and their families in these geographic areas must surely be suffering significantly as a result of this lack of rehabilitative support.

This chapter will discuss—from the perspective of patients and caregivers—the specific themes emerging in the brain tumour community in connection with rehabilitation, survivorship and quality of life so as to highlight the unique challenges we face. Policy-makers and healthcare commissioners must be aware of these challenges so that improvements can be made which will result in better outcomes for brain tumour patients based on what matters most to the people living with this disease.

17.5 Themes Reported by Patients, Caregivers and Health Professionals

To understand the issues in more depth, UK data has been gathered over a period of years from patients, caregivers and healthcare professionals, through online and offline channels. This has allowed for an accessible and open discussion, as real-world experiences and opinions have been shared, built on and contested. This evidence has provided research, stories, insights and ideas that can be provided to healthcare professionals and policy makers to help shape their thinking, as people work to collectively and collaboratively solve the issues that need addressing.

Themes that have emerged from offline and online interactions with brain tumour patients, their caregivers and healthcare professionals are the sense of isolation, lack of voice and the daily challenges they face. Patients are concerned about vitality, their identity and role, limitations, personal relationships and sexual issues, mental health and emotional wellbeing. All of these are important factors for patients.

Some of the highly challenging hallmarks of a brain tumour journey are:

- varying survivorship
- variable trajectory, even for benign brain tumour diagnoses
- high frequency of disabling complications

- high severity of disabling complications
- knowledge of increasing cognitive dysfunction
- life context—whether there is resilience or a lack of ability to cope

There is little available through the usual channels of clinicians for addressing these challenges—for example, only 43% of neuro-oncology multidisciplinary teams in the United Kingdom have access to neuropsychiatry services [19].

Catt et al. [20] have identified that, in the United Kingdom (where a substantial amount of research on rehabilitation has been carried out):

- Supportive care pathways for patients and their families differ between hospitals.
- Guidelines either omit important aspects of care and follow-up or are based on assumptions with little empirical support.
- As treatment of patients is often palliative, more efforts are needed to ensure good continuity of care.
- Current follow-up is failing to meet the psychological needs of patients and their caregivers.
- There is a need for developing innovative and integrated interventions that effectively support caregivers, such as proactive counseling or problem solving services.

These points are echoed in the findings of a crowdsourcing project undertaken by brainstrust and createhealth.io [21]. Brain tumour patients and caregivers highlighted four main themes that would improve the quality of care for them post surgery [16]:

- a desire to know what to expect
- better mentorship, home care, and personal support
- the importance of understanding and accessing long term care
- increased uniformity in standard of hospital care from place to place.

The two sentiments that were repeated more than any others were:

1. the desire to know what to expect during rehabilitation:
   - *"I now realise that stuff like memory loss, not being able to articulate what's in your head and the bone-aching tiredness that comes on without warning, are not just my symptoms. Knowledge is coping, for me."* (Patient, 60–70 years)
   - *"Community caregivers need a lot more education on the effects of brain tumours. This is an area that falls down in far too many areas."* (Patient, 40–50 years)
   - *"If doctors would continue the dialogue and engage with the patient more to build a good rapport I believe that would improve many patients' situations."* (Patient, 40–50 years)
2. calls for better mentorship, home care and personal support - this includes a more equal relationship with clinicians through more effective conversations:

- *"There should be a dedicated social worker for this client group and they should also be educated about the complexities of brain tumour patients."* (Nurse, 30–40 years)
- *"It would be nice to have a mentor or support worker allocated to each family after diagnosis. This person could visit or phone the family on a regular basis to check on how things are going, answer questions and offer pointers to further support and help."* (Caregiver, 40–50 years)
- *"Simply never happened. Went for a very thorough assessment but then kept getting appointments to see various people, physios, etc which were always postponed so that I didn't actually see anyone. After a year of this I just gave up. Resorted to speaking with colleagues and being treated by them which meant I had to share my diagnosis. Live in central London and worked in oncology for 15 years so know my way around the system well. I really feel for patients."* (Patient, 30–40 years)

Two other challenges that were identified during the crowdsourcing project were:

1. the importance of understanding the long-term effects of brain tumour surgery, and the subsequent neuro-rehabilitation required:
   - *"For me, it would have been more information about what to expect during recovery. I mean not only immediately post operative but in the months and even years after."* (Patient, 60–70 years)
   - *"I would have liked to have known about the possibilities of late effects rather than wait until they appeared."* (Caregiver, 50–60 years)
   - *"There is perhaps a place for an annual neuro-rehab MDM [multi-disciplinary meeting], where people who are 'stable' after treatment are seen in clinic once or twice per year after having an assessment to cover areas that the patient/carer feel important or lacking."* (Doctor, 50–60 years)
   - *"We didn't hear about 'late effects' until they started to become evident. We might have got on with doing some of the travelling we hoped to do while things were easier."* (Caregiver, 60–70 years)
2. the varying degree of hospital care that they receive from place to place:
   - *"All departments we visit for monitoring his condition are all different, some good, some bad, some lazy, some exceptional. The problem is that there is little to no coordination between these healthcare professionals."* (Caregiver, 40–50 years)
   - *"Having lived three separate places post diagnosis the care varies widely from place to place. We need to create minimum standards."* (Patient, 40–50 years)

The most repeated comment in the crowdsourcing project was in relation to holistic and long-term care, for example:

"It would be good to see a more holistic approach. After my treatment for a brain tumour had finished I was left to my own devices. It would be helpful to have a road map for the patient how to get back to… normality - if there is such thing. Many things required are of a fairly practical nature - moving from independent to assisted living, travel support, dietary support, exercise planning and tracking, hair dressing."
(Patient, 40–50 years)

In the crowdsourcing project, caregivers strongly supported the provision of specific neuro-psychosocial support to help with the patient's

- short term memory
- personality and behaviour changes
- difficulty in decision making
- pain management
- depression (including feelings of despondency)
- hemiparesis (and the safety issues that come with this)

Caregivers are concerned, too, about the potential for the patient to suffer falls and mobility problems. This is a limiting factor which results in caregivers feeling that they are unable to leave the patient alone at home. Whilst fatigue is mentioned, caregivers do not see this to be a particular problem, nor do they relate this to a quality of life issue. Fatigue limits the activities they could do together with the patient, but the upside is that it means that the caregiver *"could get on with things"* (caregiver of patient with a glioblastoma). Research demonstrates however, that fatigue is a significant issue for patients [22, 23].

Caregivers also feel that they have significant unmet needs and that support and rehabilitation services should address these, particularly where the caregiver is the primary source of support for the patient.

Brain tumour caregivers have confirmed that they, themselves, suffer from a wide range of emotions and mental stress [24] such as:

1. Feelings of Despondency
This includes feelings of hopelessness and fear of recurrence, fear of treatment, fear of losing a loved one and what the future holds.

"Watching your best friend's life be snatched away from under feet, and not being able to do a single thing to stop it." (Caregiver, 30–40 years)

"Watching my beautiful wife fight so hard yet slowly deteriorate over the weeks and months. My heart is breaking. Where has our life together gone?" (Caregiver, 60–70 years).

2. A Sense of Loss
This includes—but is not limited to—loss of identity and loss of normality and life as it was. Some caregivers mourn the loss of the person they loved because that person is no longer the same person they once knew.

"The tumour has changed my wife's personality so much I no longer see the person I married and love ... I feel so alone and trapped." (Caregiver, 40–50 years).

3. Lack of Psychological Strength
"I can't be strong for my family all the time. Sometimes I need a shoulder to cry on." (Caregiver, 40–50 years).

4.'Scanxiety' [25]

The agony of waiting for scans, for results, for treatment to start and to work, for recurrence.

"The worst part of having a brain tumour is waiting for things to happen with your treatment ... the waiting is mental torture." (Caregiver, 30–40 years).

5. Feeling Alone/Isolated

"...I am a mother, a daughter, a sister, an employee. I am surrounded by many, yet so alone...I'm lost." (Caregiver, 40–50 years).

6. Brain Tumours Are Unique

People may not understand that in the world of brain tumours, 'benign' does not mean harmless as in other cancers. Friends and family may assume the patient is 'cured' after treatment and that they will return to 'normal' after treatment. This is rarely the case in brain tumours. There is also a need for recognition that living with a brain tumour brings disability. Patients are also affected by epilepsy, changes in personality and other side effects unique to brain tumours.

"Knowing that my brain just doesn't work the same anymore since surgery." (Patient, 40–50 years)

"[I'm] looking for support from the government to recognise that a brain tumour is a disability and not just a condition." (Caregiver, 50–60 years).

7. Unresourced

There is not enough help in the way of support and information for patients and caregivers on the brain tumour journey.

"No follow-up after release from hospital. I had to contact a brain tumour charity to ask what happens next as hospital and GP didn't offer any help/support." (Caregiver, 40–50 years)

"Nobody from the hospital gives you any information about brain tumours when you are diagnosed. You are just left to try and find it all out for yourself and struggle through." (Caregiver, 40–50 years).

17.6 Challenges

From the perspective of patient-centred brain tumour care—which includes rehabilitation—empowerment models such as choice and entitlements are generally seen as ways of better responding to a person's needs.

The 'asset-based' community development approach is an interesting one. Originating in the United States, it takes a different starting point. It rejects the view of the citizen as principally a service user with needs that the state must meet. The citizen-as-service-user model tends to infantilise and disempower people, creating dependency cultures in which the best hope for improving a person's situation is to wait for a paid professional to step in. Instead, asset-based approaches see capabilities in everyone and seek to mobilise these. In particular they seek to mobilise people's 'relational power'—that collective impetus which achieves social change and which develops when communities come together to achieve their goals [26].

Such approaches are still generally counter-cultural in some of our health systems. But moving in the direction of shared decision-making begins at the same starting point. In particular, care planning for such services as rehabilitation under this model must start by discussing a patient's needs and aspirations—and importantly, what is of value to that person. Then there must be consideration of what resources are available to help meet these requirements, taking into account a person's own skills and capabilities, as well as resources from the local community before looking at what should be provided by the wider state.

For example, inpatient care may be very cohesive and coordinated but patients and caregivers may not know what range of services is available to them following discharge from hospital. A patient returning to the community needs to be more proactive and have a comprehensive care plan in place [27]. It's interesting to note that even in the UK (according to 2016 statistics) 74% of patients never received a care plan [18].

With regard to brain tumours specifically, there usually comes a point when additional resources are needed for the patient and caregiver due to the devastating nature of this progressive neurological disease. There can be a disconnect between what happens in hospital and what happens after discharge and once at home. At home, patients and caregivers will need to address such substantial issues as:

- speech deficits
- balance issues
- visual problems
- seizures
- swallowing issues
- challenges of daily care including bathing, insomnia, dressing, eating and physical activity

Caregivers and patients may be completely unaware of the range of rehabilitation services available to them which can diminish the impact of these issues. In many cases, there are district nurses, social services, physiotherapists, speech therapists, occupational therapists, counseling facilities and complementary therapists—to name but a few—who can help.

There is a significant shortage of rehabilitation facilities, particularly for those patients with brain and spinal cord tumours. Supportive care and rehabilitation for these people is of key importance and requires development and consolidation with commissioned rehabilitation facilities.

There are over 150 different types of brain tumours and prognoses can vary from very short term to longer-term. Access to appropriate levels of neuro-rehabilitation is vital for people with brain tumours but rapid referral for those patients with palliative and end-of-life care needs is particularly crucial. For these patients rehabilitation can be complicated by a prolonged period of physical and cognitive disability with distressing symptoms that are hard for patients and families to endure. This group of patients often requires a different rehabilitation approach, with care and support being given closer to home. Collaboration between health and social care is required to develop appropriate placements for those people who need ongoing institutional care and may have challenging symptoms.

In addition, patients and caregivers frequently have no idea how to access rehabilitation services [16]. A caregiver said:

My son (aged then 28) was told, after surgery and while still in hospital, that he was waiting for a bed in rehab and would stay in hospital until the bed was available. Then he was discharged - without warning. No rehab. No home visits. He was offered physio and OT [occupational therapy] as an outpatient but because of depression would not go. So it never happened, was never followed up. No support offered to us, as his carers, at all. And because of our ignorance at the time - we just accepted it. Bitterly regretted. I had to trawl the internet to find out what was available and was fortunate to find a good support group - that was where I learned what we needed to know.

And on a more pragmatic level, another caregiver said:

Just to advise that I had to take Natalie into hospital last Tuesday due to severe headaches etc. The scan highlighted that the tumour was active again and she had a huge one-off dose of chemo last Friday evening. The plan is to allow her to return home, however I need a certain hospital bed to fit into a downstairs room. In your list of contacts, do have anyone who might be able to help? The hospital has offered a normal size hospital bed but it is about 4 inches too long. I also need a wheelchair. What else will I need?

In addition, caregivers sometimes feel that non-specialist nursing services have little understanding of the specific needs of a brain tumour patient and that caregivers' concerns are not acknowledged.

One caregiver, Simon, was anxious to keep his wife at home when she was in the end-of-life phase but the district nurse accused him of being selfish, which led him to take extreme action at a time when he needed to be building a rehabilitation team around him. He said:

I have decided to take control. I am going to change doctors, as I should stop getting frustrated by the situation. I am going to change to a practice that is closer to home and apparently has a robust procedure for fast tracking those critically ill to either a doctor's visit or at the least a phone call…I will request that another district nurse is appointed. I am very low at the moment and do not need to be advised by the district nurse (who has only just appeared on the scene) that I am being selfish and very unkind to Jane by not allowing her to use a commode. I only read this in Jane's notes. So I am angry. A lack of tact I fear!

17.7 Future Directions

Qualitative studies [16, 24, 28, 29] show that some patients and the majority of caregivers want to be fully involved in:

- understanding their illness
- exploring their options for treatment and for living with the illness
- sourcing information, knowledge, help and advice

Following diagnosis and treatment for a brain tumour, patients will have differing trajectories which may be predicted, ranging from recovery, stable situation or progression. Research shows that neuro-rehabilitiation and neuro-psychosocial support improves outcomes for patients diagnosed with a brain tumour [30].

For improved survivorship and to plan transition points in care, close collaboration is required between clinicians involved with neuro-rehabilitation, supportive care, quality of life, psychological and palliative care. This entails coordination of different specialties and expertise—from symptom management to end-of-life care.

Furthermore, engaged patients and caregivers are better able to manage the complexity of their journey, have more resilience and a better quality of life. Patients and caregivers who are fully involved in shared clinical decision-making processes also do better. They are significantly more likely to attend screenings, regular check-ups, and much more likely to engage in healthy behaviours like eating a healthy diet [31, 32] or taking regular exercise [33–37].

Conversely, less engaged patients are significantly less likely to have prepared questions for a visit to the doctor, to know about treatment guidelines for their condition or to be persistent in asking if they don't understand what their doctor has told them [33]. They are also two to three times more likely to have unmet medical needs and to delay medical care compared with more highly engaged patients, regardless of income, education and access to care [35]. There is a straightforward moral case for empowering people in health and care—but there is an enabling case as well.

Empowerment of patients and caregivers creates a range of positive factors:

Autonomy

- Having greater control over our health and care is a good thing. Autonomy, or the ability to exercise control over the forces that affect our lives, is an essential part of a good life. In healthcare, self-directed support is only now starting to break through into mainstream services, but there are strong grounds for extending it. Healthcare services should support people to lead independent lives, rather than forcing them to fit their lives around the services on offer.

A Better Quality of Life

- Research has shown that patient 'activation' (having the knowledge, skills and confidence to manage one's own health) is strongly correlated with a broad and positive range of health-related outcomes, which suggests that improving activation has great potential' [31]. This is because patients with chronic conditions like brain tumours live with their disease 24/7 and only spend a fraction of their time visiting clinical experts. The rest of the time they have to manage their condition themselves [38]. Studies show that shared decision-making processes are more likely to result in people adhering to treatments and actions.

Patient Satisfaction

- In addition, research has shown that patients who are engaged in their health and healthcare—through health literacy, shared clinical decision-making and self-management—are more likely to say that their healthcare is of high quality, and are less likely to report experience of medical errors [39].

Saving Money

- Giving people the support and information they need to avoid getting ill, or when they have a chronic condition to self-manage it effectively, should save money by reducing demand on acute care. If people are not equipped and supported to self-manage, they are effectively left on their own and can end up with complications, health crises, preventable trips to the primary care clinician or emergency care, avoidable suffering and even premature death. Around 20% of emergency admissions to hospital are thought to be potentially preventable, and many of these involve chronic conditions [40]. In this era of cash-strapped national health services and the vital need to develop sustainable and affordable models for healthcare, this is an approach which certainly has the potential to avoid inefficiency and therefore eliminate wasting precious resources.

The most robust evaluations of empowerment programmes focused on peer support and redesigned consultations have been estimated to reduce acute care costs by 7%. Nesta (a global foundation focusing on innovation) estimates conservatively that this would save the NHS £4.4 billion a year across England [41].

The Health Foundation in the UK has found that:

- Self-management programmes can reduce visits to health services by up to 80%.
- Although shared decision-making approaches can lead to extended consultations, in the long term they are associated with higher satisfaction levels and can reduce the need for further future consultations.

17.8 Coaching: A Navigational Aid for Patients

Navigation to support decision making, improve understanding and information has been shown to be associated with better knowledge and understanding of diagnosis and treatment, better ability to cope and improved distress levels [28].

'Coaching' is a one-to-one relationship in which the patient is supported by a coach to identify, focus on and achieve what is important to that patient. Patients felt that, by preparing for consultations through coaching, a discussion of personalised key issues, broader than the prime focus of the consultation, resulted. Patients felt more informed and utilised coaching materials to aid memory, information gathering and understanding.

Clinical feedback revealed that coaching led to more effective consultations and facilitated communication within consultations by giving insight into information gaps. Telephone follow-up was effective for information and support and psychoeducation increased feelings of mastery [42]. Through a focus on achieving specific immediate goals which relate to specific areas—for example, weighing up the pros and cons of having a particular treatment, or overcoming a problem with caring—patients and caregivers can also experience a sense of healing, as they make courageous decisions about their lives and work.

17.9 Conclusion

Unsurprisingly, there are gaps in neuro-rehabilitation and neuro-psychosocial support as the evidence from patients diagnosed with a brain tumour and their caregivers reveals. The causes for this are complex; it isn't just a resource issue but is also an attitude of mind of all involved.

Preventive rehabilitation (rehabilitation that is proactive and aims to prevent problems rather than treat problems) can help maintain independence in brain tumour patients who undergo treatment and who have potential loss of function. When tumour progression causes a decline in functional skills, or the disease causes neurological deficit, rehabilitation assumes a supportive role, with goals adjusted. If patients and caregivers are more informed in advance about the progression of the disease they could be better prepared sooner with helpful interventions.

During terminal stages of illness, palliative rehabilitation can improve and maintain comfort and quality of life until the end of life. Brain tumour patients and caregivers need to be more specific and more proactive in asking for help from support services, outlining definitively what the problem is so that additional assistance can be targeted effectively. It is difficult to ask for support if you don't know what is available or where it is available.

This could so easily be addressed. A simple, key question: "What are you struggling with the most?" elicits unmet needs. Once this is articulated it is easy to clearly define what is needed.

The lack of identification of needs and the absence of documentation regarding these is worrying because funding and resource allocation follows need. Patients and caregivers should be more proactive and confident about what it is they need. They don't need to fix the problem; they just need to identify it and share it with a healthcare professional (HCP) who can fix it. HCPs need to identify for themselves the range of rehabilitation and support services offered, the uptake of services and any barriers to service use. Only then can the gaps begin to be addressed.

Brain tumour patients and their caregivers have the capacity to take control of their situation to secure the best possible outcomes. Empowering the patient and caregiver community results in autonomy, a better quality of life, more patient satisfaction, and a strong health economic argument. Everyone has capabilities and we should seek to mobilise these.

By creating the space to explore a person's needs and aspirations, their values, context and appetite for risk, resources can then be identified which meet the needs of the patient and caregiver.

This is patient-centred care.

References

1. Rarecare definition of rare cancers. http://www.rarecare.eu. Accessed online 20 Nov 2017.
2. Wirsching HG, Galanis E, Weller M. Glioblastoma. Handb Clin Neurol. 2016;134:381–97.
3. Ostrom QT, Gittleman H, Liao P, Vecchione-Koval T, Wolinsky Y, Kruchko C, Barnholtz-Sloan JS. CBTRUS statistical report: primary brain and other central nervous system tumors diagnosed in the United States in 2010-2014. Neuro-Oncology. 2017;19(suppl_5):v1–v88.

4. Brain Tumour Research. https://www.braintumourresearch.org/campaigning/stark-facts. Accessed online 20 Nov 2017.
5. Burnet N, Jefferies S, Benson R, Hunt D, Treasure F. Years of life lost (YLL) from cancer is an important measure of population burden – and should be considered when allocating research funds. Br J Cancer. 2005;92(2):241–5.
6. Lehmann J, DeLisa JA, Warren CG, et al. Cancer rehabilitation assessment of need development and education of a model of care. Arch Phys Med Rehabil. 1978;59:410–9.
7. Mukand JA, et al. Incidence of neurologic deficits and rehabilitation of patients with brain tumors. Am J Phys Med Rehabil. 2001;80(5):346–50.
8. Ibid.
9. Addario BJ, Fadich A, Fox J, Krebs L, Maskens D, Oliver K, Schwartz E, Spurrier-Bernard G, Turnham T. Patient value: perspectives from the advocacy community. Health Expect. 2018;21(1):57–63. https://doi.org/10.1111/hex.12628.
10. Albreht T, Kiasuwa R, Van den Bulcke M, CANCON. Survivorship and rehabilitation: policy recommendations for quality improvement in cancer survivorship and rehabilitation in EU Member States. Ljubljana: National Institute of Public Health; Brussels: Slovenia and Scientific Institute of Public health; 2017. https://cancercontrol.eu/archived/uploads/images/Guide/pdf/CanCon_Guide_FINAL_Web.pdf.
11. National Institute for Clinical Excellence. Improving supportive and palliative care for adults with cancer: the manual [Internet]. London: National Institute for Clinical Excellence; 2004. p. 70. [updated 2004 Mar 24; cited 2018 Jan 2]. Available from: https://www.nice.org.uk/guidance/csg4/resources/improving-supportive-and-palliative-care-for-adults-with-cancer-pdf-773375005.
12. Bottomley A. The cancer patient and quality of life, European Organisation for Research and Treatment of Cancer (EORTC). Oncologist. 2002;7:120–125. http://theoncologist.alphamedpress.org/content/7/2/120.full.pdf.
13. Ibid.
14. brainstrust. Quality of life: what the brain cancer community needs [Internet]. Cowes: brainstrust; 2015. [updated 2015 Apr 2; cited 2017 Aug 26]. Available from: https://issuu.com/brainstrust/docs/150309_what_the_community_needs_fin.
15. The Brain Tumour Charity. Finding myself in your hands: the reality of brain tumour treatment and care. Farnborough: The Brain Tumour Charity; 2016.
16. brainstrust. Quality of life: what the brain cancer community needs, p. 15.
17. brainstrust. Quality of life: what the brain cancer community needs, p. 11.
18. Quality Health. National cancer patient experience survey 2016: national results summary [Internet]. Chesterfield: Quality Health; 2016. [updated 2016; cited 2018 Jan 2]. Available from: http://www.ncpes.co.uk/index.php/reports/2016-reports/national-reports-1/3572-cpes-2016-national-report/file.
19. Rooney A. Challenges and opportunities in psychological neuro-oncology. Oncol News. 2011;6(4):133.
20. Catt S, Chalmers A, Critchley G, Fallowfield L. Supportive follow up in patients treated with radical intent for high grade glioma. CNS Oncol. 2012;1(1):39–48.
21. Fellgate T, Bulbeck H, Hill M, Jones W. Patient crowdsourcing: ideas that will improve the quality of life for people living with a brain tumour. October 2014.
22. Armstrong TS, Cron SG, et al. Risk factors for fatigue severity in primary brain tumor patients. Cancer. 2010;116(11):2707–15.
23. Armstrong TS, Gilbert MR. Practical strategies for management of fatigue and sleep disorders in people with brain tumors. Neuro-Oncology. 2012;(Suppl 4):iv65–72.
24. brainstrust Share Aware Pinboard [Internet]. brainstrust. 2013 [cited 2018 Jan 2]. Available from: http://www.brainstrust.org.uk/pinboard/.
25. Andrykowski M, Kangas M. Posttraumatic stress disorder associated with cancer diagnosis and treatment. In: Holland B, et al., editors. Psycho-oncology. Oxford: New York; 2010. p. 353.
26. For example, see the asset-based community development model: https://resources.depaul.edu/abcd-institute/publications/publications-by-topic/Documents/What%20isAssetBased-CommunityDevelopment(1).pdf.
27. NICE Improving Outcomes for People with Brain and Other CNS Tumours 2006.

28. Shepherd SC, Cavers D, Wallace LM, Hacking B, Scott SE, Bowyer DJ. Navigation' to support decision making for patients with a high grade brain tumour. A qualitative evaluation. Neuro-Oncology. 2012;14(2):4.
29. Cavers D, Hacking B, Erridge S, Kendall M, Morris P, Murray S. Social, psychological and existential well-being in patients with glioma and their caregivers: a qualitative study. Can Med Assoc J. 2012;184(7):E373–82.
30. Bartolo M, Zucchella C, Pace A, Lanzetta G, Vecchione C, Bartolo M, et al. Early rehabilitation after surgery improves functional outcome in inpatients with brain tumours. J Neuro-Oncol. 2011;107(3):537–44.
31. Greene J, Hibbard J. Why does patient activation matter? An examination of the relationships between patient activation and health-related outcomes. J Gen Intern Med. 2012;27(5):520–6.
32. Hibbard J, Stockard J, Mahoney E, Tusler M. Development of the Patient Activation Measure (PAM): conceptualizing and measuring activation in patients and consumers. Health Serv Res. 2004;39(4p1):1005–26.
33. Fowles J, Terry P, Xi M, Hibbard J, Bloom C, Harvey L. Measuring self-management of patients' and employees' health: Further validation of the Patient Activation Measure (PAM) based on its relation to employee characteristics. Patient Educ Couns. 2009;77(1):116–22.
34. Becker E, Roblin D. Translating primary care practice climate into patient activation. Med Care. 2008;46(8):795–805.
35. Hibbard JH, Cunningham PJ. How engaged are consumers in their health and health care, and why does it matter. Health Syst Chang Res Briefs. 2008;8:1–9.
36. Hibbard J, Mahoney E, Stock R, Tusler M. Do increases in patient activation result in improved self-management behaviors? Health Serv Res. 2007;42(4):1443–63.
37. Mosen DM, Schmittdiel J, Hibbard J, Sobel D, Remmers C, Bellows J. Is patient activation associated with outcomes of care for adults with chronic conditions? J Ambul Care Manag. 2007;30(1):21–9.
38. National Voices. Supporting self-management: summarising evidence from systematic reviews, 2014.
39. Edgman-Levitan S, Brady C, Howitt P. Partnering with patients, families, and communities for health: a global imperative – report of the Family Engagement Working Group 2013 [Internet]. Ar-Rayyan: World Innovation Summit for Health; 2013. [updated 2013; cited 2018 Jan 2]. Available from: http://dpnfts5nbrdps.cloudfront.net/app/media/387.
40. Blunt I. Focus on preventable admissions: trends in emergency admissions for ambulatory care sensitive conditions, 2001 to 2013 [Internet]. London: The Health Foundation and the Nuffield Trust; 2013. Available from: http://www.qualitywatch.org.uk/sites/files/qualitywatch/field/field_document/131010_QualityWatch_Focus_Preventable_Admissions.pdf.
41. Nesta. The business case for people powered health [Internet]. London: Nesta; 2013. [updated 2013 Apr 8; cited 2017 Aug 26]. Available from: https://www.nesta.org.uk/sites/default/files/the_business_case_for_people_powered_health.pdf.
42. Piil K, Juhler M, Jakobsen J, Jarden M. Controlled rehabilitative and supportive care intervention trials in patients with high-grade gliomas and their caregivers: a systematic review. BMJ Support Palliat Care. 2014;6(1):27–34.